Behaviour Problems in Small Animals
Practical Advice for the Veterinary Team

Jon Bowen, BVetMed MRCVS DipAS(CABC)

Veterinary Behaviourist, Hove, East Sussex, UK

Sarah Heath, BVSc MRCVS Dip ECVBM-CA

Veterinary Behaviourist, Chester, Cheshire, UK

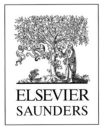

ELSEVIER
SAUNDERS

EDINBURGH   LONDON   NEW YORK   OXFORD   PHILADELPHIA   ST LOUIS   SYDNEY   TORONTO   2005

ELSEVIER
SAUNDERS

First published 2005

ISBN 0702027677

British Library Cataloguing in Publication Data
A catalogue record for this book is available from the British Library

Library of Congress Cataloging in Publication Data
A catalog record for this book is available from the Library of Congress

Notice

Knowledge and best practice in this field are constantly changing. As new research and experience broaden our knowledge, changes in practice, treatment and drug therapy may become necessary or appropriate. Readers are advised to check the most current information provided (i) on procedures featured or (ii) by the manufacturer of each product to be administered, to verify the recommended dose or formula, the method and duration of administration, and contraindications. It is the responsibility of the practitioner, relying on their own experience and knowledge of the patient, to make diagnoses, to determine dosages and the best treatment for each individual patient, and to take all appropriate safety precautions. To the fullest extent of the law, neither the publisher nor the author assumes any liability for any injury and/or damage.

The Publisher

Printed in China

The
Publisher's
policy is to use
**paper manufactured
from sustainable forests**

Contents

Preface

Behavioural medicine is an important branch of both human and veterinary medicine. When we are unwell friends or family members may notice that we have become moody, irritable or depressed, while work colleagues may pick up on a drop in our performance or concentration and these behavioural, rather than physical signs may be the reason that medical assistance is sought. Once we have been successfully treated our mood often lifts and our behaviour returns to normal. In some circumstances we may consider it perfectly acceptable to use illness as an excuse for our own bad behaviour while in others we may be acutely aware of the need to mask our illness and put on a show of strength in order to conceal our vulnerabilities.

In a veterinary context things are not so different and when companion animals are ill they often obtain medical help primarily because their owner has noticed a change in their behaviour. Owners often refer to general signs of illness such as mood changes, irritability and depression and as vets we are frequently presented with animals that are reportedly unwell on the basis of these general signs. It is up to us to investigate the cause. In other cases more specific medical symptoms may be reported, such as polydypsia and lameness, but these are merely behavioural adaptations that enable the animal to continue to function despite the presence of pathology, so once again behavioural medicine is involved. The expression of signs of illness is very dependent on the ethology of the species and in a social species, such as the dog, it can be potentially risky to show signs of vulnerability that might affect rank within the group, so signs of illness are often concealed. One possible result of this is that the ill individual may become more aggressive in order to deter competition that may reveal weakness. In companion dogs this might translate into increased aggressive reactions towards other dogs in the home, unfamiliar dogs met on a walk, children or the adult owner. Direct signs of the physical cause of the change in aggressiveness may be suppressed, but there is still a very obvious change in behaviour and this may be the only reason why an owner approaches the veterinary surgeon for advice.

This strong link between behaviour and disease makes it essential that we ask questions about behaviour as part of our routine consultations and investigate potential medical causes when behavioural symptoms are presented. Unfortunately behavioural medicine forms only a tiny part of the curriculum for most universities and colleges that teach veterinary medicine or nursing and it is easy to be overwhelmed at first by the range and type of behavioural problems that clients bring to us in general practice. Certainly there may be some that could be referred straight away but in most cases the vet will feel obliged to offer some first line advice and this stage of dealing with a behaviour case is vitally important since mishandling can lead to serious consequences in terms of animal suffering, human injury or litigation.

In this book we have adopted a particular style and layout that we hope will make it more accessible for readers in a busy practice environment. For example, key information on problem prevention and immediate advice to give to clients is placed into easily located text boxes within each section. We deliberately chose not to break up the text with references because we wanted the text to be easily read but further reading suggestions are included for those who wish to expand their behavioural knowledge and look at some of the primary research in this fascinating field.

Acknowledgements

I would like to thank my wife, family and friends for continuing to offer support and advice throughout every foul mood I experienced whilst writing my sections of this book. I would particularly like to thank my mother, Jo Bowen, for her incredibly diligent and patient proof reading. Without her contribution my sections of the book would never have been completed.

Jon Bowen

Thanks to my two sons, Matthew and David, and to my parents. Without their support this book would certainly not have been written. Thanks also to all of the staff at the practice for their support and to Jon's mum for her much appreciated proof reading.

Sarah Heath

We would both like to thank Elsevier for giving us the opportunity to produce this book and hopefully encourage the study of behavioural medicine in a veterinary context.

PART 1

Practice tips

PART CONTENTS

Chapter 1

Providing a practical behavioural service

DEALING WITH BEHAVIOURAL ISSUES

When considering the incorporation of behaviour into general practice, veterinary surgeons are often concerned about the level of time commitment that will be required to deal with individual cases. They are also concerned about the lack of education that they received at undergraduate level in the field of companion animal behaviour and are aware of the need to be familiar with the natural behaviour patterns of the common companion animal species, as well as with the possible link between human behaviour and inappropriate animal responses. These concerns often prevent practices from pushing behaviour to the top of their agenda, but dealing with specific behavioural cases is only one aspect of providing a behavioural service and veterinary practices can significantly improve their service to their clients by offering behavioural advice in a variety of other ways. Providing a behavioural service has numerous benefits both for the clients and the practice; in particular it can:

- improve the quality of life for animal and owner alike and so increase client appreciation of the practice
- make life easier in the consulting room and increase job satisfaction for both vets and nurses
- provide a valuable extension of the veterinary nurse's role
- encourage a greater rapport with clients
- be financially rewarding, either directly through offering behavioural consultations or indirectly by decreasing the possibility of euthanasia of otherwise healthy young pets.

An obligation to be involved

The high incidence of behavioural problems in the domestic pet population is highlighted by research which suggests that the primary reason for euthanasia in young, physically healthy animals is concern over an aspect of their behaviour. The welfare concerns that such research raises lead to an obligation on the part of the veterinary profession to be involved in the prevention and treatment of behavioural disorders and in the education of those that breed, rear, and own domestic pets.

PROVIDING A PRACTICAL BEHAVIOURAL SERVICE

Although behavioural consultations with clients already experiencing problems with their pets is often highlighted as the main emphasis of behavioural practice, this is not necessarily the case and a more holistic view of behavioural medicine is needed within general practice. Providing a behavioural service involves a number of elements including:

- making clients aware that behavioural issues are taken seriously within the practice
- providing pet selection interviews and literature to assist prospective owners in choosing their pet
- providing a behavioural advice service for breeders
- providing behavioural advice for new owners
- organising kitten information evenings and puppy parties
- offering informed referral to a veterinary behaviourist or behaviour counsellor
- providing behaviour-based information clinics and literature for clients
- offering behavioural consultations for individual clients and their pets.

Increasing owner awareness of the behavioural service

It is necessary to take every opportunity to inform the clients of the behaviour services that the practice has to offer.

Simply by mentioning behaviour during a consultation, and by showing interest and concern about the issues that owners face, the veterinary practice can help clients to recognise where there may be a problem and encourage them to seek suitable advice. Waiting room space is often sadly underused and there are a number of ways in which this area can be utilised to demonstrate that the veterinary practice has a positive attitude to behavioural issues.

Posters can be a useful way of getting the message across, and perhaps provoking discussion between clients as they wait. They can advertise the fact that the practice acknowledges behavioural problems and can offer help with their solution, which will often be enough to encourage clients to mention their concerns to both the vet and the nursing staff, thereby opening up the possibility of taking the subject further.

Merchandise such as books on companion animal behaviour and a range of behaviour-related products (for example, headcollars, clickers, and bitter apple spray), in the reception area will often quietly increase the profile of behaviour within the practice and make clients more aware of the services the practice can offer. It can also provide an

opportunity for the reception staff to mention behavioural topics as they sell the items, which can often lead to owners feeling able to discuss specific behavioural issues.

Booklets and magazines with a behavioural message can be left on the tables in the waiting room. Most owners are grateful for something interesting to read or look at while they are waiting for an appointment and the presence of literature with a behavioural slant increases awareness that the practice is interested in behavioural issues. Practice copies of the booklets that are stocked as merchandise can help to promote sales by allowing clients time to leaf through them.

Handouts and information sheets are used in many practices to convey important messages to clients on a wide variety of subjects, including dental care, worming and vaccination. It is easy to include behaviour in these handouts and, by leaving them in the waiting room for clients to help themselves, the very common problem of people being reluctant to admit that they are concerned about their pet's behaviour can be overcome. The practice address and telephone number should be clearly printed on the leaflets and, if possible, the name of a member of the practice staff who can be contacted to discuss the problem should also be given. A personal touch is extremely beneficial in behavioural cases since the owners are often at the end of their tether and many are experiencing feelings of guilt, shame and failure as a result of their pet's behaviour. It is therefore essential to offer relevant and helpful advice in a friendly and welcoming manner.

Videos can be played in the waiting room area and used not only to impart some information about behaviour, but also to inform clients that behaviour is taken seriously in this practice. Videos can then be lent, hired out or even sold by the practice.

Ideally, a receptionist should be constantly available so that any questions that the client wishes to raise as a result of seeing posters or reading behavioural material can either be answered there and then, or the client can be advised to mention the matter to the vet once they get into the consulting room.

Catering for the prospective owner

One of the most disheartening aspects of working in the field of veterinary behaviour is the fact that so many of the problems that are being presented could have been avoided. Taking the time to consider the way in which domestic pets are bred and reared is obviously important, but it is not the only possible approach in the prevention of behavioural problems and working with prospective owners can be a very rewarding exercise for the veterinary practice.

The main objective is to assist people in choosing the pet that is best suited to their requirements and which offers them the best potential for a long and mutually rewarding relationship. In order to achieve this it is worth taking time to determine the prospective owner's expectations and help them to assess the commitment of pet ownership in realistic terms. There will be a number of factors that need to be considered and it is important to steer people away from misguided choices and give clearly justifiable reasons for the selection that is advised. Many prospective owners will not have taken the time to sit down and rationally evaluate their reasons for wanting a pet and it can be very helpful to talk them through this process. Pointing out the possible considerations in terms of the species, breed, age, and sex of the potential pet can help to put the decision in perspective and can prevent distressing mismatches.

Since many owners are still unaware that veterinary practices can offer any support or guidance before a pet is acquired, it is important to increase awareness by displaying posters in the waiting room. Drawing attention to the existence of pet selection interviews can emphasise the importance of the decision-making process and encourage prospective owners to think carefully about the issues involved. These interviews are often carried out by the veterinary nurse and they offer another way in which nursing staff can make a valuable contribution to the overall preventative health care programme that the practice can provide. If the practice does not have the time to offer face-to-face interviews for this purpose, it is possible to produce handouts which can be available at the reception desk.

At pet selection interviews it is important to discuss all the factors that can influence the choice of pet, and these must include practical considerations of time and money as well as emotional factors such as personal preferences. Advice will not be limited to dogs and cats and consideration of other species should be encouraged if they are more suited to the person's personal circumstances. However, for the purpose of this book the option of only feline or canine companions will be discussed.

Cats and dogs have different attributes to offer but neither is any 'easier' to care for or any 'less trouble' than the other. Ownership of either species brings with it very real responsibilities and one of the roles of the veterinary practice is to make those responsibilities known to the prospective owner.

Some of the main considerations for the prospective owner are as follows:

- Breed : mixed breed or purebred
- Sex : male, female, entire, neutered
- Age : adult, kitten, puppy
- Source : breeder (professional or private), rescue centre

Once a selection has been made the prospective owner will need some guidelines in order to avoid the common pitfalls encountered when selecting a pet.

Advice sheets covering the most important considerations for owners who are about to take on a puppy or kitten, or give a home to an adult dog or cat, can make valuable additions to the practice literature (see Figs 1.1 and 1.2 for sample guidelines).

Advice for prospective owners electing to take on an adult.

- Carefully consider the source of your new pet. If you are taking on a rescue animal visit the rescue centre before you are actually looking for a pet and observe their facilities and ask about their re-homing policy.

- Try to ensure that your selection is ruled by your head and not your heart. Resist the temptation to take an animal home on impulse and do not base your selection purely on appearance – there is a lot of information that you need to find out.

- If possible gain as much information as possible about the animal's history. Find out as much as possible about the environment in which it lived and the human composition of its previous household.

- Be patient in the early stages after adoption, but do start as you mean to go on and consistently apply any house rules that you wish to establish.

- Expect a honeymoon period – it can take three or four weeks for behavioural problems to show.

- Do not fall into the trap of selecting an adult rather than a puppy or kitten because they are 'less work' – this is not necessarily true.

Figure 1.1   Advice for prospective owners electing to take on an adult pet.

Providing a behavioural advice service for breeders

Much has been written about the responsibility of breeders with regard to the successful rearing of pets that are suited to life in a human context and yet the preventable behaviour problems, which prohibit these animals from integrating into society, remain at an unacceptable level. Education is vital and the veterinary profession is well-placed to interface with breeders and offer practical and relevant advice regarding breeding stock selection, early socialisation, habituation, and selection of appropriate homes. The common aim of the breeder and veterinary practice should be the production of emotionally stable puppies and kittens who can adapt to whatever lifestyle they are offered and can successfully coexist with their own and other species. Veterinary practices are suitably placed to offer the necessary advice to achieve this aim, and working with breeders in this area can be very rewarding.

Providing preventive behavioural advice for the breeder will involve:

- studying the breeding programme and offering practical advice on behaviour-based selection of breeding stock
- observing current housing and advising on its effects on the behaviour of breeding bitches and stud dogs and on the behavioural development of puppies

---

Advice for prospective owners electing to take on a puppy or kitten.

- Carefully consider the choice of pet. The species, breed, age and sex are all important. Be realistic in expectations concerning financial and time commitments. Do not underestimate the work involved in caring for a new puppy or kitten.

- Do not consider obtaining a kitten or puppy from a pet shop or from an outlet that claims to sell a range of different breeds which are not connected in any logical manner.

- Take the time to locate a reputable breeder or visit a reputable rescue organisation. If necessary be prepared to travel.

- Ask to meet the dam and, if possible, the sire.

- Spend time observing the litter at play and watching just how they interact.

- Look for a litter where all of the puppies or kittens are outgoing and confident.

- Observe the behaviour of other animals at the breeder's premises, or visit owners of dogs and cats from previous litters, as this will give an indication of the success of socialisation and habituation programmes carried out by the breeder.

- Observe reactions to novel stimuli in their environment, such as a new toy, and to strange and unexpected sounds such as the gentle rattling of car keys. In an ideal situation, the puppies or kittens should appear surprised but quickly recover and go to investigate.

- Handle the puppies or kittens and see their reaction to strange people. The way in which a young animal responds to being handled and examined gives a good indication of the success of socialisation.

- Once you have selected a kitten or puppy, arrange to visit it as often as possible prior to collection in order to build up a relationship with your new pet.

- Do not be too impressed with immaculate and clinically clean premises if they are totally devoid of stimulation. Cleanliness is important, but so too is habituation.

Figure 1.2 Advice for prospective owners electing to take on a puppy or kitten.

- assessing current rearing methods and offering advice on socialisation and habituation programmes.

These aims can be achieved through a variety of means including:

- Providing access to suitable literature through a practice library system
- Preparing advice sheets for breeders on major issues
- Setting out socialisation and habituation programmes for breeders
- Organising evening meetings with outside speakers who are of particular interest to breeders.

The major issues for most breeders are the selection of breeding stock, the social and physical environment for rearing of puppies and kittens and the communication with new owners to ensure the continuation of socialisation and habituation in the new home. Veterinary practices need to be prepared to spend time getting alongside breeders and understanding their criteria before being able to offer advice which is tailor-made for that breeder and their specific circumstances. The production of client information sheets with advice for breeders (Fig. 1.3) is one way in which the subject of behavioural considerations in breeding establishments can be raised. These can act as a springboard for more in-depth conversations and the delivery of more specific advice.

However, puppies and kittens are not only reared and sold through commercial enterprises and veterinary prac-

tices also need to be involved in offering practical advice and support to owners who decide to have one-off litters from family pets. This is more of an issue in a canine context since human control over breeding of domestic cats is often limited and the number of non-commercially reared pedigree cat litters is minimal. The provision of advice regarding the suitability of bitches for breeding is a very important area of behavioural problem prevention where veterinary practices can easily become involved. It is impossible to prevent someone from using an unsuitable bitch for breeding, but many errors are made through ignorance (rather than deliberate irresponsibility) and education of owners as to the heritable nature of fear-related behaviour and the importance of using only emotionally stable individuals in breeding programmes cannot be overemphasised.

There are numerous opportunities to give advice about breeding programmes but vaccination appointments – both primary and booster – are particularly useful times to consider the issue of breeding. For owners of new puppies the prospect of allowing their bitch to give birth, or their dog to have one taste of the good life and sire one litter may seem like the kindest thing to do, but practical considerations regarding the responsibility of rearing and finding homes for a number of lively young pups may not have been made.

By raising this subject at the time of the first vaccination and providing a client handout with guidelines for people considering using their pet dogs for breeding (Fig. 1.4), the

Advice for breeders.

- When deciding on breeding programmes, temperament of both dam and sire need to be considered. This is especially relevant in feline breeding where the paternal effect on the behavioural characteristic of boldness is well documented.

- Once a litter has arrived ensure that the puppies and kittens become accustomed to being handled. Handling must take place in an appropriate manner and it is important to take care not to distress the dam.

- Gradually increase the amount of contact with people. Start with people known to the dam and gradually introduce less familiar people as well as a wide range of individuals: old and young, male and female. Of course, it is essential that adequate precautions are taken at all times to prevent introduction of disease.

- Encourage new owners to come and visit their pet in the breeding environment as often as possible before they take it home.

- Introduce the puppies and kittens to a wide range of environmental stimuli, including everyday household noises such as washing machines. Ideally, there should be an opportunity for the puppies and kittens to experience home life as early as possible, even if it is only for a few hours a few times a week. Where it is totally impossible to do so, use tape recordings of common sounds, such as children playing, doorbells, vacuum cleaners and tumble driers, which can be played in the breeding area in those crucial early weeks.

- Provide a wide range of stimulation through provision of species-appropriate toys and activities, as well as exposure to human-related stimuli.

- Design breeding establishment buildings to take into account not only disease prevention and ease of management but also behavioural considerations.

- Inform prospective new owners of the importance of continuing the socialisation and habituation process in the new home.

Figure 1.3   Advice for breeders.

General guidelines for clients considering using their pet dogs for breeding.

- Question the motivation for wanting a litter – only go ahead if the motivations are clear, identifiable and justifiable.

- Consider the issue of re-homing – is there a suitable and available market for the puppies?

- Remember that the sire will influence the behaviour of his pups even if he never meets them, and consider the temperament of the stud dog as well as the bitch.

- Carry out a small behavioural test on prospective breeding dogs and bitches to determine their level of suitability for breeding.

- Remember that it is not only the actual level of fear responses that an individual exhibits that is significant but also the recovery time when the fear-inducing stimulus is either removed or is proven to be non-threatening.

- Do not consider breeding from a nervous or aggressive bitch or dog.

- Be prepared for the phenomenal commitment involved in providing a suitable physical, social and emotional environment for the rearing of young puppies.

Figure 1.4   General guidelines for clients considering using their pet dogs for breeding.

veterinary practice can help to improve the level of thought that is given to the subject and perhaps dissuade owners from breeding from pet bitches who are unsuitable for the purpose.

If clients are determined to go ahead with the breeding programme and they have given due consideration to the commitment involved, it is important for the veterinary practice to be on hand to offer advice and practical support. The most important considerations are:

- selection of dam and sire
- provision of appropriate health care
- provision of suitable physical housing, which provides for the five basic freedoms: freedom from thermal and physical distress, freedom from pain and injury, freedom from hunger and malnutrition, freedom from fear and stress and freedom to express most normal behaviour
- provision of a social and emotional environment that supports the behavioural development of the puppies and kittens and maximises the emotional stability of the animals reared
- establishment of a socialisation and habituation programme which is started at the breeder's premises and is then continued by the new owner in the new home. Tick chart checklists can easily be constructed by the practice and distributed to breeders but the availability of commercially prepared socialisation and habituation checklists for breeders of puppies and kittens makes this unnecessary. Ideally one of the practice staff should be available to explain how these charts should be used, but booklets, which accompany these products, can be self-explanatory.

For those clients who are in the process of rearing litters of puppies or kittens, it is useful to provide guidelines as to the most important experiences for those animals while they are still on the breeder's premises (Box 1.1).

> **Box 1.1   Important experiences for puppies and kittens while still on the breeder's premises**
>
> - Interaction with other dogs. The dam and littermates will be the first contacts and other dogs on the premises, possibly including the sire, can also be incorporated into the socialisation programme.
> - Introduction to people including men, women and children. Varying appearances, clothing and activity should be included in these introductions.
> - Auditory, visual and tactile stimulation. This can be provided through the use of toys and games, and by exposure to normal everyday human activities.
> - Introduction to the concept of solitude. There should be very short and controlled periods of being alone.

The new owner

Once owners have acquired their new pet, the veterinary practice has an essential role in providing preventive behavioural advice. It is a good idea to advise clients on how to socialise and habituate their puppy or kitten successfully as soon as they contact the practice, and while they are at a very receptive stage in their relationship with their pet. It is important to emphasise that these vital processes can begin while the vaccination programme is in progress and that a high percentage of behavioural problems can be prevented if puppies, kittens, and young of other companion animal species are given the correct experiences early in life. However, socialisation and habituation are not the only behavioural issues of interest to new owners and veterinary practices are called on to give advice on topics ranging from house-training puppies to teaching kittens to use a cat flap and from teaching puppies to cope with being alone to introducing suitable forms of play between owner and cat (Boxes 1.2 and 1.3).

> **Box 1.2   Examples of behavioural issues that need to be raised with new puppy owners**
>
> - Providing suitable introductions to people and other animals
> - Providing a complex environment and introduction to a variety of experiences
> - Introducing suitable toys and games
> - Using successful house-training techniques
> - Reinforcing appropriate behaviours when greeting people and other dogs
> - Teaching basic obedience, including sit, stay and recall
> - Preventing specific behaviour problems such as play biting
> - Introducing the puppy to the experience of being alone

> **Box 1.3   Examples of behavioural issues that need to be raised with new kitten owners**
>
> - Providing suitable introductions to people and other animals
> - Accustoming the kitten to appropriate human handling
> - Providing a complex environment and introduction to a variety of experiences
> - Providing suitable litter facilities to facilitate litter training
> - Introducing suitable games and toys
> - Teaching the kitten some basic behaviours such as coming when called
> - Introducing the kitten to using a cat flap and wearing an appropriate collar
> - Preventing specific behaviour problems such as indoor scratching

Socialisation and habituation

The importance of these two processes in the preparation of puppies and kittens for life in a domestic environment has been highlighted over recent years and far more is now known about the effects of early-life experiences on future behaviour.

The most sensitive period of behavioural development in terms of socialisation and habituation is from 2 to 7 weeks in the kitten and from 4 to 14 weeks in the puppy (with particular emphasis on the period from 4 to 8 weeks). It is important to understand that this is a sensitive period rather than a critical one and therefore preferences can be formed and altered outside of these boundaries, but receptivity to socialisation and habituation is at its maximum at this stage of development and it is therefore advisable to take advantage of this biological window of opportunity.

The issue of socialisation and habituation has been most widely publicised within the canine context but cats also need to experience suitable socialisation and habituation if they are to develop into family pets and respond to the ever-changing demands that are made of them in terms of their role as companion animals.

Socialisation: The process whereby an animal learns how to recognise and interact with its own species and the species with which it cohabits.

Kittens and puppies need to be introduced to a wide range of people and other animals during their socialisation period (Fig 1.5). In the case of kittens, it has been shown that introduction to at least four different people is needed before there is a generalised acceptance of human company, and it is recommended that these people represent a range of ages, sexes and appearances in order to maximise the beneficial effects of the socialisation process. For the domestic cat, the aim is for them to be able to have a mutually beneficial relationship with their owners and to

One of the main aims of the socialisation process is for pet dogs and cats to be better-equipped to cope with life in a human context and to be able to fulfil their owner's expectations of a companion animal. For the dog this is relatively straightforward since it is a pack animal with an inbuilt desire for social interaction. It also has a hierarchical structure to its society, which is not dissimilar to our own, and this enables it to integrate into human social structure relatively easily. In contrast, the cat comes from a very different social background and has no ultimate need for physical interaction with its owners. It is a social animal but the basis of its social behaviour in the wild is the cooperative rearing of young and, when it comes to ultimate individual survival, the cat is a solitary creature. These fundamental differences in ethology have important implications for the socialisation of kittens and, in order for domestic cats to appreciate and even value human company, they need exposure to social contact, which prepares them for the expectations of their owners. One of those expectations is close physical interaction and during the socialisation period kittens need to be lifted frequently, gently restrained and touched gently all over their bodies. Such handling prepares them for the cuddling interaction that many owners desire but which is totally alien to a species in which flight is the primary form of defence and the act of being restrained with all four feet off the floor is inherently threatening.

Habituation: The process whereby an animal becomes accustomed to non-threatening environmental stimuli and learns to ignore them.

Kittens and puppies need to be introduced to a variety of environments during their primary socialisation period and also need to encounter those experiences that are part and parcel of life in a domestic environment (Fig 1.6). For the dog, habituation is particularly important because they will encounter a wide range of environments and experi-

---

Recommended socialisation experiences.
Meeting a variety of people:

- Men
- Women
- Young people – babies, children, and teenagers
- Elderly people
- Delivery people – milkman, postman
- People of varying personal appearance – wearing glasses, with and without a beard
- People in a variety of clothing – everyday clothes, uniforms, veterinary practice clothing
- People with various modes of transport – walking, riding a bicycle, on a skateboard, jogging, pushing a pram or pushchair

Meeting a variety of animals:

- Cats
- Dogs
- Livestock
- Horses
- Small domestic pets, e.g., rabbits, guinea pigs, caged birds

When different species are being introduced, it is important to remember the role of prey and predator and to avoid unnecessary stress for either species.

Figure 1.5   Recommended socialisation experiences.

be able to cope with the normal range of human visitors to the home and interact with them without fear. When socialising puppies, it is important to remember that dogs need to cope not only with the family and their visitors but also with delivery people who approach the home and with the vast range of human appearances that they may encounter when they are taken away from the home for exercise. It is therefore important to pay attention to varying appearances when implementing socialisation programmes for puppies and to include people with beards, glasses, walking sticks, people in wheelchairs and those carrying boxes or other heavy loads.

Recommended habituation experiences.

Introduction to a variety of environments
- Veterinary clinic
- Other people's houses
- Railway stations
- Bus stations
- Built-up areas
- Rural areas
- Recreation areas, such as playgrounds and parks
- Highways

Introduction to a variety of novel objects
- Children's accessories, including pushchairs, cots, highchairs, prams
- Household appliances, such as vacuum cleaners, dishwashers, tumble driers
- Human toys, including bicycles, dolls, soft toys
- Animal toys such as chew sticks, squeaky toys
- Traffic

Introduction to a variety of novel sounds
- Aeroplanes
- Gunshots
- Fireworks
- Thunderstorms
- Traffic
- Children and babies

Introduction to a variety of experiences
- Grooming
- Exercise
- Veterinary examination
- Going inside lifts and up and down escalators
- Travelling in a car and on public transport

Figure 1.6   Recommended habituation experiences.

ences as adults and their behaviour is likely to impact on other members of society as well as on their owners. In the past, habituation for cats has been overlooked but, as the cat becomes expected to fulfil a role as a primary companion animal, the number of objects, environments and experiences it is likely to encounter in adulthood are increasing. Fear-related behaviour problems are known to be very prevalent in the feline population and, while many owners never seek professional help for these animals, the welfare implications of poor habituation for kittens cannot be overlooked. The range of experiences that are necessary for puppies and kittens are obviously slightly different and not all the examples in Fig. 1.6 apply to both species!

DEALING WITH BEHAVIOUR CASES

Advice on dealing with common behavioural problems, such as house-soiling in cats and separation-related problems in dogs, is an essential element of preventive behavioural medicine and can prevent minor problems from escalating into serious issues. It can also form an important part of the information offered by the veterinary practice, either as a first-aid approach or as a prelude to referral in established behavioural problems. Specific behavioural conditions are dealt with in the latter parts of this book but at this point it is worth considering the way to approach a behaviour case if the practice decides to offer a more formal behavioural service and carry out behavioural consultations within the practice (Box 1.4).

The behavioural consultation

Due to the nature of behavioural problems and the inevitable relationship between the animal's environment and its behaviour, it is useful to have as many of the people who live with the animal present during the behavioural consultation as possible. This may mean a ratio of as many as one to four for the counsellor and there can be no doubt that increased numbers of people present can make history-taking all the more difficult. It is likely that there will be disagreements between the members of the family but, as long as these stay within control and do not become too heated, such discussion can be helpful in developing a truer picture of the animal's individual circumstances and problem.

Taking a behavioural history

The ability to take a good history is central to all aspects of veterinary work and is arguably the most important skill for a veterinary surgeon to possess. It is essential to be able to differentiate between peripheral information and crucial details. Many veterinary surgeons find the differences between the approach for a medical and a behavioural case somewhat daunting and the sort of information that needs to be obtained and the techniques that are used to obtain it can make history-taking in a behavioural context something of a challenge. However, the aims of a medical and a behavioural consultation are basically the same and behaviour should be seen as a natural extension of veterinary medical practice.

Gathering the relevant information

Many people find it useful to work from some form of questionnaire in order to ensure that all the vital information is received, but it is important to tailor the exact format of any consultation to the individual requirements of the particular client. It is essential to guard against the situation where regimented questions prevent the owner from expressing feelings freely and also to avoid the use of leading questions which will provoke an expected, but not necessarily accurate reply.

Keeping things on track

Although the aim is to put the client at ease, it is also important to remember that you need to gain the maximum amount of information in the time available and that there should be some structure to the consultation in order to avoid rambling conversations that get nowhere (Box 1.5). A combination of a questionnaire approach and casual dialogue is likely to give the best results.

Determining the client's perception of the problem

At the start, it is important to determine what the problem is from the client's point of view and how they expect you to be able to help. In many cases, the client will identify more than one problem and it is useful to determine which of these problems is the most troublesome and focus attention on that in the first instance.

Box 1.4   The aims of a behavioural consultation

- Investigate potential medical causes of the behavioural change
- Reach an accurate diagnosis through observation and questioning
- Get alongside the client
- Communicate the diagnosis and prognosis to the client
- Prescribe a treatment regime if appropriate
- Encourage the client to adhere to the treatment plan via aftercare support

---

Box 1.5   During the consultation the aim is to collect all of the pertinent information about the following areas

- The Pet
- The People
- The Environment
- The Problem

Don't just focus on the problem

In addition to the obviously important details in terms of signalment and clinical history, it is essential to build up a picture of the animal and its environment, both physical and social. Details about the early life experiences of an individual, together with their genetic makeup, can be highly relevant to a behavioural problem and if the owner has information about the behaviour of other related animals, such as littermates or sire or dam, then this may also be useful. In the case of dogs, details about any initial training may also provide an insight into the owner–pet relationship and information about previous behavioural therapy will be relevant for any species (Box 1.6).

Turning attention to the animal's present situation, it is important to gain as clear a picture as possible of the way that the family concerned operates and how the pet fits into that unit. Details of the daily routine will give vital clues and it is important to ask about the pet's reactions to the routine of the owners as well as about its own routine: for example, exercise, play sessions and sleep patterns. Diet and feeding regime also need to be considered since the way in which pets are fed can certainly affect their relationships both with each other and with their owners. However, there is a lack of sound scientific research to support the anecdotal reports of a clear link between diet and behaviour and far more work is needed in this area.

The next area that needs to be explored is that of the human–pet interactions within the family unit. It is useful to ask the client to describe in their own words their relationship with their pet and its relationship with them. This will often give a very good idea of the basis of the bond between them and may provide a vital clue as to the cause of the specific problem in question. It is increasingly being recognised that the way in which owners interact with their pets, and even with each other, can have marked effects on an animal's behaviour and it is not uncommon for there to be a direct link between tensions within the home and development of behavioural problems in pets.

The animal's temperament is obviously of fundamental importance and information can be gained both by asking the client to give a description of it, as they perceive it, and by using observational skills during the consultation to draw your own conclusions. Equally important is information about any alterations in temperament that the owner has noticed over recent weeks and any situations that the owner believes to trigger such alterations.

Getting down to the problem

Obtaining an accurate description of the specific behaviour problem is often difficult but it is a key step toward a diagnosis. Obviously, any description given by the client is going to be dependent upon their personal interpretation of the problem and this does provide room for error. Misinterpretation of the animal's posture and facial expressions may easily lead to confusion as to the motivation for the behaviour and, although much of the information that the counsellor requires can be obtained by talking extensively with the client, additional (and often vital) details will be obtained by careful observation of the animal's behaviour. First hand observation of the specific behaviour is obviously ideal but video footage can also be extremely useful. There is a great deal of benefit to be derived from comparing the information acquired by observation and that provided verbally by the owner and, if there is extreme conflict between the two, it may be necessary to alter the interviewing technique in order to obtain a more accurate picture (Box 1.7).

As well as a description of the behaviour itself, it is also necessary to find out about the circumstances surrounding the onset of the behaviour and any external factors which may have acted as catalysts for the problem. The frequency with which the behaviour is exhibited, as well as the way in which it appears to be developing, are also important factors to be considered. Predictability can be a useful factor in determining prognosis and it is important to remember that a behaviour that is a logical consequence of some trigger perceived by the animal may appear to the owner to be random and unpredictable.

Finally, the client's response to the behavioural problem needs to be considered since this can be of crucial significance, not only with regard to the perpetuation of a problem through some form of reward, be it accidental or intentional, but also when considering the triggering of a specific problem. Any implication that the owner may have contributed to the problem will only serve to make them defensive and hamper the consultation process, so the way in which this area is investigated can be crucial to success.

Box 1.6	General Behavioural History
Animal's details	Genetic influences
Client's details	Early experiences
Relevant clinical history	Daily routines
Present medication	Diet and feeding regime
Previous behavioural therapy	Human–pet interactions
Initial training	Genetic makeup
Previous training	Animal's overall temperament

Box 1.7	Relevant information about the specific problem
Detailed description	
Onset	Frequency
Development	Predictability
Client's response	

Beginning to realise that your own actions may have unwittingly contributed to the problem is very different from feeling that you are being accused of being responsible for your pet's behaviour.

Making the diagnosis

Once all the information has been gathered, you should be in a position to start analysing that information and reaching your diagnosis. As with any veterinary treatment, the aim is to deal with the causes of the problem and not simply the symptoms and, therefore, exploring why the behaviour has developed is an integral part of the consultation (Box 1.8).

Box 1.8   Possible causes of behavioural problems

- Normal species-specific behaviour in an inappropriate context
- Inappropriate learned responses
- Behavioural changes resulting from physical or mental illness
- A combination of the above

Providing informed referral

In some cases, the practice may be able to offer the necessary expertise to deal with the case in-house; but it is not unusual for practices to consider referral for behavioural cases and, when this option is favoured, it is important to ensure that the referral is beneficial to all involved.

Referral in a behavioural context is no different from the process in any other veterinary discipline and appropriate transfer of information from the referring veterinary surgeon to the behaviourist involved is essential. When the referral is to a veterinary behaviourist, it is best to provide a full copy of the animal's medical history over the previous 12 months, together with any significant health information from before that. The results of any medical investigations that have been performed should also be supplied. **Veterinary surgeons are reminded that they do need to obtain the consent of the owner to provide this information to a third party**. If referral is being made to a non-veterinary behaviourist, a written summary of the animal's relevant medical history should be provided.

Informed referral involves a basic level of understanding of behavioural medicine and, just as a veterinary surgeon referring a complex orthopaedic case would be well aware of the surgery required to deal with the problem, so the veterinary surgeon referring a behavioural case should do so with some level of knowledge and understanding, rather than seeing it as an easy option for difficult patients.

Referral involves the transfer of a patient to another party for further investigation of a behavioural problem,

but this does not exclude the primary practitioner from carrying out the initial veterinary examination and health check. Animals presenting with behavioural symptoms should always be examined for potential physical causes and thorough physical examination is the minimum input required prior to referral. In many cases, basic haematology and biochemistry screens will also be useful prior to referral and, in the case of house-training problems and indoor-marking behaviours in cats, urinalysis should be carried out before a behavioural referral is sought.

In order to assist the veterinary surgeon in referring behaviour cases, the Companion Animal Behaviour Therapy Study Group has produced a printed referral form, which has been compiled in consultation with the Royal College of Veterinary Surgeons. This form provides space for all the essential information required in behavioural referrals and encourages a more systematic approach to the referral process. A copy is available in Appendix 1, and an electronic version may be downloaded from http://www.cabtsg.org.

Making the link with disease

One of the most important roles of veterinary involvement in the workup of individual behavioural cases is the exclusion of potential links between systemic disease and behavioural symptoms. Providing suitable medical care for the patient exhibiting behavioural symptoms is the first step in providing a behavioural service, and knowledge of the medical differential diagnoses for the commonly presented behavioural symptoms enables the practice to investigate those symptoms in the most comprehensive way. Details of medical conditions that present with behavioural symptoms can be found in mainstream veterinary medicine textbooks, and examples of medical differentials will be highlighted in the relevant sections of this book.

When investigating a behavioural case, it is important to obtain a thorough medical history, together with the results of a full physical examination. If a medical condition is suspected, it may be necessary to obtain further information such as the result of a basic neurological examination or the results of additional tests, including biochemistry, haematology, urinalysis and, sometimes, radiography (Box 1.9). More specialised tests such as electrocardiograph (ECG), electroencephalograph (EEG), magnetic resonance imaging (MRI), computed tomography (CT) scanning or cerebrospinal fluid (CSF) analysis may be required but are most likely to be requested following behavioural consultation with a veterinary behaviourist rather than carried out prior to referral (Box 1.10).

Although medical differentials should be considered in any behavioural case, those situations in which a medical workup is of specific relevance are as follows:

1. Those involving a change in the personality of the animal, with the onset of aggression or the development of a generally irritable disposition.

> **Box 1.9   Screening profile for behavioural disorders**
>
> - History and clinical examination
> - Basic neurological examination
> - Haematology, to include: PCV, white blood cell count, cell morphology
> - Biochemistry, to include: urea, creatinine, total protein, albumin, bilirubin, bile acids, cholesterol, glucose, ammonia, ALT, AST, ALK, BSP retention, calcium, sodium, potassium, thyroxine, thyroid-stimulating hormone (thyrotropin) stimulation test
> - Urinalysis, to include: blood, protein, SG, pH, bilirubin, bacterial culture and examination for crystals

2. Those involving symptoms related to urinary or gastrointestinal tract function.
3. Those involving dermatological symptoms.

In situations where the appearance of behavioural symptoms does not seem to coincide with any external factors (such as changes in social or physical environment or alterations in the relationship with the owner), where the owner reports the behaviour to be unpredictable and inconsistent, and where the development of the behaviour does not appear to be consistent with the theory of learning, it is especially important to consider medical differentials and provide a thorough medical workup of the case (Box 1.11).

> **Box 1.10   Additional tests as required**
>
> - Cortisol/adrenocorticotropic hormone (ACTH) stimulation test
> - Radiography
> - Assay of sex hormones
> - Skin scrapings and/or biopsies
> - Cultures – swabs or faecal material for bacterial culture, hair samples for fungal culture
> - Myelography
> - Ultrasound/CT/MRI scanning
> - CSF analysis
> - Toxin assays
> - Hearing tests
> - Coomb's test/antinuclear antibody (ANA)/LE cells
> - ECG
> - Malabsorption tests/TLI
> - Allergy tests/exclusion diets
> - Rectal examination
> - Microscopic examination of urine for neoplastic cells or crystals
> - Water deprivation and urine SG
> - Parasitic egg counts

> **Box 1.11   Potential medical causes of inappropriate, abnormal or unacceptable behaviour**
>
> - Cardiovascular disease
> - Congenital/inherited conditions
> - Degenerative conditions
> - Gastrointestinal disease
> - Hormonal disorders
> - Immune/inflammatory conditions
> - Infectious disease
> - Metabolic disease
> - Neoplasia
> - Neurological disorders
> - Nutritional disorders
> - Orthopaedic conditions
> - Pain
> - Toxic conditions
> - Trauma
> - Urogenital disorders

Offering options

The individual nature of behavioural problems not only accentuates the importance of accurate history-taking but also necessitates the careful tailoring of treatment plans to the specific needs of both the animal and its owners. There may be more than one possible approach to the problem and factors such as the severity of the problem, the owner's feelings toward the animal, and their motivation to put any advice into practice, will all need to be considered. The necessary outlay for the owners in terms of money and commitment will also need to be balanced against a realistic prognosis.

Guidelines to dealing with behavioural problems and offering behavioural advice

1. There are no magic injections available for behavioural problems and owners need to be aware of the long-term nature of treatment regimes. Unrealistic expectations will lead to frustration and will rapidly decrease the level of owner motivation that is so crucial to the potential success of treatment.

2. There can be no guarantees since we are always dealing with individual living creatures, each of whom can react differently in any given situation. As Robert Holmes, veterinary behaviourist in Australia, has said, 'Euthanasia is the only way to guarantee that a behaviour will stop'.

3. When dealing with behavioural issues it is essential not to apportion blame but rather to establish the cause, or causes, of the problem by careful questioning of the owners and observation of the animal.

4. It is important to make the client aware of their own role in the modification of their pet's behaviour and to emphasise that success depends on cooperation between themselves and the behaviour counsellor. The counsellor will, hopefully, be able to reach an accurate diagnosis and offer appropriate treatment regimes but it is up to the owner to put the treatment into practice and to keep in touch with the counsellor afterwards to assess progress.

5. Behavioural consultations are always substantially longer than their medical counterparts and hence they will also be correspondingly more expensive. However, the comparison between a clinical consultation and a behavioural consultation is unrealistic. It is more accurate to compare the behavioural consultation with a thorough workup of a complicated medical condition. The difference is that the workup in the case of a dermatological or orthopaedic condition takes place away from the owner while the animal is hospitalised for the day and is in the form of skin scrapes and X-rays. Behavioural workups take place in the presence of the client and take the form of in-depth discussion since the client holds the majority of the information that is necessary to reach a diagnosis.

All part of the service

Preventive treatment and behavioural therapy have a very important place in veterinary practice and by increasing the awareness of behaviour problems within the practice and working closely with behaviourists where necessary, it is possible to offer both patients and clients an excellent service in this field (Box 1.12). The benefits of doing so are enormous for pets and their owners and, indeed, for veterinary practices and their staff.

Box 1.12 Promoting a behavioural service in veterinary practice

- Talk about behaviour during routine consultations.
- Display posters in the waiting room advertising the behavioural service.
- Stock behaviour-related merchandise in the practice.
- Put booklets and magazines with a behavioural message on the tables in the waiting room.
- Play videos in the waiting room area that not only impart some information about behaviour but also to inform clients that behaviour is taken seriously in your practice.
- Pick up on clients' comments, either over the telephone or whilst popping in to buy dog food, and take every opportunity to discuss behaviour.
- Organise talks at your local school – children are very effective at getting the message across to their parents.
- Use practice newsletters and client evenings of talks and seminars to make clients aware of behavioural topics.
- Run puppy parties and kitten information evenings.
- Arrange referrals to someone with a specific interest in behaviour.
- Offer behavioural consultations at the practice.

Chapter **2**

Running puppy classes and kitten information evenings

INTRODUCTION

One very practical way in which veterinary practices can be involved in preventive behavioural medicine is through the provision of puppy parties, puppy classes and kitten information evenings.

The idea behind these ventures is that owners of new puppies and kittens are encouraged to come to the practice for specific sessions during which the major behavioural principles can be introduced and explained, the client and patient can familiarise themselves with the practice, and the practice can bring to the attention of their clients the many services that they have to offer.

PUPPY PARTIES

Puppy parties are the simplest version of these client and patient-centred events and are the easiest to provide. They are one-off events which are usually held on one evening a month and are intended as a foretaste of the more structured puppy socialisation classes. Puppies usually attend 'parties' at between 9 and 12 weeks of age and up to eight puppies can usually be accommodated at each party. Since the puppies are between their first and second vaccinations, it is important to prepare the room adequately by disinfecting the area and to ensure that owners realise the importance of keeping poorly puppies at home. If a puppy is noticeably off-colour it is not sensible to bring it along and no puppy should attend a party on the same day as its vaccination.

Puppies only attend one party and they are sent home with a goody bag packed full of information about the practice and the services that are available. These goody bags can also contain information about important issues such as insurance, but it is important for practices to scan the small print on the policies that they are recommending and advise clients to obtain the most comprehensive cover that they can afford. Edible treats for the puppy can also be included but be careful to ensure that the treats you provide do not, in any way, undermine or contradict your previous advice! The party will usually last for approximately 1 to 2 hours and it is common practice to ensure that it is free to the clients. The practice provides safe, suitable toys and tiny titbits for the puppies and often will provide drinks and light refreshments for the owners. All the family are invited and it is useful if children are encouraged to attend since the presence of a wide range of age-groups will help to provide valuable socialisation for the puppies. However, it is important to remember that 2 hours can be a long time for children to concentrate and the provision of some form of child-orientated activity, such as a colouring table or reading corner, is worthwhile.

In the limited time that is available at puppy parties it is important to prioritise the information that is given and to emphasise the fun element of the evening. The idea is for owners and puppies to have a pleasant evening within the veterinary practice premises, to meet staff in a relaxed and informal manner and to teach some basic behavioural principles which will put the owner on the right road in their relationship with their dog.

There is no set format for these evenings and practices need to develop a plan that works for them, but dividing the evening up into three sessions can be a useful way of ensuring that the important points are covered.

1. An informal introduction.
2. An educational section.
3. A practical session involving introducing the puppies to the consulting room.

During the informal introduction owners should be encouraged to introduce themselves to the other puppies in the group and a game of 'pass the puppy' can certainly help to break the ice. Interaction between the puppies can also take place in this session and practice staff need to be on hand to supervise this 'playtime' and ensure that it is beneficial for all of the puppies that are present. If a very nervous puppy has an aversive experience during a puppy party, it can do more harm than good so identification of strong boisterous individuals and shy timid pups should be done as the clients enter the premises at the start of the evening and, if necessary, the release of puppies for 'playtime' should be staggered. During the informal play session, it is important to take the opportunity to teach owners the importance of playing the right games with their puppies and of ensuring that interaction with other dogs is always under their control.

During the educational section of the evening there are a variety of topics which practices may wish to discuss. Time is limited so it is important to make sure that the most important points are emphasised and, if necessary, other information can be covered in handouts which are included in the goody bag which every puppy gets to take home.

Possible topics to include in the educational section of the puppy party include:

- prevention of common behaviour problems
- neutering
- parasite control
- vaccination
- nutrition
- insurance

In the third part of the evening the individual puppies are taken into the consulting rooms and introduced to the veterinary surgeon or veterinary nurse who offers the puppy titbits as it is standing on the examination table. The aim is to form pleasant associations with the consulting room and make consultations in the future far less traumatic for pets and their owners, as well as for the veterinary surgeon! While each puppy is being given its personal introduction to the examination table, the veterinary nurses can be giving the other puppy owners some more information about health issues or practice facilities.

While the owners are in the consulting room the veterinary surgeon or nurse can teach them how to give their pet a very basic health examination and can emphasise the importance of training their puppy to accept daily inspections of its feet, teeth, eyes and ears. This early training is not only beneficial in teaching puppies to accept veterinary clinical examinations but is also helpful in ensuring that the administration of first-aid will not be a problem should it ever become necessary.

Cost of providing puppy parties

Some practices are reluctant to consider providing puppy parties because of the costs involved but it is worth remembering that the benefits of puppy parties can be seen on three fronts, with owners, pets and practice staff reaping the benefits of this early investment (Box 2.1).

Clients value the opportunity to build a stronger relationship with the practice and to receive valuable advice about how to care for their pets. Practices gain a chance to inform clients of the many services that they have to offer and to educate their clients to take advantage of them. They also have an opportunity to lay good foundations in terms of client interactions with their pets and to pave the way toward better-behaved animals in their consulting rooms. Pets in turn benefit from better education and training from their owners, from increased opportunities to socialise with people and other dogs and from the chance to form positive associations with the veterinary practice environment and staff.

In cases where practices are reluctant to cover the entire costs of these evenings, sponsorship is often a viable alternative and many companies will welcome the opportunity to introduce their products to receptive new puppy owners. In return for sponsorship, the company will be able to distribute literature to clients and to increase the profile of their name in the minds of new owners.

PUPPY SOCIALISATION CLASSES

Although puppy parties are a valuable addition to the services that practices have to offer, they are not long enough to allow in-depth discussion of behavioural or health-related

Box 2.1   Benefits of providing puppy parties within the practice

Pets gain:

- an opportunity to socialise with other people and other dogs
- the chance to go to the veterinary practice for a positive experience
- an opportunity to meet practice staff in a positive atmosphere
- an increase in the level of their owner's understanding of their needs.

Practice staff gain:

- the chance to inform clients of the varied practice facilities and services
- the opportunity to form closer relationships with clients
- an improvement in the standard of behaviour of patients in the consulting room.

Owners gain:

- the opportunity to meet with other puppy owners
- the chance to discuss their concerns with veterinary practice staff
- valuable education about their pet's behavioural and physical needs
- a better behaved pet who is a pleasure to own

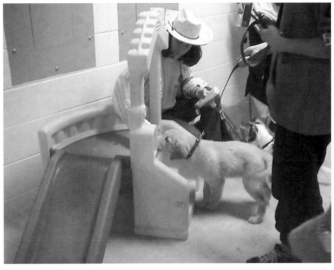

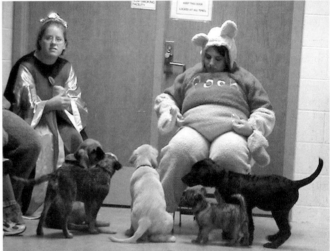

Figure 2.1   The range of novel stimuli encountered by puppies at socialisation classes may be expanded by the use of costumes and props.

issues and owners are advised to follow on with more socialisation and training by enrolling their puppies in a puppy socialisation class.

In contrast to the puppy party, the socialisation class spans 4 to 6 weeks and takes the form of a course in early training, appropriate socialisation, and responsible pet ownership. There is a greater opportunity to provide the puppies with exposure to novelty in the form of play equipment, different domestic items brought from the owners' homes and people dressed differently so that the puppies have experienced a really wide range of people, including children and the elderly (Fig. 2.1)

Some veterinary practices have the facilities and the manpower to set up puppy classes at their own premises. This is ideal since it offers extended opportunities to educate owners and improve client relations and the puppy class in a veterinary context can include education on health-related matters as well as behaviour. Unfortunately, however, it is simply not possible for all practices to provide this service and, in these situations, it is important for practice staff to make it a priority to find out about the nearest puppy socialisation classes that are available and to encourage clients to take their puppies along. Those classes that are held at training schools rather

than veterinary practices will obviously be more focused on behaviour and training but, provided that they are well run, they offer a vital opportunity for puppies to socialise with people and other dogs and to set owners on the right path in terms of training techniques. In some areas it may be necessary for owners to travel considerable distances to get to a puppy class but an investment in time and money in order to attend will more than pay for itself if the result is a well-mannered dog who is a pleasure to own for the next 15 years. By giving owners the information about puppy classes and telling them how to find one, the veterinary practice is providing as much of a behavioural service as one that has the facilities to offer classes on its own premises. See Figure 2.2 for guidelines for the format of puppy socialisation classes.

Potential pitfalls of puppy classes

Veterinary practices are in an ideal position to explain the potential benefits of puppy classes and their recommendation will be seriously considered by any new owners who

---

Suggested format for a 4-week puppy socialization class within a veterinary practice.

At each session (excluding week one) there is the opportunity for a session of controlled play, a short 'training session' and introduction to the consulting room. Each session ends with a short question session.

WEEK ONE
- Owners come to the practice without their puppies!
- This gives the opportunity for owners to concentrate on the information that is being given without being distracted by their puppies
- Videos can be used to educate owners about canine communication and pack structure
- The importance of socialisation and habituation is highlighted
- The aims of the puppy class are explained and any important questions answered

WEEK TWO
- Puppies and owners are welcome
- Discuss basic principles of learning theory
- Introduce the concept of the use of a food lure and hand signals in teaching puppies to sit
- Discuss ways to overcome common problems such as play-biting and house-training
- Give information about diet and exercise

WEEK THREE
- Introduction to basic veterinary examination to encourage acceptance of handling
- Introduce the concept of clicker training and use to teach 'down' command
- Discuss dental issues
- Give information about identification and neutering

WEEK FOUR
- Discuss need for routine vaccination and parasite control
- Teach basic first aid for dogs
- Discuss legal implications of dog ownership
- Explain the benefits of pet insurance

Figure 2.2   Suggested format for a 4-week puppy socialisation class within a veterinary practice.

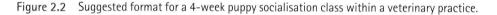

are keen to do the very best for their new pet, so it is vital that the practice has first-hand knowledge and experience of the class before it starts to recommend that its clients attend. As with dog training classes, there are good and bad puppy classes and, whilst the advantages of socialisation classes are undoubted, the way in which those classes are run is crucial to their success. Socialisation and habituation are vitally important but they need to be carried out correctly if they are to be beneficial and inappropriate techniques can result in an experience which is totally counterproductive. For example, periods of off-lead socialisation need to be controlled and small numbers of puppies should be allowed to interact at a time. Free-for-alls with large numbers of puppies being let off to 'enjoy themselves' can do more harm than good. Instead, owners should stay in control and, periodically throughout the 'playtime', puppies should be called back to their owners in order to learn that human instruction is always more important than uncontrolled fun. The temperaments of the puppies present need to be taken into account and nervous and withdrawn individuals need to be given the opportunity to explore without being overwhelmed by others. Inappropriate experiences at this stage can lead to the development of behaviour problems, rather than their prevention and the products of unsuccessful puppy classes will often find their way into behavioural clinics later in life with problems relating to inappropriate communication with other dogs.

ESTABLISHING LINKS WITH TRAINERS

It is well established that even the best programme of socialisation and habituation in early puppyhood needs to be maintained if it is to have lasting effects and, for owners who have attended appropriate puppy socialisation classes, it is important to follow this early education programme with ongoing and appropriate training.

Basic obedience training is an important factor in maintaining a good dog–owner relationship and it has a strong role to play in the prevention of behavioural problems. Obviously, it is neither possible nor appropriate for veterinary surgeries to offer training classes at their premises, but owners will often look to veterinary practice staff for guidance as to which training school to select. Many practices do not wish to be seen to endorse any particular trainer, but the desire to remain impartial can lead to the practice of veterinary surgeries displaying the business cards of every training club in the area! This is not helpful to the clients and may even be detrimental to the animals. If telephone numbers have been obtained from a veterinary surgery most clients will assume that the training club is in some way approved by the practice and, especially for new dog owners who have nothing to compare, such recommendation is heavily relied upon. It does not take long for a member of the practice staff to visit the local training classes while they are in action and this gives them the opportunity to see what training methods are being employed. Inappropriate training techniques can do immeasurable damage both in the short and the long term and, therefore, practices owe it to their clients to only suggest training classes that they know something about.

KITTEN EVENINGS

Until recently the emphasis in terms of preventive behavioural medicine has been on the provision of adequate socialisation and habituation for puppies but, as the cat takes over the number one slot as the most popular companion animal, the importance of preparing kittens for life in a human context is also increasing. Many practices are now finding that they have a higher percentage of cats on their books than dogs and yet kitten owners often receive a fraction of the help and support that is on offer to puppy owners in terms of their pet's behaviour (Fig. 2.3).

There has been a lot of interest in the programme of Kitten Kindergarten, which has been pioneered in Australia by veterinary surgeon Dr Kersti Seksel and involves inviting kitten owners to bring their kittens to the veterinary hospital in order to attend two 1-hour classes held 1 week apart. Dr Seksel stresses that these classes are not simply feline versions of the puppy party since cats and dogs are two very distinct species and the methods used to train and socialise dogs cannot simply be transferred to the feline world.

The aims of the classes according to Dr Seksel are to:

- increase the knowledge of owners about cats
- have better behaved adult cats
- prevent behaviour problems
- build a strong bond between the veterinary practice and the client.

In the Australian programme, the classes accommodate kittens of 12 to 14 weeks of age, with classes being limited to 3 to 6 kittens. Kittens older than 14 weeks are excluded as they may simply learn to fight rather than play, unless the classes are very well controlled. In the UK there has been some resistance to the provision of classes for kittens and their owners owing to concerns over the fact that the kitten's socialisation period runs from 2 to 7 weeks of age and, therefore, the benefits of actual social interaction with other kittens during the class may be limited. Obviously, the limitations of vaccination mean that classes at an earlier age are not possible on health grounds and, therefore, a compromise has been established whereby owners of young kittens are invited to come along to the practice without their pets for a 'kitten information evening'.

These evenings can be highly successful as a public relations exercise and they offer the opportunity for practice staff to pass on crucial information about kitten development and health care. If the practice has an adult cat or demonstration kitten that can be on site for the evening, it is possible to demonstrate the various training techniques and handling skills and then encourage owners to go home and practice with their own pet. Until the contentious issues regarding face-to-face feline socialisation classes are explored in more detail the 'kitten evening' is the perfect compromise and illustrates to clients that cats are valued by the practice as much as dogs (Fig. 2.3).

Suggested format for a 2-week course of kitten information evenings within a veterinary practice.

WEEK ONE
- Discussion about the origins of the cat and the history of its relationship with man
- Explanation of the social structure of feline society
- Overview of feline communication systems
- Explanation of the importance of play in feline development and the selection of appropriate toys
- Discussion about dental care and nutrition

WEEK TWO
- Introduction to the basics of learning theory, illustrated by teaching the demonstration cat to give a paw!
- Discussion about the appropriate use of rewards and discipline
- Explanation of the importance of environmental enrichment, especially for totally indoor cats
- Discussion about routine vaccination and parasite control
- Explanation of the benefits of pet insurance

Figure 2.3   Suggested format for a 2-week course of kitten information evenings within a veterinary practice.

PART 2

Basic tools in behavioural medicine

PART CONTENTS

Chapter 3

An overview of canine social behaviour and communication

INTRODUCTION

In order to understand the way in which dogs relate to their owners, to people outside the family, to other household pets and to dogs that they meet out on walks, it is essential to have a basic knowledge of canine social behaviour and communication. It is generally accepted that the domestic dog is descended from the wolf, although the process of domestication is believed to have occurred in more than one location and despite the time that has elapsed and the significant level of selective breeding that has occurred, the dog still shows many of the behaviour patterns that are exhibited by its ancestor species.

WOLF SOCIAL BEHAVIOUR

The wolf is the largest and the most social of all canids. Characteristically, wolves live in a pack of related individuals but, in common with most canids, they display significant flexibility in their social organisation depending upon the availability of food. Under normal circumstances only one male and one female within the pack breed at one time and these individuals are referred to as the 'alpha' or top-ranking pair. Their role is to ensure the continuation of the pack through breeding and in order to achieve this, they provide leadership for the group, control access to shared resources and suppress breeding in other pack members. The remaining lower-ranking members of the pack assist in the rearing of young and all members of the group cooperate in hunting in order to increase the size and range of prey that can be caught. Individuals only remain associated with the pack as long as it is advantageous to them. When food becomes plentiful during the summer months the members of the pack often disperse and then reunite in the autumn when it becomes necessary to hunt larger prey.

The individuals who obtain the most personal benefit from their pack membership are the alpha male and alpha female since their fellow pack members help to feed and protect their cubs, so increasing the cub survival rate and the chances of the alpha pair successfully passing on their genetic material into the next generation. The nature of aggression within the pack reflects this fact and the alpha female in particular is very aggressive towards other females during the mating season. Studies have shown that through persistent attacks they will cause the cubs being carried by a lower-ranking female in the group to be miscarried. The alpha male, contrastingly, is most aggressive towards strangers that attempt to associate with the pack and this is presumably to ensure that no other unrelated wolf sires cubs that he will then help to raise.

Interestingly, the lower-ranking members of the group tend to be sociable to other wolves, both inside and outside the pack, and to demonstrate an inherent need for social interaction.

DOG SOCIAL BEHAVIOUR

Although many similarities are seen between the natural behaviour of the wolf and the behaviour of the domestic dog, it is important to remember that the close association between the dog and man has had a profound effect on canine social behaviour and communication. The fact that most dogs are kept within a predominantly human-orientated environment and have only brief opportunities to interact with other members of their own species in a social context means that few dogs have a chance to set up stable social relationships free from human influence. Studies which have investigated the effects of domestication on the social behaviour of the dog have primarily focussed on feral and free-roaming dogs and have shown that packs are formed in which some individuals are able to gain plenty of access to resources over others. This supports the concept of relative status within the group and the existence of some form of dominance hierarchy. Unlike wolf packs, however, little cooperative hunting and rearing of the young is seen and communication between individuals appears to be more limited than within wolf packs. Nonetheless, many of the same signals have been demonstrated in feral or free-roaming dogs and more research is required to investigate their significance.

COMMUNICATION

Within a social system, effective communication is essential for the formation and maintenance of relationships and dogs, like wolves, have three main methods of communication. These involve the use of auditory, visual and olfactory signalling and a basic awareness of the significance of these signals can hold the key to understanding many of the commonly presented behavioural problems in veterinary practice.

Auditory communication

Auditory signals are used to communicate in a variety of different contexts over a range of distances. Studies have described a range of signals given by dogs that have also been recorded in wolves. Sounds include grunts, whines, yelps, screams, coughing, tooth snapping, growling and barking. The message conveyed by these sounds seems to vary according to the context (Fig. 3.1).

The information conveyed by the vocalisation is supplemented with information about the whereabouts of the messenger and vocal signalling can take on specific significance when vision is impaired, for example, by thick vegetation or at night.

One of the most striking differences in terms of auditory signalling in dogs and wolves is in the frequency of barking and levels of this particular form of canine communication are believed to be higher in the domestic dog than in any other canid. Certainly, adult wolves rarely bark unless they are doing so to alert the rest of the pack to some potential danger or offer some form of challenge to a wolf from outside of the social group. It is this second function of defending the social group and calling attention to potential threats that is believed to have been selected for in the breeding of domestic dogs, but this is not the whole story and barking is also believed to have been advantageous in the guiding of human hunters during the pursuit of prey.

Barking is also believed to be more frequent in juvenile canids than in adults and the selection of juvenile characteristics in dogs through the process of neotenisation is believed to have included selection for more frequent barking. As this has happened, the function of the bark has

SOUND	BEHAVIOUR
Whimper/whine	Appeasement Defence Greeting Pain Attention-seeking
Teeth-chatter	Play Defence Warning General Excitement Anticipation
Grunt	Greeting Sign of contentment
Growl	Defence warning Threat/play signal
Bark	Defence Play Greeting Call for attention Warning
Howl	Call for attention To announce presence

Figure 3.1 Meanings of different canine vocalisations.
(Adapted from J. Serpell 1995 The domestic dog. Cambridge University Press, Cambridge, UK)

altered to the point where it now serves no function except to attract attention to the animal and any visual signals it may be displaying. It is certainly not possible to gain any additional information about an individual as a result of its bark, other than the fact that it is in a raised state of arousal.

Visual communication

Within and between wolf packs visual communication is central to conveying information about social status and emotional state and is particularly useful for controlling aggression during social interactions. Whole body postures, together with facial expressions and tail postures, are used to convey the likelihood of conflict and to offer the opponent an opportunity to signal that confrontation is unnecessary (Figs. 3.2–3.5).

In wolf society, a high-ranking individual is characterised by an upright, high body posture with head, tail and ears held erect, while less confident, lower-ranking individuals adopt a lower, more crouched, body posture with tail and ears held low and close to the body. The impression created by the higher-ranking individual is one

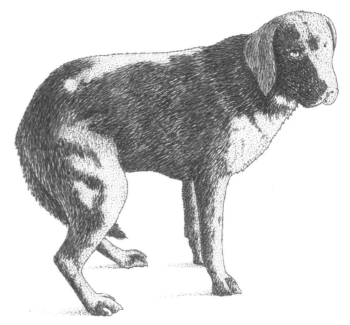

Figure 3.2　Labrador retriever showing posture typical of fear. This posture decreases the animal's apparent size in order to reduce the threat it poses. Tail is tucked under and head is carried low.

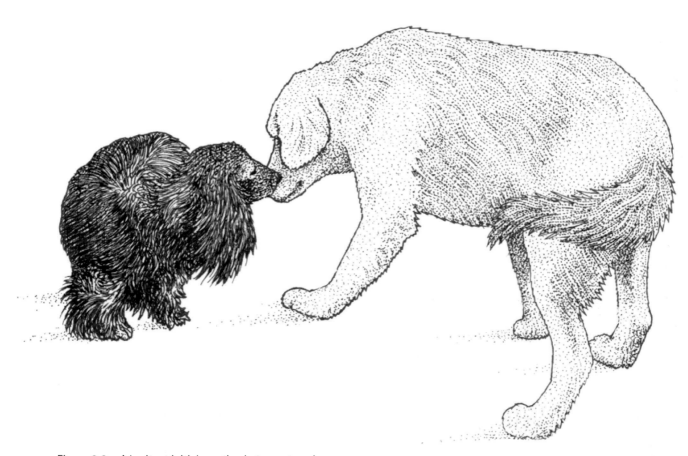

Figure 3.3　A hesitant initial greeting between two dogs.

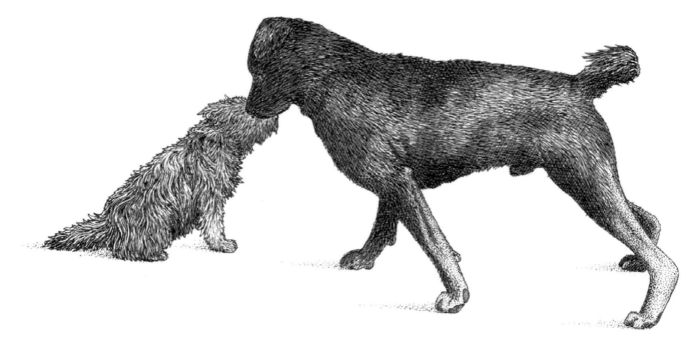

Figure 3.4   The dog on the right is more bold, showing a more upright body posture and higher tail carriage.

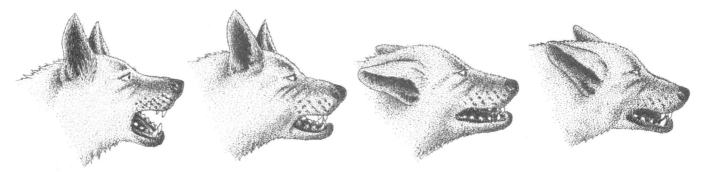

Figure 3.5   Aggressive facial postures in the dog. To the left is a typically dominant facial posture, with increasing subordinate or fearful posture displayed rightwards. Note the ear position, facial tension, eye closure, and shift from front teeth being displayed to side teeth being displayed.

of confidence and control while the lower-ranking animal uses posture to make it look smaller and less significant than it really is.

Signals of aggression and fear, or appeasement, are used to exaggerate these basic postures and to avoid direct confrontation but as the distance between the individuals lessens, so the need for more honest signalling is seen. A confident wolf that is intending to use aggression to resolve the situation, if necessary, will use postural signals to make its body appear larger. These might include raising the hackles and tail, leaning forward toward the animal which is being threatened and staring intently, baring its teeth, curling its lips and flicking its tongue in and out to draw attention to the oral weaponry on display. As the aggressive encounter continues, the aggressor will move closer to its opponent and show its strength by attempting to physically push or displace the other, but this will not occur until some subtle communication on the part of the lower ranking individual has taken place. A fearful wolf that is trying to stop any further escalation in aggression will attempt to do so by decreasing its perceived physical size through cringing, tucking its tail between its legs and holding its head down and demonstrating its desire to appease by avoiding eye contact and displaying a submissive grin in which the corners of the mouth are pulled back. If the aggressor fails to respond to these signals and the threat of out-and-out physical confrontation continues, these fearful individuals will roll on their back and display the anogenital area as a sign that they are giving up any attempt at defence. This passive submission is sometimes accompanied by urination. A more confident subordinate will adopt a slightly different strategy and engage in active submission whereby it approaches the aggressor with its body held low and its tail wagging. It will often attempt to lick and nuzzle the face of the opponent in a parallel to the food-begging gestures shown by cubs and will respond to attempts to physically displace it.

In view of the fact that outright physical confrontation runs the risk of injury to either party, the wolf has developed an elaborate communication system and when two wolves meet one another and both are interested in gaining the same resource, such as a piece of food, they will exchange a display of visual signals which are designed to avert conflict. Through the signals each is able to assess its likelihood of success in a physical fight. The signals that are first shown are usually ones that can be exchanged at a distance and the least aggressive of these signals is the stare. If an animal decides to proceed no further in its aggression it can end the conflict by looking away. As the competition progresses the signals escalate in intensity and the individuals move closer to one another, so increasing the chances of physical injury occurring. As the intensity of aggressive signalling increases, so too does the intensity of appeasement which is needed to stop the conflict and the postural signals become more and more exaggerated. The only circumstances in which overt damaging aggression will occur are when two animals are so well-matched that neither is able to determine which is physically stronger, or when both are equally motivated to fight in order to protect a resource of significant value.

Another socially significant posture in wolves is the play-bow (see Figure 3.6 for an example in the domestic dog), which indicates a willingness to play. This is shown by the wolf lowering its fore-quarters whilst keeping its hind legs erect. Prior to this, the wolf may have made several exaggerated approaches to the individual it wishes to play with and have withdrawn rapidly while wagging its tail. Often the mouth is held open and exaggerated panting occurs. These behaviours are designed to ensure that there is a level of understanding between the individuals as they engage in play and to signal that any aggressive signals encountered during the impending interaction are not to be taken seriously.

The degree to which a domestic dog uses visual signalling depends to a large extent on the breed since selective breeding for particular colourings and certain morphological characters, such as drooping ears, long fur, heavy jowls and short tails, have made it difficult for some breeds to accurately signal their emotional state. An Old English Sheepdog, for example, is unable to significantly raise its

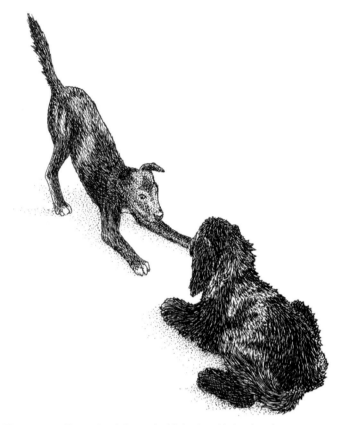

Figure 3.6   Example of the typical 'play bow' behaviour between two puppies.

hackles, has great difficulty in signalling with its tail and ears and finds it impossible to use eye contact effectively. For such breeds the only type of aggressive signals they can display are the more intense ones and, since this limits their options for warning other dogs off, it becomes more likely that they may get involved in physical fights. Studies done at the University of Southampton have indicated that the range of aggressive and submissive behaviours shown by a breed is closely correlated to their physical appearance. For example, breeds that resemble juvenile or neonatal wolves more than adults, such as the Pekingese, show fewer and more intense agonistic signals than more adult wolf-like breeds such as Huskies. Interestingly, it is the breeds of more juvenile appearance which are more likely to interact with other dogs in a juvenile manner and, since juvenile interactions are often more physical (and hence aggressive), this explains why many of the small companion breeds have a reputation for being aggressive.

Olfactory communication

Scent signals are often overlooked by humans since they are of very little significance in their own social communications but wolves and dogs show a similar ability to communicate via smells and odours and their importance should not be underestimated.

In the canine world, the deposition of faeces, urine, and anal sac secretions around the animal's environment is an important aspect of social communication and the distinctive body odour of individuals is believed to convey important information about a number of issues, including identity, sex and sexual receptiveness. In addition, a combination of scent signals are used to indicate information about ownership of an area, the frequency of its use and how recently an animal has passed through it.

One of the major advantages of olfactory signalling over other forms of communication is the fact that the messages remain in the environment for a long time and can signal even when the depositor is not present. This is particularly useful when encounters between individuals are best avoided and when animals are entering into a territory for the first time and run the risk of meeting with a hostile reception.

Faeces

Faeces do appear to have a particular significance as a form of scent communication in wolves, with pack members leaving their faeces where they are likely to be located by other wolves. They are believed to act as a marker of residency without the need for the territory owners to be present and it is certainly true that scent marks are deposited at greater densities along the edges of territories and especially if a foreign scent is encountered. In contrast, dogs show much less interest in faeces, and defecate most commonly when off the lead and when the owner is not present. This is possibly due to the inhibitory effect of training methods used during the house-training process but there is little evidence that faeces play much of a role in olfactory communication in dogs apart from notifying an individual, by the freshness of the dung, that another dog has passed by.

Urine

Unlike faeces, urine appears to be equally important to both wolves and dogs as a method of communication and urine marks are eagerly investigated by both species. The strength of the odour of urine marks decay over time as volatile chemicals in the urine evaporate and this enables animals to use these signals to determine how recently a dog has passed by and left a mark. Regular overmarking of scent marks indicates to others that an individual wolf or dog uses the area frequently.

In addition to supplying dogs with temporal information, urine marks can also give information about sex and sexual receptivity and status. In oestrus, females produce urine that is rich in social odours that indicate sexual receptivity and they increase their frequency of urination during oestrus to spread the odour-rich urine over a wider area so as to increase their chances of attracting a mate.

It is not only the odour of urine marks that conveys important information between wolves. Location is also believed to be significant. Alpha males and females cock their leg when they urinate and information about status is believed to be conveyed in the relative positioning of urine signals, with higher-ranking individuals depositing their marks higher off the ground than lower-ranking members of the pack.

In dogs, status seems to affect the method of leaving scent marks less significantly, but males will generally deposit urine by raising a leg in a cocking motion while females more commonly squat to urinate. Prominent objects are usually selected to urinate on, presumably because they act as visual cues to encourage investigation of the presence of any olfactory marks.

Anal sacs

All canids possess anal sacs which are paired reservoirs either side of the anus that produce apocrine gland secretions. The contents of the anal sacs are discharged during defecation and variation in the composition is believed to reflect changes in daily diet. The significance of the anal gland secretions in canine communication is the subject of some debate, but studies have shown that individuals differ in the chemical constituents of their anal sac secretions and they are therefore thought to be important in individual recognition. In wolves, the highest-ranking individuals within a pack present their anogenital area for inspection during greeting rituals but subordinates cover it with their tail and try to avoid being sniffed. Such behaviour appears to be mimicked when two strange dogs encounter each other and in many cases both dogs seem to behave like subordinate wolves, eager to collect scent information but unwilling to give any away.

General odours

These are produced by a variety of skin glands situated around the head, anal region, upper surface of the base of the tail and the perineum. These glands are thought to provide each dog and wolf with an individual odour and to be important in the recognition of members of the same social group. Detection of these odours is therefore important in greeting rituals and this explains why dogs usually engage in head-to-head or head-to-rear end communication when they first meet.

Chapter 4

An overview of feline social behaviour and communication

INTRODUCTION

Many of the behaviour problems commonly presented in the domestic cat arise as a consequence of the constraints of domestic life on an animal that is not truly domesticated and from human misinterpretations of natural feline behaviours. It is therefore important for anyone dealing with the prevention and treatment of these problems to have an understanding of feline social structure and of the communication systems that are central to the maintenance of an effective feline society.

In the wild, cats live together in groups of related individuals and they have very little contact with outsiders. They hunt alone and when they are out on hunting expeditions they aim to limit their interaction with other felines. For these reasons, most feline language is designed to increase distance between individuals and those signals that are intended to encourage interaction are usually reserved for members of the same social group.

SOCIAL STRUCTURE AND BEHAVIOURS

Feline society is matriarchal in nature, with related females living together in highly cooperative groups, sharing the rearing of each other's offspring and defending each other from potential intruders. In order for a society to function it is necessary for interactive behaviour patterns to signal group identity and structure and in many species, including dog and man, these patterns are related to some kind of hierarchical organisation within which an individual's position can be determined by observation of its interactions with other members of its group. Some of the most significant of these patterns are those indicating submission but within the feline world no such pattern has been identified and their reaction to hostile interactions is one of defence rather than submission. Without the presence of a hierarchical framework, the stability of social groups relies on the presence of cooperative behaviours and in the case of feline society, it appears that the affiliative social behaviours of allogrooming and allorubbing hold the key to social harmony. These mutual behaviours appear to be important in confirming the social relationship between individuals and in establishing and maintaining a common scent profile within the social group.

Allogrooming

In the case of allogrooming the behaviour appears to be reciprocal in nature. It often coincides with resting and therefore it is most commonly seen between cats that rest together (Fig. 4.1). In addition to its role in reinforcing bonds between closely related individuals and providing stability within the social group, allogrooming is also believed to facilitate reconciliation between two members of a social group that have recently been antagonistic towards one another.

Allorubbing

Allorubbing is believed to act not only as a means of mixing scents between individuals (Fig. 4.2) but also as a means of exchanging tactile signals and, unlike allogrooming, this behaviour appears to be asymmetrical in nature with one individual noticeably taking the initiative in the interaction. Indeed, it is often possible to detect a pattern of rubbing within a social grouping which suggests some hierarchical significance to this behaviour as it progresses from kittens, which rub frequently on all cats except adult males, through juveniles, which rub on adult females, to the adult females themselves, which rub on each other and, occasionally, on adult males. Of all of the feline social behaviours rubbing is the one with most significance in the cat–owner relationship and when cats rub on their owner's legs it is usually interpreted as a sign of affection. However, observation of the behaviour between cats suggests that it is used when the relationship is slightly one-sided and is usually initiated by the weaker individual. Cats do not live in a structured hierarchy but they do have respect for one another and, while rubbing may not be classed as a submissive behaviour, it

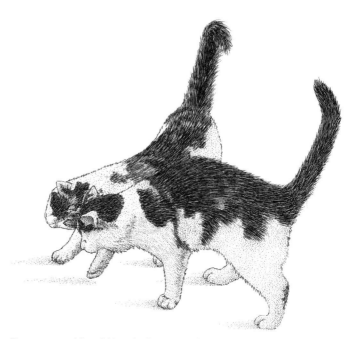

Figure 4.2   Allorubbing during a greeting between two cats.

does appear to be important as a means of acknowledging status. Immediately before a rubbing interaction the initiator will raise its tail as it approaches the other cat and this gesture appears to be a significant signal of intent to rub. What happens next appears to depend on the reaction of the recipient and in situations where it responds with a raised tail signal, the rubbing appears to continue as a mutual and simultaneous behaviour whereas recipients that do not use a tail-up response will either rub after the initiator has rubbed, or not at all. Within the context of cat–owner interactions, rubbing appears to be a means of acknowledging owner status, confirming the relationship between the two species and also exchanging scent signals in order to establish a common scent which can then be used to identify members of the same social group and reassure individuals that they belong. It is also a behaviour that is reinforced in most domestic cats by the response of the owners and for many individuals it has been conditioned as a behaviour which results in the human response of opening another tin of cat food!

COMMUNICATION CHANNELS

In common with canine communication, the methods that cats use to convey information fall into the three main categories of visual, vocal and olfactory signalling, but transferring knowledge of dog communication into the feline world simply does not work and trying to do so can lead to unnecessary confrontation. Feline visual signals are often subtle in nature and can be difficult to interpret whereas olfactory communication, which plays such a vital role in feline society, is simply a mystery to human beings. Vocalisation is a highly conditioned form of communication in the domestic cat and, while information is available about the function of the major vocal signals, it should be remembered that some of the signals used by individual

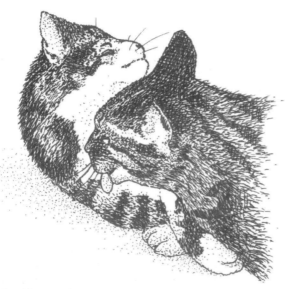

Figure 4.1   Allogrooming

cats within households are learned responses to the interactions of those around them. These signals are used by cats to initiate social interaction with owners and to direct people to perform certain tasks, such as feeding the cat or opening doors and windows to allow access to outdoors.

Olfactory communication

Although cats are social creatures, they retain an element of independence and when it comes to the process of hunting they act alone. Important consequences of this solitary hunter status are the need to maintain personal fitness, to avoid unnecessary conflict and risk of injury and to secure and protect a hunting territory. In order to fulfil these objectives the cat needs to be able to communicate with other cats from a distance and to signal its occupancy of its territory without risking direct physical interaction with total strangers. It is for this reason that olfactory communication, which provides a signal that lasts over a period of time and gives a message to other cats remotely, is so important in the feline world. Indeed, the cat is highly adapted to send and receive scent signals through the presence of special scent-producing glands in various locations around the body and through the use of the Jacobson's or vomeronasal organ to receive and interpret scent messages. The major areas of scent production are the face, the flanks and the tail base but cats also have glands on the paws, which deposit scent signals during the process of scratching. The scent that the individual produces is believed to be unique and helps to identify it to other cats both within its social group and in the wider community. It is also important to realise that scent signals can be used as a means of self-directed communication and can be deposited as signals to the depositor regarding the familiarity of the environment and the level of security that it offers. The depositing of scent signals, or marking behaviour, is therefore essential to feline communication and social behaviour and within the context of domestic cat behaviour it takes four main forms.

Rubbing

In addition to the social behaviour of allorubbing, cats use the glands on the face, flank and tail base to mark items within their territory. They will rub their face along twigs and fence posts in the garden and along items such as shopping bags and new furniture that are brought into the house. Owners will often comment that their cat rubs its face along their shoes when they return home and this appears to be a reaction to the multitude of different scent signals that are carried on the surface of shoes. Although little is known about the behavioural significance of many of the social odours produced from the range of scent-producing glands on the cat's skin, there has been extensive research into the constituents of some of the facial scent glands and the scents that are deposited during the act of facial rubbing seem to be highly correlated with the solicitation of social interaction and with familiarisation with the environment.

Commercially produced analogues of the F3 (Feliway) and F4 (Felifriend) fractions are used in the prevention and treatment of certain behavioural problems in cats.

Scratching

When cats scratch they are engaging in a very natural and complex behaviour which has both functional and marking components. As the front claws are pulled downward in that familiar stropping action, the blunted outer claw sheath is removed and a glistening new claw is revealed. In addition to preparing the claws for hunting, scratching also enables cats to stretch their front legs, shoulders and back and exercise the muscles and tendons involved in claw protraction, thereby ensuring swift action when prey is detected. Although the maintenance of hunting prowess is a priority for cats, scratching is also an important behaviour in terms of communication and the glands between the pads of the cat's feet deposit a special scent signal as the cat scratches. This scent message is in addition to a visual signal: the vertical scratch marks which are left in the surface.

Urine marking

The use of urine as a marker is common practice in feline circles and the act of urine spraying is usually performed from a standing position. The name *spraying* comes from the very characteristic position that cats adopt as they back up against the scent post and squirt very small amounts of urine in a horizontal stream onto the vertical surface. They usually have their back slightly arched during the behaviour and will tread with their hind feet while the tip of their tail quivers (Fig. 4.3). Most cats appear to concentrate while they are depositing their signal and a vacant expression on the face is common. Although spraying is the most common form of urine marking, it is not the only one and some cats will mark with urine that they deposit from a squatting position. Whichever position they adopt, all cats engage in urine marking at some point in their lives and most do so on a very regular basis in their outdoor territory. This is not a behaviour that is limited to tomcats and cats of either sex will still urine-mark when they are neutered. One of the purposes of urine-marking as a form of communication in the outdoor environment is to operate a very elaborate time-share system which ensures that the available territory is not overhunted. It also minimises the risk of unfamiliar individuals coming into contact and potential confrontation.

Although spacing between cats appears to be one of the most important functions of feline marking behaviours, it is important to remember that urine marking has the opposite function when it is performed by entire males and females as a means of informing neighbouring cats that they are ready and available for mating. In this situation the urine of oestrous females appears to carry important information regarding her sexual status and level of receptivity and tomcats pay a great deal of attention to the marks of these females. It is this sexual component of spraying

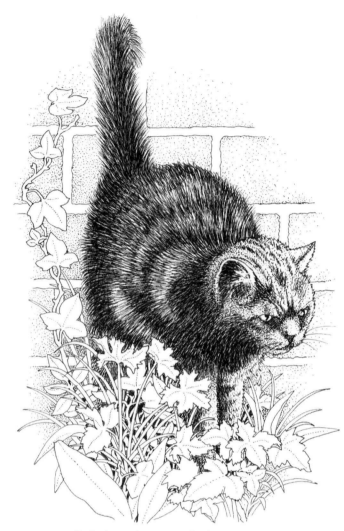

Figure 4.3   Typical spraying posture in the cat.

behaviour which is affected by neutering and, therefore, the likelihood of developing problems associated with this form of marking can be reduced by ensuring that cats of both sexes are neutered prepubertally.

In many cases within the domestic environment, urine marks appear to act as a self-directed signal and a means of reassuring the cat that the territory is their own or of signalling that a particular location is associated with potential danger. Indeed, the locations of indoor spray marks are often those that are associated with something unpleasant, such as threat from outside cats. Spraying can also occur as a redirected activity when other forms of social interaction are frustrated, or even as a learnt attention-seeking activity to gain social contact with owners. It has also been reported as a passive manifestation of aggression in situations of social tension between cats in the same household.

Middening

As well as using urine as a marker, cats can use their faeces to communicate with other cats and when they deposit faeces in deliberate locations in order to get a message across to their fellow felines this is called *middening*. This behaviour is usually seen at the boundaries of the cat's territory and piles of faeces which are found in exposed locations such as the middle of a well-mown lawn, the tops of fence posts and the ridges of roofs are more likely to have been deposited as deliberate markers than be the product of normal elimination behaviour.

Vocal communication

Although cats do use vocalisation in order to communicate this is probably the form of feline communication that we know least about. Cats are generally considered to be at their most vocal while they are kittens and a lot of vocal signalling in the cat is associated with greeting and with social contact. There are thought to be at least 16 different distinct vocal signals but research is still being carried out into exactly what each of these signals means. The picture is also complicated by the fact that many cats use vocal signals that are unique to themselves; owners of more than one cat will often comment on the fact that they know which cat is approaching by the type of miaow. It is well-recognised that cats are very good at training their owners to respond to their vocal demands and the development of the individual noises is probably connected with the timing of the owner's response.

In general terms, cat sounds can be divided into three groups. The first includes those noises that are produced with the mouth open and gradually closing, in a similar way to our own speech, and examples include the miaow which is used in greeting and the female and male calling signals used during the mating process. Their aim is to incite social interaction and this group of sounds is associated with amicable encounters.

In the second category there are sounds that are produced with the mouth closed and these include the purr and the trill or chirrup. The purr is a very characteristic feline sound and the situations in which it occurs are many and varied. The old myth that all purring cats are happy is easily dispelled when you listen to purring road traffic accident victims and cats that purr loudly as they are examined on the veterinary consultation table. This form of communication is commonly associated with mothers and kittens and certainly kittens do use the purr to communicate during nursing. However, it is also used in play and during social interactions with owners and it appears that the purr is either associated with periods of actual interaction between cats or with people or in situations where social contact is desired.

The loud vocal signals that make up the third category are produced when the cat holds its mouth open in a fixed position and they have been called strained-intensity calls. Examples include the hiss, the spit, the growl and the snarl and their use is limited to situations of defence and aggression. One specific example of this sort of call is the pain shriek which is designed to startle an attacker into loosing its grip and anyone who has had to handle a cat against its will understands just why it is classed as a shriek!

Body language

Sound and smell are obviously very important in the feline world of communication, but body language is also used to get messages across and it is important for those involved in dealing with feline behaviour problems to understand how cats use both their whole body posture and their facial expressions to communicate. As a result of its solitary predator role the cat needs to have very clear and unambiguous signals in order to prevent misunderstanding with the strangers it encounters when away from home. The lack of any pack structure means that an injured cat is very vulnerable and therefore most of the cat's communication signals are designed to avoid conflict rather than incite it.

The position of the body and its readiness to flee from the situation give the best indications as to the intention of the cat and, although the facial signals are undoubtedly the most important in fine-tuning the cat's message, it is the body posture that gives the first impression to an approaching cat (Fig. 4.4). Cats are renowned for bluffing their way out of conflict and raising the hairs along the back and on the tail is often combined with arching of the back and standing sideways on to a potential opponent in order to make the cat look twice its actual size. The theory is that a large cat will scare away any would-be attackers but in some situations the bluff fails and, when it does so, the cat will slowly retreat by moving sideways out of range. The slow movement is very important in order to prevent inciting the attacker to chase and the sideways movement allows the cat to keep its adversary in view, just in case there is a last minute change of tactic.

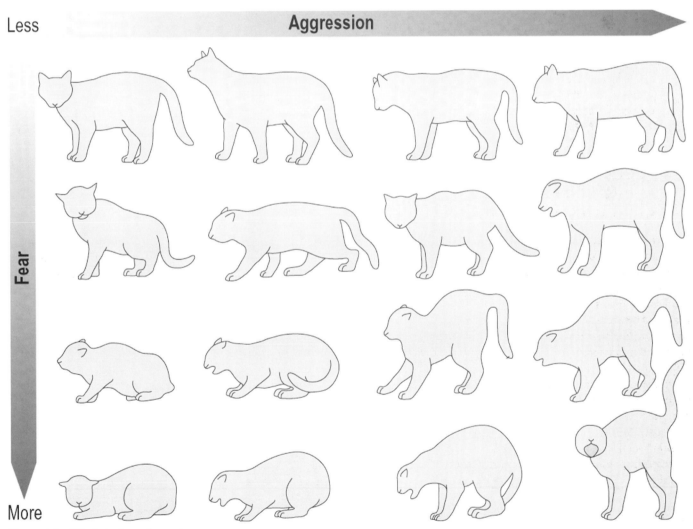

Less   **Aggression**

Fear

More

Figure 4.4 Whole body postures.
In this grid of body postures aggression increases from *left* to *right* and fear from *top* to *bottom*. So the cat in the bottom right corner is the most aggressive and fearful.
(Adapted from P Leyhausen 1979 Cat behaviour. Garland STMP Press, New York)

Bluffing is not always considered an appropriate response and when cats are very frightened they will often shrink to the smallest possible dimensions and try to hide. It is in these situations that the feline maxim of 'I can't see you so you can't see me' really comes into play. In the end, all cats would prefer to avoid conflict if possible and this explains why flight is seen as such a desirable option when a cat finds itself in a situation where it feels threatened.

Facial expressions

Cats use the position and shape of the ears, the eyes and the position of the whiskers as rapid vehicles of communication and, although overall body posture gives important information, it is the face that is most useful in the fine-tuning of feline communication and is the most important part of the cat to watch for clues as to what it is going to do next (Fig. 4.5).

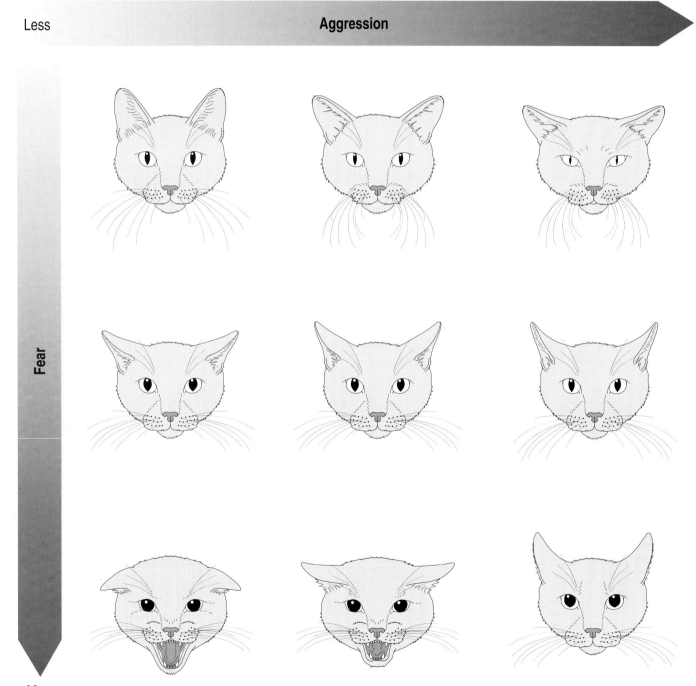

Figure 4.5 Facial postures. In this grid of facial postures aggression increases from left to right and fearfulness from top to bottom. (Adapted from P Leyhausen 1979 Cat behaviour. Garland STMP Press, New York)

The eyes can hold information about the emotional state of the cat, with dilated pupils being commonly associated with fear and narrow pupils being regarded as a sign of contentment. However, it is important to read these signals in association with all the body language that is being displayed since large pupils can also be associated with high arousal unconnected with fear and with poor light levels. Blinking can be used in communication between cats and even from cats to people and it is believed to signal that the cat is seeking reassurance in a tense environment. Staring on the other hand is the sign of a very assertive individual and prolonged eye contact is used to intimidate an opponent, so it is important to avoid such signals when meeting a cat for the first time. The fact that people who like cats are more likely to look at them and try to approach them leads to the paradoxical behaviour of cats in the company of people who dislike them and the tendency for them to head for the one person in the room who finds cats unpleasant to be with.

Ear positions can be useful indicators of feline emotion and of the intention to interact but serious confusion can arise if these signals are confused with ear positions in canine communication. Ears that are folded sideways and downwards indicate that the cat is trying to avoid confrontation and is preparing to defend itself from an approaching threat whereas the cat whose ears are flattened against the head with a backwards rotation is getting ready to attack. Ear positions can be altered very quickly and during any encounter it is not unusual to see cats alter their ear position several times as though these small movements are being used to test out the reaction of their opponent.

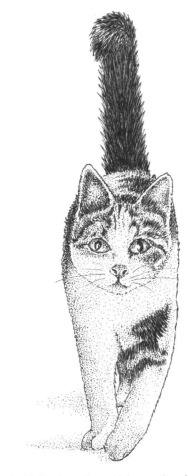

Figure 4.6   Typical 'tail up' greeting which precedes affiliative interaction.

The role of the tail in feline communication

The tail of the cat is often one of its most striking features and its role in the balance and agility of the cat is well recognised. However, the role of the tail in communication is sometimes overlooked and in the past the only comments regarding the tail have related to the belief that the wagging tail of the cat indicates anger and the potential to attack. In fact, the rapid movement of the tail simply indicates that the cat is agitated and is in a state of emotional conflict. Obviously, this may well lead to aggression if the warning goes unheeded but this does not necessarily show that the cat is bad-tempered. In addition to wagging, cats can use their tails to indicate a range of emotions and to assist in their overall communication.

During greeting cats will approach with their tail in an upright position and when this tail posture is associated with cats approaching their owners, it appears that the cat is offering a greeting and an invitation to be stroked and played with. In encounters between cats the raised tail signal is usually given before a cat rubs on another cat and this is important as a means of avoiding conflict (Fig. 4.6). Rubbing is a behaviour associated with relative status and if a cat just waded in and rubbed without asking permission he might find himself in trouble, so the raised tail is a friendly gesture used to test out the potential reaction of the other individual and to avoid rejection.

Other tail positions have been associated with sexual communication in particular with the signalling of female receptivity and the 'bottlebrush' tail is usually associated with fear and defence (Fig. 4.7). Aggressive cats may also use their tail to indicate their intentions, and both the concave and the lowered tail positions are commonly associated with conflict.

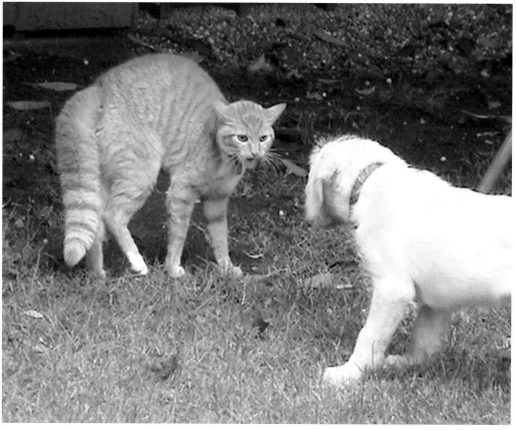

Figure 4.7 This cat displays a vertically hanging 'bottlebrush' tail that indicates fearfulness as it encounters an unfamiliar dog.

Chapter 5

Learning theory and behaviour modification

CHAPTER CONTENTS

INTRODUCTION

Before beginning to tackle the treatment of behavioural problems or starting to offer advice to owners on these subjects, it is necessary to have a basic knowledge of how animals learn since it is this information which will be used in the formation of treatment programmes. Learning theory is a complex subject and further information can be obtained by referring to relevant textbooks (see Further reading).

The two methods of learning that are of most importance to veterinary practices involved in behavioural medicine are:

- Classical conditioning
- Instrumental (operant) conditioning.

CLASSICAL CONDITIONING

The best-known example of this form of learning is to be found in the famous experiment involving Pavlov's dogs when a neutral sound stimulus was paired with the stimulus of food until it elicited the response of salivation in the absence of food.

The two main features of classical conditioning as a learning process are that it involves involuntary or reflex responses and it does not rely on the presence of external reward (Fig. 5.1).

Step one:

A stimulus known as an unconditioned stimulus (US) in this case food naturally provokes a reflex or unconditioned response (UR) in this case salivation.

Step two:

The US is associated with another previously unassociated stimulus (in this case a neutral tone). The previously unassociated stimulus is termed the conditioned stimulus (CS) and this is repeatedly presented to the animal at the same time as the US.

Continued

Step three:

Eventually the CS alone will evoke the reflex response, which we now term the conditioned response (CR). So, in this example, we reach the situation where the dogs salivate (CR) whenever they hear the neutral tone (CS) regardless of the presence or not of any food.

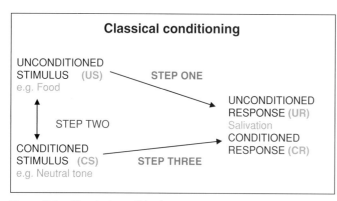

Classical conditioning

UNCONDITIONED
STIMULUS   (US)   STEP ONE
e.g. Food

                                            UNCONDITIONED
                                            RESPONSE (UR)
        STEP TWO   Salivation
                                            CONDITIONED
CONDITIONED   RESPONSE (CR)
STIMULUS   (CS)   STEP THREE
e.g. Neutral tone

Figure 5.1   Classical conditioning.

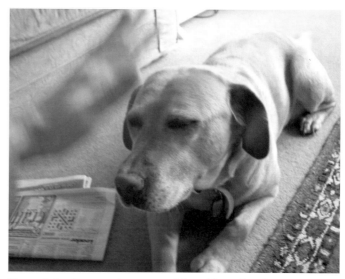

Figure 5.2   Dogs can learn a conditioned fear of a raised hand after a single incident involving physical punishment. This can continue to affect the animal's reaction to other forms of hand contact including petting, grooming and play.

Everyday examples of classical conditioning include the conditioned fear of a raised hand after an animal has previously been hit (Fig. 5.2) or the sound of a syringe or needle packet being removed before an injection is given. Classically conditioned fears of this kind are highly important in the maintenance of fear and aggression problems.

There are numerous ways in which classical conditioning influences the behavioural responses of domestic cats and dogs but one of the most common and easiest to understand is that of house-training young puppies (Fig. 5.3).

The key to successful classical conditioning is to ensure that at all times, as far as is possible, the desired conditioned stimuli occur at the same time as the unconditioned stimuli. If this is not the case there is a danger of unintentional conditioning taking place and the unconditioned stimuli becoming associated with extraneous unrelated stimuli. In the case of house-training, examples of unintentional conditioned stimuli include carpets and newspaper.

One of the obstacles to successful house-training is the fact that it can be difficult for owners to predict when the unconditioned stimuli are present and therefore it is not easy to ensure that a puppy is outside when they occur. In order to overcome this situation, it is necessary to look for signs that are predictors of a full bladder or full bowel and use these as a guide to timing the coincidence of being outside and needing to eliminate.

Predictors of the need to eliminate in a young puppy:

- Recent meal
- Recent period of sleep
- Sniffing around in search of scent marks
- Period of boisterous play

Step one:

An US (in this case the internal sensations that are mediated via the nervous system and which communicate to the brain the need for the animal to either urinate or defecate) naturally provokes a reflex or UR (in this case elimination).

Step two:

The US is associated with another previously unassociated stimulus (in this case environmental stimuli associated with being outdoors), again termed the CS. This CS is repeatedly presented to the animal at the same time as the US. In most cases of housetraining a generalised association with outdoors is all that is required, but if owners so wish they can make the CS more specific and train dogs to eliminate in response to more specific stimuli such as a certain substrate or a certain area in the garden. If so desired the CS can be as specific as a verbal command of 'be quick' or 'hurry up.'

Step three:

Eventually the CS alone will evoke the reflex response, which is the CR. That is, we reach the situation where the dog will urinate or defecate (CR) whenever it encounters the environmental stimuli associated with being outdoors (CS), regardless of whether the bowel or bladder are completely full.

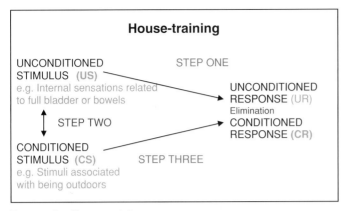

House-training

UNCONDITIONED   STEP ONE
STIMULUS **(US)**
e.g. Internal sensations related   UNCONDITIONED
to full bladder or bowels   RESPONSE (UR)
                                        Elimination
↕   STEP TWO   CONDITIONED
                                        RESPONSE (CR)
CONDITIONED
STIMULUS **(CS)**   STEP THREE
e.g. Stimuli associated
with being outdoors

Figure 5.3   House-training

Box 5.1   Clicker introduction

- The clicker is a reliable and easily reproducible signal that can be used as a consistent signal of reward.
- The first step is to deliver the sound of the clicker immediately prior to the arrival of a valuable resource, such as a food treat.
- Within a few repetitions the dog will react to the sound of the clicker with anticipation of the arrival of the reward.
- After many repetitions the sound of the clicker elicits the same emotional response as the arrival of a food reward and the clicker is now acting as a conditioned reinforcer of that emotional response.

In most cases house-training in respect of defecation is achieved more rapidly than training in relation to urination. This is due to the fact that there are fewer incidents of defecation within a 24 hour period and, therefore, there is greater chance that the puppy will be outside on each of these occasions and will rapidly associate the sensation of a full bowel with the presence of external environmental stimuli.

The fact that house-training is based on classical conditioning means that there is no need for an external reward but the process can be accelerated by the addition of reward, provided that the timing is accurate. No-one would claim that house-training is easy, but in many cases the process is made unnecessarily more tiresome because owners fail to realize that classical conditioning holds the key to success and that punishment of failure is counterproductive.

During the process of house-training there are two important rules to convey to puppy owners:

- Maximum opportunity to get it right
- Minimum opportunity to get it wrong

Puppies should never be punished when they make a mistake since they can only do so if the opportunity arises and, if it does, the owner is the one to take the blame.

Box 5.2   Using conditioned reinforcers in behavioural modification

- The conditioned reinforcer must only be encountered during the exhibition of an appropriate behavioural response.
- The conditioned stimulus will need to be periodically associated with the unconditioned stimulus to prevent extinction of the association and loss of the reinforcer status of the conditioned stimulus.

Application of conditioned stimuli in the process of behavioural modification

One of the most frequent applications of classical conditioning in the treatment of behavioural problems is the development of a conditioned stimulus that can then be used in the reinforcement of appropriate behavioural responses; that is, a conditioned reinforcer. There are various examples, including hand signals, whistles and specific praise commands, but one conditioned reinforcer which has attracted a great deal of interest within the dog world is the clicker (Boxes 5.1 and 5.2, Fig. 5.4). Once the clicker has been introduced and has taken on its status as a conditioned reinforcer, it may be used to assist in the instrumental conditioning of certain behaviours, but the initial introduction is done through a process of classical conditioning.

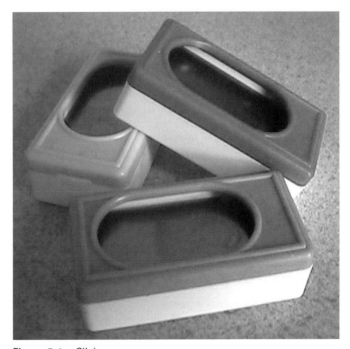

Figure 5.4   Clickers

INSTRUMENTAL (SKINNERIAN, OPERANT, TRIAL AND ERROR) CONDITIONING

In order for instrumental conditioning to occur there has to be integration of three events; namely a stimulus, a response and a consequence. The nature of the consequence in terms of its effect on the animal will determine the likelihood that the response will occur again if the same stimulus is presented.

If the behaviour is more likely to occur in future the consequence is described as a *reinforcer*; if the behaviour is less likely to be repeated the consequence is described as a *punisher*. Technically, all consequences of behaviour in instrumental conditioning are forms of reinforcement and to be absolutely accurate it is better to speak about *appetitive* reinforcement and *aversive* reinforcement, but the terms reinforcement and punishment are commonly accepted. Unfortunately, however, there is often confusion over the use of these terms and when people start to consider the issues of negative and positive forms of both reinforcement and punishment the situation can become very complicated.

In a simplified form, the consequences of a behaviour can be divided into those that **increase** the probability of a behaviour recurring (the **reinforcers**) and those that **decrease** the probability of a behaviour recurring (the **punishers**).

In order to understand the terms 'positive' and 'negative' in this context it is important to remember that they do not relate to the behavioural outcome under consideration but rather to the manner in which the reinforcer or punisher is delivered.

Definitions

Reinforcer: An event which increases the probability of a response. It can be negative or positive.

Positive reinforcement: An increase in the frequency of a behaviour when a positive reinforcer (something pleasant) is presented.

Negative reinforcement: An increase in the frequency of a behaviour when a negative reinforcer (something unpleasant) is removed (or avoided).

Punisher: An event which decreases the probability of a response. It can be negative or positive.

Positive punishment: A decrease in the frequency of a behaviour when a positive punisher (something unpleasant) is presented.

Negative punishment: A decrease in the frequency of a behaviour when a negative punisher (something pleasant) is removed.

An aversive or unpleasant consequence can therefore be described as a negative reinforcer or a positive punisher, depending on whether it is being presented or withdrawn as a consequence of the behaviour. Likewise, a pleasant or appetitive consequence can be described as a positive reinforcer or a negative punisher, depending on the manner in which the consequence is applied (Fig. 5.5). Some examples that illustrate different situations involving punishment and reinforcement are found in Table 5.1.

Table 5.1   Situations involving punishment and reinforcement

		Reinforcement	Punishment
POSITIVE	Canine example	Giving food reward when dog sits	Smacking a dog for jumping up
	Human example	Giving child a gift for good achievement at school	Shouting at a child for misbehaving
NEGATIVE	Canine example	Removal of adverse effects of rain by coming inside from the garden	Withdrawing attention when a dog misbehaves
	Human example	Child not having to go to bed at usual time because they are well-behaved	Child being denied toy or pocket money as a consequence of bad behaviour

The principles of instrumental conditioning form the basis of animal training and much of behaviour modification, but they are also involved in the unintentional learning of inappropriate responses. We need to remember that dogs are continually learning. Provided a stimulus and a response occur in conjunction with some form of consequence then learning will take place; in this way a lot of so-called problem behaviour is inadvertently learned. For example:

Dogs that bark incessantly when in the car

Stimulus:	Travelling in the car
Response:	Barking
Consequence:	Car continues on its journey and reaches a pleasurable destination
Dog's perception:	Positive reinforcement of barking

Dogs that jump up at people when they greet them or are generally over-enthusiastic when visitors call

Stimulus:	Visitors call
Response:	Jumping up
Consequence:	Social interaction, however negative that may appear (e.g., shouting)
Dog's perception:	Positive reinforcement of jumping up

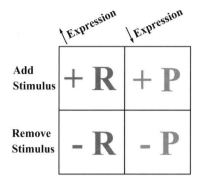

Figure 5.5   Diagram of the different forms of positive and negative punishment and reward.

Training classes

It is generally a good idea to encourage owners to take their dogs to some form of formal training programme, but there are four important messages for the veterinary practice to convey to their clients:

1. **Inappropriate training techniques can do immeasurable damage** and many behavioural problems are caused or exacerbated by exposure to such techniques. Selection of a training club is a very serious process and owners should take time to visit clubs before they take their puppy along. Training classes which rely on the use of positive punishment techniques and excessive dependence on negative reinforcement should be avoided. Owners need to look for classes where the emphasis is on positive reinforcement and negative punishment techniques.

2. **Any situation has potential for learning** and the fact that instrumental learning is occurring all the time means that, although training classes are often very useful for organising a routine of training, the learning process is not confined to one particular night of the week in the village hall.

3. **The maintenance of behaviour taught in training classes relies on the consistent application of the reinforcement techniques at other times.** If alternative behaviours are inadvertently reinforced outside the training class situation they can become established in preference to the behaviours being taught at 'school'.

4. **Behaviours that are taught in the training class location will be specific to that venue unless they are reproduced and reinforced consistently in a number of other situations** because dogs are contextual learners. It is therefore vital that owners 'do their homework' and apply the same training techniques when the dog is at home and out on walks.

The need for patience

A dog will learn more readily if both the required response occurs spontaneously and the required stimulus and con-sequence can be arranged to occur in conjunction with it than if the response is forced. Obviously this will make training a slow process. The use of clicker training, in which the dog is reinforced for performing a particular behaviour which it has selected itself, and of lure training in which the dog is persuaded into performing a behaviour and is then reinforced for doing so, are both positive forms of training but require a great deal of patience on the part of the owner.

The clicker is intended as a training tool and not as a permanent method of reinforcing appropriate behaviour. Transfer from clicker training to alternative long-term methods of reinforcement is known as 'fading the clicker'. Introduction of an alternative long-term conditioned reinforcer, such as specific verbal praise ('good dog'), will depend on associating this new consequence with the clicker until the verbal praise alone is acting as the reinforcer of the response.

Important points to remember in application of instrumental learning

Correct application of reinforcement (be that appetitive or aversive, negative or positive) is central to the success of instrumental learning. There are a number of important factors to consider including:

- the nature of the reinforcer or punisher
- the timing of application of the reinforcement
- the intensity of reinforcement
- the schedule of delivery of reinforcement.

Nature of the reinforcer or punisher

In order for something to act as a reinforcer or punisher it must be perceived as being appetitive or aversive by the individual animal concerned. When using positive reinforcement techniques it is sensible to use as wide a variety of reinforcers during training as possible since the response is then less likely to become focused onto one particular reward (which may not be available at all times). It also makes sense to use the most effective reward in any given situation and owners need to be reassured that within the context of training their dog there is no such thing as bribery. Whereas in some circumstances praise from the owner is sufficient reward, there are times when a tasty food reward is most definitely the reward of choice. The use of positive punishment is not recommended; in fact it is to be discouraged at all times. One of the obstacles to the effective use of this method of reinforcing responses is that selection of suitable positive punishers is extremely difficult. The aim is to select something that is mildly aversive to the animal and not one that causes fear. This selection will depend on the species, breed and individual characteristics of the animal and there is huge potential for error.

EXAMPLE: TEACHING A DOG TO SIT

Response required: Dog sits
Stimulus required: Verbal command from owner
Ultimate consequence: Praise from owner

Training methods

Lure training

Stage one
Lure into sitting using food treat placed just above nose and gently moved upwards and backwards, resulting in dog entering into sit position.
As the dog sits, and **not before**:

Stimulus: Give 'Sit' command
Response: Dog already in sit position
Consequence: Give food treat and verbal praise while dog is in sit position
Dog's perception: Positive reinforcement of being in sit position

Stage two
Repeat stage one several times.

Stage three
Once dog sits as it sees the hand raise it is time to use the stimulus (voice command or hand signal) as a predictor of the behaviour. Now the command should be given while the dog is still standing:

Stimulus: Give sit command or raise hand (as if with treat inside)
Response: Dog enters sit position
Consequence: Give food treat and verbal praise as sit position is achieved
Dog's perception: Positive reinforcement of entering sit position

Stage four
Once the dog will reliably enter the sit position on hearing the verbal command or on seeing the visual hand signal, it is important to teach the dog that it is required to stay in the position until instructed to do something else. In order to achieve this the time delay between entering the sit position and receiving the reinforcement needs to be gradually extended. Failure to do this will result in a dog that bobs in and out of the sit position believing that it is the act of entering the position that yields reward rather than remaining in the position.

Stimulus: Give sit command or raise hand (as if with treat inside)
Response: Dog enters sit position
Consequence: Wait for a very short time before giving food treat and give verbal praise while dog is still in sit position. (The time between entering the sit and receiving the reinforcement should be very gradually extended.)
Dog's perception: Positive reinforcement of remaining in sit position

Final stage:
Stimulus: Give sit command or raise hand (as if with treat inside)
Response: Dog enters sit position
Consequence: Wait for a very short time before giving food treat and verbal praise, while dog is still in sit position
Second stimulus: Give release command (gesture to dog to come toward owner and as it leaves the sit position give release command e.g., 'enough')
Response: Dog leaves sit position
Consequence: Give food treat and verbal praise as dog leaves sit position
Dog's perception: Positive reinforcement of entering sit position on command, remaining in sit position and leaving position on command

Clicker training

Remember that the clicker must be introduced and established as a conditioned reinforcer before it can be used. The clicker can be incorporated into the lure training method as the conditioned reinforcer, which is used as the positive consequence of the required response, or it can be used alone without the incorporation of a lure. The main difference between clicker training (without a lure) and lure training lies in stages one and three of the process. In clicker training there is no stimulus involved in stage one since this method starts by reinforcing the dog's own spontaneous behaviour and there is no need for stage three since the clicker can be used to reward the act of sitting in stage one.

Stage one
Response: Dog spontaneously enters sit position
Consequence: Clicker is heard as dog enters sit position and food reward follows
Dog's perception: Positive reinforcement of entering sit position

Stage two
Repeat stage one several times.
Stages four and five are the same as for lure training, except for the use of the clicker as the reinforcer for the appropriate behaviour.

Reinforcers and punishers can be primary or secondary in nature. 'Primary' refers to the fact that they are inherently appetitive or aversive while 'secondary' refers to those consequences of behaviour which are inherently neutral but have acquired reinforcing properties by contiguous association with a primary reinforcer or punisher (Table 5.2).

Table 5.2   Appetitive versus aversive reinforcers for dogs

	Appetitive reinforcers	Aversive reinforcers
PRIMARY	Food Play Canine or human social interaction (assuming successfully socialised)	Pain Surprise or shock Social isolation Fear
SECONDARY	Specific verbal praise, e.g., 'Good dog' Clicker	Verbal reprimands, e.g., 'No' Training aids which induce pain or fear, e.g., shock collar or freedom fence

In order for secondary reinforcers or punishers to be effective they have to be highly-predictive of an appetitive or aversive outcome and this predictive value is referred to as contingency. For example:

High level of contingency: The sound of a clicker used as a reinforcer when it is always followed by the arrival of a treat and is never encountered in any other situation.

Low level of contingency: The sound of a rattling bunch of keys used as a punisher when the dog hears the keys being picked up and rattled at a variety of times with inconsistent results.

Timing of application of the reinforcement

Successful timing is crucial to the instrumental learning process. Reinforcers or punishers must be delivered at the same time as the response, or immediately afterward, if they are to be effective. A delay of even 1 second can weaken the effect or even result in inadvertent reinforcement of a response other than the one which was intended. The relationship in time between the reinforcer and the behaviour is referred to as *contiguity*. Events that are contiguous occur at the same time. Poor timing of application of appetitive or aversive reinforcers is at the heart of many a behavioural problem.

It is worth reminding owners that interaction with their dog influences whatever the dog is doing at that time and so they need to pause and ask themselves, 'Is what my dog is doing at this precise moment something which I wish him to continue doing?'. If the answer is 'yes' then go ahead and interact with him with some form of appetitive reinforcement, but if the answer is 'no': STOP!

Intensity of reinforcement

When using positive reinforcement methods, it does not always follow that the more intense a reward the more effective it is. In some circumstances it is necessary to use a very intense reward in order to increase the level of motivation to perform the behaviour or to compete with other

---

EXAMPLE: HOUSE-TRAINING A DOG

Example 1 (✗)

Desired response:	Toileting in garden
Actual behaviour:	Toileting in house
Consequence:	Food treat and verbal praise
Timing:	Delivery of reward as dog comes back into house from garden
Dog's perception:	Positive reinforcement of entering home
Effect:	No effect on location of toileting; increased anticipation of reward when entering house from garden

Example 2 (✗)

Desired response:	Toileting in garden
Actual behaviour:	Toileting in house
Consequence:	Use of verbal or physical reprimand
Timing:	Delivery of punishment when dog caught toileting in house
Dog's perception:	Positive punishment of toileting in front of owner
Effect:	No effect on location of toileting; increased anticipation of toileting in front of owner, resulting in dog not toileting if owner is present, even when in garden!

Example 3 (✔)

Desired response:	Toileting in garden
Actual behaviour:	Toileting in house
Consequence:	Verbal praise
Timing:	Delivery of reward as dog is in the act of toileting in garden
Dog's perception:	Positive reinforcement of toileting in garden
Effect:	Enhancement of classical conditioning of being outside and toileting

potential reinforcers within the environment; for example, training a dog to respond to commands in the presence of distracting stimuli (teaching a recall in the park when there are discarded chip papers under the bushes).

However, when circumstances call for the dog to respond calmly then a reward that is highly intense can have the opposite effect by inducing too high a level of excitement and preventing the dog from performing the desired behaviour. In these situations it is important to use a low level of reward intensity. An example is teaching a dog to greet visitors at the door calmly. Use of a highly rewarding food treat in the hand of the visitor may encourage the dog to be excitable and to jump up. Calm verbal or tactile interaction may be more beneficial.

When considering the use of positive punishment methods the punisher must be applied at the first presentation and at a sufficient strength to stop the behaviour. This fact makes the application of positive punishment very difficult to achieve and is one of the many reasons why it is an unsuitable method of training in the hands of inexperienced trainers and owners. The intensity of the punisher needs to be exactly correct in order to avoid the situation where the punishment is too weak to have any effect or so strong that it induces fear or even aggression. The optimum level is the minimum required to be effective in suppressing the response.

This optimum punishment level will depend on the individual animal, the reaction varying with its species, breed, temperament and previous experience. What has no effect on one dog may severely frighten another. Gradual increases in intensity from an initial low level may be ineffective because the dog will adapt to these increases and eventually need an even greater intensity of punishment to suppress the behaviour.

The intensity of punishment will also be related to the type of behaviour which is involved since the more motivated an animal is to perform a behaviour the more intense the punishment will have to be in order to stop it. It is also worth bearing in mind that, where punishment is repeated, the dog is likely to become habituated to it. Thus a punishment that was effective in stopping the behaviour the first few times may become gradually less and less effective, resulting in a situation where the owner finds themselves using steadily more severe forms of punishment to achieve the same result.

Schedule of reinforcement

Reinforcement can be delivered on a continuous or partial schedule. While an animal is learning to behave in a new way, it will learn most quickly if its responses are reinforced on each and every occasion; this is described as a continuous schedule of reinforcement.

When applying positive reinforcement in order to increase the occurrence of a new behaviour, it is important to tailor the schedule of delivery to the stage of learning. In other words, behaviour that is continuously reinforced will be quickly incorporated into the behavioural repertoire but it is also highly susceptible to extinction (the removal of a behaviour from a behavioural repertoire) since the failure to deliver the reinforcer will be readily noticed. Therefore, once the behaviour is established it is important to vary the schedule of reward and employ partial reinforcement schedules which improve the maintenance of the response and result in higher rates of response and greater resistance to extinction. Intermittent and irregular reward is the most effective way of making any behaviour resistant to extinction and this is the basis of the gambling habit in humans. Whilst this is very useful in the maintenance of wanted behaviour, it can also lead to problems in the treatment of behavioural problems since an unwanted behaviour that has been intermittently rewarded, often unintentionally, can take some considerable time to extinguish.

When applying positive punishment techniques in order to decrease the occurrence of an unwanted behaviour, the process is most effective when the punisher is administered on a continuous schedule and every occurrence of the unwanted behaviour is punished.

Partial reinforcement schedules can be either fixed or variable and can be determined by time intervals or by ratios of responses.

When using partial schedules, it is important to ensure that there are sufficient occurrences of the reinforcement for learning to occur. If the intervals are too long or the ratios too high then the behaviour will be prone to extinction.

Animals tend to work harder to perform the desired behaviour when reinforcements are:

- relatively few and far between
- relatively irregular and unpredictable.

BEHAVIOURAL MODIFICATION TECHNIQUES

Extinction

The removal of a behaviour from a behavioural repertoire is termed 'extinction' and it is an extreme form of negative punishment. Every time a behaviour is performed reward is taken away or withheld. Extinction needs to be applied on a continuous schedule and ensuring that a behaviour is never rewarded is the safest and most reliable method of removing that behaviour from the animal's repertoire.

It is important to remember that behaviours can be rewarded internally as well as externally and therefore application of extinction as a means of modifying a behaviour can have limitations. Behaviours which are inherently rewarding to the animal will continue even if the external rewards, that is those rewards which are under the influence of the owner, are removed. In addition, the removal of external reward must be complete for the process of extinction to be effective and in households with more than one family member there is a risk that reward may still be available from one source and so lead to failure of the extinction process.

One of the main difficulties that owners experience when attempting to implement an extinction programme is related to the 'frustration effect'. When a behaviour has been previously reinforced and that reinforcement is abruptly removed, the animal will respond to the resulting frustration by performing the behaviour more frequently and more intensely in an attempt to gain access to the reward. Persistent withdrawal of reinforcement is therefore essential since transfer onto an intermittent schedule of reinforcement will prolong the process of extinction.

Shaping

In some situations the required response in training or in behaviour modification is so far removed from the animal's present behaviour that it is impossible to make the change in one step. When this is the case, it is possible to use a learning process whereby the animal is positively reinforced for performing successive and increasingly accurate approximations of the target behaviour. This process is called *shaping*. The command or cue for the target behaviour is not introduced until the animal has succeeded in performing that response in its entirety.

The process begins by reinforcing whatever aspect of the animal's behaviour is closest to the desired response. Once this behaviour occurs more often, the trainer withholds reinforcement until some closer approximation to the desired response occurs and this series of steps continues until the desired response is achieved.

The most notable use of this technique is in the training of performance animals; for example, in television adverts or films. However, shaping can also be useful in modifying an animal's response.

Systematic desensitisation

Systematic desensitisation is a method used to gradually reduce an animal's response to a stimulus until the animal remains in a neutral emotional state when the stimulus is presented. It is achieved by gradually exposing the animal to increasingly intense forms of the stimulus while the animal is relaxed. Systematic desensitisation is commonly used in the treatment of fears and phobias and it is important to identify the separate elements of a fear-inducing situation and present these components to the animal separately so that it can learn to relax in their presence. It is also important to present the fear-inducing stimuli in a diluted form in the early stages of treatment in order to avoid the induction of a fear response. This is easy to achieve with sound stimuli since CDs and cassette tapes enable the owner to effectively dilute the stimulus and gradually increase the volume. Visual stimuli on the other hand can

---

EXAMPLE: A DOG THAT BEGS AT THE TABLE

Stage one

Stimulus:	Family eating food at table
Response:	Dog begging and salivating at table
Consequence:	Food given to dog by various family members
Dog's perception:	Positive reinforcement of begging behaviour

Stage two
(Decision made to try to change dog's behaviour)

Stimulus:	Family eating food at table
Response:	Dog begging and salivating at table
Aim:	Stop dog begging at table
Consequence:	No food given to dog at table
Dog's perception:	Need to work harder for previously continuously delivered reinforcement
Result:	Dog makes more deliberate begging action and starts to bark at people for food while they are at table. One family member gives in and feeds dog
Dog's perception:	Positive reinforcement of begging behaviour

In order to improve the success of extinction as a behavioural modification technique it is useful to teach an alternative and incompatible behaviour in the same context as the behaviour being extinguished.

Stage one

Stimulus:	Family eating food at table
Response:	Dog begging and salivating at table
Consequence:	Food given to dog by various family members
Dog's perception:	Positive reinforcement of begging behaviour

Stage two
(Decision made to try to change dog's behaviour)

Stimulus:	Family eating food at table
Response:	Dog begging and salivating at table
Aim:	Stop dog begging at table
Consequence:	No food given to dog at table but reward given if dog sits in bed while family eating at table
Dog's perception:	Positive reinforcement of 'being in bed' behaviour
Result:	Dog elects to sit on bed while family eat, in anticipation of reward

be harder to dilute, but introducing items in miniature toy form or from a distance are both possible approaches to this problem.

One of the limitations of desensitisation is that its best result is an animal that has no emotional reaction to the stimulus and this leaves the possibility that the problem behaviour can re-emerge or generalise.

If a desensitised animal is exposed to the full-blown form of the stimulus unexpectedly, it can easily be sensitised again because desensitisation is a reversible process. In order to avoid such problems in behavioural practice, the process of systematic desensitisation is usually combined with counterconditioning in any treatment protocol.

Counterconditioning

This is the process by which an animal's emotional or behavioural response to a stimulus is altered by conditioning a response which is incompatible with the unacceptable behaviour or emotion that currently exists. It is possible for counterconditioning to be carried out in either a classical or an operant manner. Operant counterconditioning is also referred to as 'response substitution'.

Classical counterconditioning

This is used in the treatment of fears and phobias and involves association of the fear-inducing stimulus with a stimulus that evokes a positive emotional state. The aim is to repeatedly present the stimulus in association with something that the dog is known to enjoy, such as food or play. In order for this technique to be effective, it is essential that the association between the pleasant stimulus and a positive rewarding emotional state is stronger than the association between the fear-inducing stimulus and the unpleasant emotional reaction. (The strength of the association is depicted in Fig. 5.6 by the size of the arrows.) If this is not the case, there is a risk that the previously pleasure-inducing stimulus will become associated with an emotional state of fear. It is therefore beneficial to begin with a programme of systematic desensitisation to reduce the intensity of the fear reaction before commencing the counterconditioning.

A common example of this is seen when people offer food treats to fearful dogs in an attempt to decrease their fear of strangers. If the fear of strangers is stronger than the positive reaction to the food treat, the dog may become frightened of the act of being offered food treats. It is therefore beneficial to reduce the intensity of the fear reaction by diluting the perceived threat from the person and this can be achieved by asking the stranger to drop food treats onto the floor, but not speak to or look at the dog while this is done. This is sometimes referred to as a 'no strings' approach as the pleasant experience in the presence of the stranger does not rely on any behavioural response from the dog and there is no pressure for the dog to approach the person directly or cope with an approach from them.

When it is carried out successfully, classical counterconditioning has a blocking effect that reduces the chance of resensitisation and generalisation occurring when the animal encounters the fear-inducing stimulus in the future.

Systematic desensitisation and counterconditioning therefore complement one another and work to reduce and replace the conditioned emotional response of fear.

Figure 5.6 Classical counterconditioning.

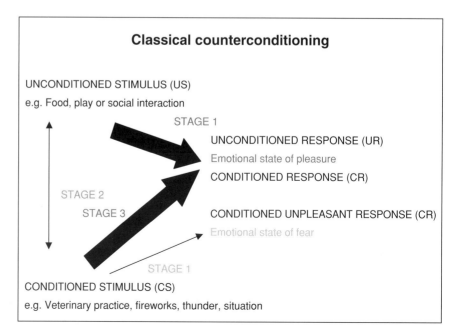

Response substitution

When counterconditioning involves replacing an unwanted behaviour with an acceptable conditioned response, it is referred to as response substitution. The new response must be incompatible with the old one and, in order for this technique to be effective, it is essential that the motivation to perform this new incompatible behaviour is greater than that for the unwanted behaviour. The first step in response substitution is to condition the 'new' behaviour and this should be done in a context that is unrelated to the problem behaviour and in which there are few distractions. It is important to develop a strong association between the conditioned stimulus, or 'cue', and the conditioned response. A high level of contingency will assist in increasing the motivation to perform this new behaviour when the process of response substitution is carried out within the problem context.

Once the new behaviour has been conditioned, it can be introduced to the dog in the presence of the stimulus which triggers the undesirable response. It is helpful to present the stimulus in a diluted form to begin with and then gradually work up to the situation where the full-blown stimulus is presented.

EXAMPLE: DOG REACTS TO CERTAIN THEME MUSIC ON TELEVISION BY JUMPING ONTO FURNITURE

Stage one
Teach dog to sit on a designated 'bed' area by using clicker training at times when the television is switched off.

Stage two
When the dog sits on the bed reliably introduce a cue command such as 'on your bed' and reinforce the response by using positive reinforcement techniques as described earlier.

Stage three
When the dog will sit on the bed readily in response to the command make a tape recording of the theme music and, in the presence of ever-increasing volumes of the theme music from the tape recorder, give the dog the command 'on your bed' and reward it for responding. Remember to ensure that the dog is rewarded while it is in the bed location.

Stage four
When the dog has successfully completed stage three, the television should be switched on at the correct time for the theme music but with the volume control set very low. While the music is playing the dog should be commanded to go 'on your bed.' Gradually, over a period of a few days the volume should be increased.

Stage five
In this stage the 'on your bed' should be faded out. While the theme music is playing the command 'on your bed' should be given in a steadily decreasing volume until there is no command at all and the dog is responding to the onset of the theme music (the conditioned stimulus) by going to its bed (counterconditioned response).

A GLOSSARY OF TERMS USED IN ASSOCIATION WITH LEARNING THEORY

Blocking: where the learning of a conditioned stimulus as a predictor is blocked by the pre-existence of a conditioned stimulus that is a better predictor.

Classical conditioning: when a neutral stimulus precedes and becomes a predictor of the unconditioned stimulus, eliciting a response even in the absence of the unconditioned stimulus.

Conditioned response: the response to a conditioned stimulus.

Conditioned stimulus: a neutral stimulus which, through pairing, becomes the predictor of the unconditioned stimulus.

Contingency: the predictive value of a reinforcer.

Contiguity: the relationship in time between a reinforcer and a behaviour.

Counterconditioning: where the response to a conditioned stimulus is altered by associating it with a new unconditioned stimulus to condition a new response incompatible with the first.

Discriminative stimulus: a signal with a high level of contingency.

Extinction: removal of a behaviour from the behavioural repertoire of an individual.

Flooding: exposure to a noxious stimulus without the opportunity to escape.

Frustration effect: An increase in vigour of a behavioural response immediately following the non-reinforcement of a previously reinforced response.

Generalisation: the triggering of a behavioural response by stimuli that are decreasingly similar to the original trigger.

Habituation: the process whereby an animal becomes accustomed to non-threatening environmental stimuli and learns to ignore them.

Instrumental conditioning: a type of associative learning in which an important event follows a response, resulting in a change in the probability of the response.

Latent inhibition: exposure to a stimulus without significant aversive consequences such that subsequent aversive effects of exposure to that stimulus have minimal effect on the animal's behaviour.

Learned helplessness: a failure to learn an avoidance or escape response to an aversive stimulus due to previous experience where the subject could not escape from the noxious experience.

Operant conditioning: another term for instrumental learning.

Pavlovian conditioning: another term for classical conditioning.

Punishment: a consequence which decreases the probability of a response.

Reinforcement: a consequence which increases the probability of a response.

Secondary conditioning (Second order conditioning): pairing a stimulus with a previously conditioned stimulus.

Sensitisation: where the arousal caused by one stimulus causes greater reactivity to presentations of another.

Systematic desensitisation: reduction of the response to a noxious stimulus by relaxation rather than the introduction of a second unconditioned stimulus.

Shaping: a form of training where approximations to the desired behaviour, becoming increasingly specific over time, are reinforced.

Stimulus: that which an organism senses.

Trial-and-error learning: another term for instrumental learning.

Unconditioned stimulus: a stimulus that elicits a response without any training.

Unconditioned response: the response elicited by an unconditioned stimulus.

Chapter **6**

The role of pharmacology in behavioural medicine

INTRODUCTION

The drugs that are relevant to specific behavioural conditions are discussed in the relevant chapter in this book; this chapter is designed to give an overview of the classes of medication that can be used in behavioural medicine. The drugs covered in this book are those that are most likely to be used by a general practitioner treating behavioural cases; information about other medications that may have a place in specialised behavioural medicine practice can be found in other texts (see Further reading). Full monographs for each of the medications described here are available in veterinary formulary publications (see Further reading).

PSYCHOPHARMACOLOGY – SPECIAL CONSIDERATIONS

The majority of the drugs used in the field of behavioural medicine are unlicensed for veterinary use and will be used in an extra-label fashion. Clients must be made aware of this fact and informed consent forms should be used. The use of human medical preparations also raises the issue of potential client abuse and this should not be overlooked. Requests for frequent repeat prescriptions should be viewed with suspicion and it is advisable to limit dispensing to 1 month's supply at a time, with a revisit and re-examination being necessary before repeat prescriptions can be given.

One very important consideration when contemplating the use of psychoactive medication is the need for client cooperation over administration. Many of the drugs take a considerable time to take effect and owners need to understand the need for relatively long-term administration (months rather than weeks).

More than one dose is listed for some drugs in view of the fact that there are multiple doses cited in the literature and, since research into the use of psychoactive medication in animals is ongoing and dosages are prone to alteration, it is highly recommended that veterinary surgeons consult the most recent publications in the field for the current dosage regimes. Where possible, the lowest effective dose should be used and in most cases gradual withdrawal of medication is recommended.

Drugs are not a substitute for behavioural workup

The use of pharmacological intervention without an adequate behavioural workup is bad practice and medication should be used as a combination therapy alongside behavioural modification techniques. Concomitant behavioural therapy is needed in order to deal with the learned component of the behavioural problem and also to address the cause of the condition as well as the symptoms. Where the veterinary surgeon concerned is not able to offer appropriate behavioural therapy advice, the case should be referred for this aspect of treatment. Where possible, referral of cases involving the use of psychoactive medication should be made to a veterinary behaviourist but where this is not possible, referral to a non-veterinarian for provision of behavioural therapy is encouraged. However, the medical care of the patient remains the responsibility of the referring veterinary surgeon and queries regarding the use of psychoactive medication should be directed to a veterinary behaviourist. Prescription of medication for behavioural cases should follow the same principles as prescription in any other field of veterinary medicine and should be based on a sound diagnosis of the cause of the symptoms seen (Box 6.1).

NEUROTRANSMISSION

Before using psychoactive drugs it is necessary to understand the principles of neurotransmission. This holds the key to understanding the action of drugs on the brain, the effects of disease on the central nervous system (CNS) and the behavioural consequences of psychoactive drug treatment for animals.

There are a number of agents that act as neurotransmitters within the body and new ones are being discovered on an almost daily basis. This is a very dynamic science and an area of active research. The most important neurotransmitters in behavioural medicine are:

- Serotonin (5HT)
- Dopamine
- γ-aminobutyric acid (GABA)
- Norepinephrine (noradrenaline)

Box 6.1 Pharmacological intervention

- Relies on sound diagnosis
- Relies on client cooperation over administration
- Is open to client abuse
- Is very rarely sufficient alone
- Needs concomitant behavioural therapy

When considering the use of psychoactive medication, it is important to understand the manner in which neurotransmitter action is terminated. The most common methods are:

- Re-uptake
- Enzymatic destruction

The commonly used psychoactive drugs act on these two systems and thereby modify the availability of neurotransmitters within the CNS.

Detailed information regarding mode of action is outside the remit of this book and veterinary surgeons are advised to consult a comprehensive text on psychopharmacology in order to increase their knowledge in this area (see Further reading).

MANAGING PSYCHOACTIVE DRUG THERAPY

Case selection

When considering drug usage in behavioural medicine cases, there are some important steps that need to be taken. A complete medical and behavioural history is required in all cases and all patients must undergo a full medical and behavioural examination.

Prior to commencing drug treatment, it is advisable for all patients to undergo a basic haematology and biochemistry screen. Tests for hepatic and renal function are advisable, as is monitoring of cardiac function (Box 6.2).

There are three main reasons for good medical pretreatment workup:

- Detection and/or exclusion of potential medical conditions that could responsible for the behavioural symptoms
- Detection and/or exclusion of potential medical conditions that could affect the use of psychoactive medication (e.g., medical contraindications for particular drug classes)
- The setting of a baseline normal of biochemical and haematological parameters for the particular individual to facilitate patient monitoring during long-term drug administration.

Caution is always needed when considering drug therapy in cases where the animal:

- is old
- has metabolic or cardiac abnormalities
- is or has been receiving other medication.

Although there are very few drugs that are specifically licensed for behavioural indications in veterinary medicine, there is an extensive range of medications that are potentially useful in behavioural cases. When considering drug therapy, the main considerations are the ability to reach an accurate diagnosis and the selection of a drug that is appropriate.

Box 6.2   Selecting cases for drug therapy – some criteria

- The behavioural diagnosis
- The duration of the problem
- The severity of the symptoms
- The risk of euthanasia/rehoming and resulting need for quick results

Monitoring

In view of the fact that medication in behavioural cases is likely to be given for periods of months rather than weeks, it is important to consider the issue of patient monitoring. A complete medical examination and blood workup should be carried out every 6 months if patients are staying on drugs long term and owners must be informed of any known potential side-effects. Dosages should be adjusted according to development of the case and terminated when satisfactory results have been achieved (Box 6.3).

Box 6.3   Potential risks involved with drug therapy in behaviour cases

- Medical side-effects
- Behavioural side-effects
- Sedation interfering with learning ability
- Owner reliance on medication
- Lowered compliance with behavioural modification
- Masking behavioural symptoms without dealing with the underlying cause

Termination of treatment

When the time comes to remove medication in behavioural cases, the withdrawal should be made gradually. If another class of psychoactive medication is thought necessary there should be a 2-week washout period during which no medication is given.

Accurate diagnosis is central to the appropriate use of veterinary psychopharmacology in behaviour modification.

CLASSES OF PSYCHOACTIVE DRUG

Neuroleptics

This group of drugs is also referred to as antipsychotic agents in human psychiatry and the most commonly used class of drugs within this group is the phenothiazines. The value of neuroleptics within veterinary behavioural medicine is rather limited and although high potency neuroleptics, such as haloperidol and perphenazine are discussed in the behavioural literature, their use is largely restricted to specialised behavioural practice.

Phenothiazines are routinely used in general practice for the purposes of sedation and restraint and the most commonly used member of this class, acepromazine, has a specific application in premedication. Traditionally, this drug has been used in the treatment of behavioural problems associated with car travel and in the management of fears and phobias, particularly related to fireworks and thunderstorms, but its use in these conditions is now considered to be outdated and inappropriate.

Acepromazine exerts its therapeutic actions by blocking dopaminergic receptors in the brain. Its action is not selective and therapeutic effects cannot be achieved in isolation from CNS depression. While sedation may be desirable in short-term management of fear-related problems, acepromazine has been associated with increased sensitization to noise which makes it a poor choice in the treatment of sound phobia.

A major disadvantage of acepromazine is the blocking of motor responses while leaving sensory perception unaffected. The animal is therefore aware of the fear-inducing stimulus but limited in its ability to react. This can result in worsening of the phobia over time and treatment with acepromazine for firework phobias can be associated with increasing severity of the phobic reaction from year to year.

The major behavioural contraindication for phenothiazine use is aggressive behaviour, since acepromazine can lead to behavioural disinhibition. In addition, there are medical contraindications including epilepsy, brachycephalic breeds, history of respiratory depression, hepatic dysfunction, renal compromise and hypotension. Use of acepromazine in geriatrics (over 8 years of age) carries particular medical concerns in terms of hypotensive effects.

If acepromazine is to be used, it is advisable to carry out a pre-treatment biochemistry screen to assess renal and hepatic function.

The use of acepromazine as a treatment in behavioural cases has decreased significantly in recent years and its relevance to behavioural medicine is severely limited. In most cases, other drugs should be considered in preference.

Azapirones

The only member of this class that is used to any extent in veterinary behavioural medicine is buspirone. It has been advocated for the treatment of mild anxiety-related problems and, within the primary literature, most references to its application in a veterinary context relate to the treatment of urine spraying in cats. It is reportedly ineffective when the animal is exposed to intense fear-inducing stimuli and is therefore not advised in cases such as sound phobia or separation anxiety in dogs.

The exact mode of action of azapirones is not known but their primary action appears to be as serotonin agonists,

Table 6.1 Azapirones

Indications:	Dose:	Contraindications and special notes
Treatment of mild to moderate anxiety-related behaviour problems in dogs and cats. Treatment of urine spraying in cats when associated with mild anxiety.	**BUSPIRONE** **Dog:** 1 mg/kg 2 to 3 times daily **Cat:** 0.5–1.0 mg/kg 2 to 3 times daily For urine spraying – 5 mg/cat 2× daily for 1 week; if patient responds continue treatment for 8 weeks and then gradually withdraw. If no response, cease treatment.	Contraindicated in states of renal or hepatic impairment and in epileptics. May take 2 weeks to take effect. May cause behavioural disinhibition and increased friendliness (in cats). Contraindicated in multi-cat households due to potential paradoxical increase in intraspecific aggression.

although they are also reported to have noradrenergic and dopaminergic effects and may also suppress cholinergic pathways.

Specific advantages to buspirone use are that it does not interfere with learning and it causes minimal problems on withdrawal. However, onset of action can be between 1 and 3 weeks and administration two to three times a day can be limiting in terms of its practical application in behaviour cases.

Physical side-effects of busprione are minimal and reports have mainly related to mild gastrointestinal disturbance in the early days of administration. The main behavioural consideration when using buspirone is that it may cause a paradoxical increase in aggression in some cats and therefore its use in multi-cat households is not recommended (Table 6.1).

Benzodiazepines

The two most commonly used drugs in this class are diazepam and alprazolam. Other benzodiazepines mentioned in behavioural medicine literature include clorazepate, lorazepam, oxazepam and temazepam. The main indication of this drug class is for the treatment of anxiety-related behaviour problems in dogs and cats, and their indications in the literature have been far ranging. In cats, the most common indication has been for the treatment of urine spraying, but in recent years their use has been superseded by the use of antidepressants such as clomipramine. In dogs, the primary indication is as a short-term therapy for phobias, including sound phobia such as fireworks, and in these cases the side-effect of interference with short-term memory is beneficial. However, in other behavioural cases memory-blocking activity can be limiting and the use of benzodiazepines on a long-term basis is not advisable in situations where concurrent behavioural modification is required.

In cats, one of the main concerns relating to the use of benzodiazepines is the risk of idiopathic hepatic necrosis, which has been reported in clinically normal cats within 7 days of oral administration of diazepam. This reaction is rare but can be irreversible and fatal and should therefore be taken into consideration in any case where diazepam administration is being considered. Monitoring of hepatic

Table 6.2 Benzodiazepines

Indications:	Dose:	Contraindications and special notes
Treatment of anxiety-related behaviour problems in dogs and cats. Short-term treatment for phobias including sound phobias, e.g., of fireworks.	**DIAZEPAM** **Dog:** 0.55–2.2 mg/kg po q 6–24 hours **Cat:** 0.22–0.4 mg/kg po q 12–24 hours **ALPRAZOLAM** **Dog:** 0.01–0.1 mg/kg po q 8–12 hours **Cat:** 0.12–0.25 mg/kg po q 12 hours **CLORAZEPATE** **Dog:** 0.01–0.1 mg/kg po q 8–12 hours **Cat:** 0.125–0.25 mg/kg po q 12 hours	Contraindicated in states of hepatic impairment. May cause paradoxical excitation or anxiety – should be tested in presence of owner on first administration. Caution in cats, especially if longer term use being considered. Do not allow cats treated with benzodiazepines access to outdoors due to limitation of depth perception. Interferes with short-term memory, therefore long-term use limited. Alprazolam: more rapid onset of action and considered preferable for feline cases. May cause disinhibition of aggressive behaviour.

function in cats prior to the use of diazepam and within 1 week of the commencement of therapy is strongly recommended. In dogs, the benzodiazepines are generally well-tolerated but reports of sedation, ataxia and muscle relaxation soon after oral administration are common. Reduction in these side-effects is usually seen within a few days but the onset of paradoxical excitation or anxiety should result in withdrawal of the medication, and it is recommended that the first dose of a benzodiazepine is always administered when the animal can be carefully observed and monitored for such a reaction. The risk of behavioural inhibition prohibits the use of benzodiazepines in cases of canine aggression. The current thinking is that benzodiazepines are best suited to short-term use in the management of acute anxiety episodes but in cases where they have been used on a long-term basis, care should be taken over their withdrawal. So-called 'discontinuation syndrome', which is characterised by resurgence of the initial behavioural symptoms and an onset of nervous behaviour, and even seizures, has been reported in the literature following sudden withdrawal of benzodiazepine therapy. In order to avoid this, it is recommended that the dose is gradually tapered and that abrupt termination of therapy is avoided.

The potential for human abuse of these drugs should not be underestimated. Strict control of drug dispensing is needed and it is recommended that prescriptions are limited to 1-month's supply of medication at a time in order to facilitate effective monitoring of drug usage (Table 6.2).

Tricyclic antidepressants (TCAs)

This drug class is one of the most widely used within behavioural medicine and the variety of indications reflects the subtle differences in the mode of action of the various drugs within it. The TCAs effect their antidepressant action by blocking the re-uptake of serotonin and norepinephrine, but the proportional effects on these two neurochemicals varies considerably between the individual drugs within the group. In addition, TCAs commonly produce effects related to their activity at other receptors such as muscarinic and antihistaminic sites and these may be manifested as unwanted side-effects or potentially useful therapeutic effects, depending on the drug in question. Sedation is a common side-effect of medication with the TCAs and appears to be most pronounced in the early stages of treatment. The level of sedation is usually dose-dependent and reports in cats are often linked to unintentional overdose in that species. Dry mouth, urinary retention and constipation are commonly reported but are usually transient and not severe. Antihistaminic side-effects may be considered beneficial in conditions which include some pruritic effect and doxepin has been specifically indicated for the treatment of canine acral lick dermatitis for that reason.

Concerns have been raised over the potential for cardiac side-effects when using TCAs but the literature suggests that such effects are benign when the drugs are administered to healthy individuals and within the recommended therapeutic range. However, cardiac assessment is recommended prior to instituting treatment with TCAs since conduction disturbances may occur in predisposed animals and the use of these drugs is therefore contraindicated in any individual exhibiting a cardiac arrhythmia.

Probably the most well-known TCA in veterinary use is clomipramine, not least because it is one of the rare drugs which carries a veterinary licence for a behavioural indication. Marketed by Novartis Animal Health, Clomicalm ® is licensed for the treatment of separation anxiety in dogs but, at a practical level, the product is used for a far wider range of indications, including canine compulsive disorders and feline urine spraying.

Table 6.3   Tricyclic antidepressants (TCAs)

Indications:	Dose:	Contraindications and special notes
Treatment of anxiety-related behaviour problems in dogs and cats. Clomipramine is licensed for treatment of separation anxiety in dogs and indicated for urine spraying in cats and feline hyperaesthesia. It has also been advocated for the treatment of compulsive disorders in both dogs and cats. Amitriptyline is indicated for behavioural problems in cats secondary to idiopathic cystitis	**CLOMIPRAMINE** **Dog:** 1–3 mg/kg po q 12 hours **Cat:** 0.25–0.5 mg/kg po q 24 hours **AMITRIPTYLINE** **Dog:** 1–2 mg/kg po q 12 hours **Cat:** 0.5–1.0 mg/kg po q 24 hours **DOXEPIN** **Dog:** 3–5 mg/kg po q 12 hours **Cat:** 0.5–1.0 mg/kg po q 24 hours	May cause disinhibition of aggressive behaviour. Mild sedation is common in the first days of treatment and appears to be dose dependent. Therapeutic effects may not be seen for between 3 and 4 weeks after commencing treatment. Contraindicated in animals with urinary retention or any history of cardiac arrhythmias.

Amitriptyline is also widely referenced in the literature and its use is specifically advocated in the treatment of behavioural consequences of idiopathic cystitis in cats. These include excessive grooming, particularly on the ventral abdomen and medial thighs, associated with the pain of the underlying medical condition and inappropriate urination which can result from negative associations between pain and litter facilities.

On a practical note, administration of TCAs is usually in tablet form and some owners may experience difficulty when using fractions of tablets due to the bitter taste of the compound and the resulting hypersalivation in some individuals. In cats, where accurate dosing at relatively low levels is required, the use of a syrup form of clomipramine has proved to be beneficial (Table 6.3).

Selective serotonin re-uptake inhibitors (SSRIs)

As their name suggests, these drugs differ from the TCAs in that they selectively block the re-uptake of serotonin and as a result are specifically recommended for the treatment of behavioural conditions which involve a component of impulsivity.

The onset of action of the SSRIs is similar to the TCAs, with therapeutic effects being reported between 3 and 4 weeks after commencement of treatment. However, maximum therapeutic effect in cases of compulsive disorders may not be seen for as long as 8 weeks into the course of treatment.

The most commonly used SSRIs in veterinary behavioural medicine are Fluoxetine, Sertraline and Fluvoxamine and the main canine indications for their use include compulsive disorders, anxiety-related competitive aggression and panic disorders in dogs. In cats, SSRIs have been advocated for the treatment of urine spraying and for compulsive disorders, but careful monitoring of elimination behaviour is recommended due to the risks of urinary retention and constipation.

Reports of gastrointestinal side-effects in association with SSRI therapy are relatively common and can include inappetence, anorexia, diarrhoea and nausea. In order to reduce the risk of these effects it is recommended to administer a lower loading dose for 1 to 2 weeks before increasing to the relevant therapeutic dose. In contrast to the TCAs, cardiovascular side-effects are not reported with SSRIs (Table 6.4).

Monoamine oxidase inhibitors (MAOIs)

In the field of veterinary behavioural medicine it is only the selective monoamine oxidase B inhibitors that are of clinical significance and selegiline is the only example of this drug class that is used for the treatment of behavioural disorders in companion animals. It carries a veterinary licence in a number of countries but the labelled indications vary. In the USA the product is licensed for the treatment of canine cognitive dysfunction while in the UK it carries a very broad licence advocating its use for the treatment of disorders of an emotional origin. Clinically, selegiline is used in a wide range of behavioural disorders including cases of canine fears and phobias and canine cognitive dysfunction. Research in the UK has suggested that the wide-ranging applications of this product may be the result of a dopamine-mediated increase in reward-motivated activity and a resulting enhancement of cognitive ability. Certainly, the action of selegiline is complex and, whilst inhibition of monoamine oxidase B activity is one of its main therapeutic actions, it is also reported to affect the metabolism of phenylethylamine, enhance the activity of the free radical scavenger superoxide dismutase and exert neuroprotective activity within the CNS.

There are few reports of unwanted side-effects related to the administration of selegiline in dogs or cats, but combination therapy with other drug classes can result in very serious side-effects and should be avoided. In particular, administration with drugs acting on the serotonergic system, such as TCAs and SSRIs, can be associated with

Table 6.4 Selective serotonin reuptake inhibitors (SSRIs)

Indications:	Dose:	Contraindications and special notes
Treatment of compulsive disorders and anxiety-related conditions in dogs and cats. Indicated in conditions of anxiety-related competitive aggression in dogs. Fluoxetine is indicated for treatment of urine spraying in cats	FLUOXETINE Dog: 0.5–1 mg/kg po q 24 hours Cat: 0.5–1 mg/kg po q 24 hours SERTRALINE Dog: 1–2 mg/kg po q 12 hours FLUVOXAMINE Dog: 1–2 mg/kg po q 12 hours	Careful monitoring is essential in cases involving canine aggression and advice should be given, related to the avoidance of any potential injury to individuals. Barrier methods such as muzzle training, appropriate restraint and careful supervision should be recommended. Therapeutic effects may not be seen for between 3 and 4 weeks after commencing treatment. A loading dose is recommended at the start of treatment in order to minimise gastrointestinal side-effects.

Table 6.5 Monoamine oxidase B inhibitors

Indications:	Dose:	Contraindications and special notes
Treatment of behavioural problems of an emotional origin in dogs. Examples include fears and phobias. Treatment of age-related behavioural disorders in dogs and cats.	**SELEGILINE** **Dog:** 0.5 mg/kg q 24 hours **Cat:** 1.0 mg/kg q 24 hours	Do not administer in combination with serotonergic acting drugs such as TCAs and SSRIs or with phenothiazines, alpha-2 agonists or opiate analgesics. Do not administer to pregnant or lactating individuals. Therapeutic effects may not be seen for 6 weeks after commencing treatment for emotional disorders but onset of action is usually shorter in cases of cognitive dysfunction.

CNS toxicity and the onset of the potentially fatal condition *serotonin syndrome* and is therefore contraindicated. In addition, administration of phenothiazines, opiate analgesics and alpha-2 agonists is contraindicated in patients receiving selegiline. The use of selegiline in pregnant or lactating individuals is also prohibited (Table 6.5).

Beta-blockers

The use of beta-blockers in the treatment of human anxiety-related disorders is well-documented. In veterinary behavioural medicine their use is primarily related to the treatment of situation-specific anxieties in which somatic symptoms such as tachycardia and tachypnoea are preva-

lent. Their use is contraindicated in animals with cardiac disease, hypotension or bronchospasm. The most commonly prescribed beta-blocker in behavioural medicine is propranolol but pindolol, which has a more significant effect on serotonin receptors, is also discussed in the literature. Since beta-blockers are most frequently used for situational conditions they are usually administered on an as-and-when basis. The animal should be in a relaxed state when the drug is given and treatment is therefore recommended before the anticipated situation occurs (Table 6.6).

Antiepileptics

The use of anticonvulsant therapy within behavioural medicine is primarily indicated in those cases where epileptic activity is involved in the aetiology of the condition. Limbic or temporal lobe epilepsy has been implicated in cases of compulsive behaviour, such as tail-chasing, and in aggressive behaviour which was previously referred to as 'rage syndrome'. Breed predispositions have been suggested in both cases, with the bull terrier breeds being over-represented in the tail-chasing cases and the solid-colour cocker spaniel being associated with aggressive responses related to limbic epilepsy. Monitoring of phenobarbitone medication in these cases should take the same form as in any neurological case, and combination with potassium bromide therapy (at neurological dose rates) may be considered beneficial in some cases. Collaboration between veterinary surgeons working in the fields of behaviour and neurology is recommended when assessing these cases.

Table 6.6 Beta-blockers

Indications:	Dose:	Contraindications and special notes
Treatment of situational anxieties in dogs and cats.	**PROPRANOLOL** **Dog:** 0.5–3.0 mg/kg q 12 hours or as required **Cat:** 0.2–1.0 mg/kg q 8 hours or as required **PINDOLOL** **Dog:** 0.125–0.25 mg/kg q 12 hours	Contraindicated in cases of cardiac disease, hypotension or bronchospasm. Primarily used to deal with the somatic effects of anxiety and fear.

Table 6.7 Antiepileptics

Indications:	Dose:	Contraindications and special notes
Treatment of behavioural consequences of limbic epilepsy in dogs and cats. Carbamazepine has been indicated in cases of tail-chasing or spinning in dogs and cats as well as aggression in cats.	**PHENOBARBITONE** **Dog:** 1–8 mg/kg q 12 hours **Cat:** 1–2.5 mg/kg q 12 hours **CARBAMAZEPINE** **Dog:** 4–8 mg/kg q 12 hours **Cat:** 25 mg q 12 hours	Monitoring of therapeutic levels is important in successful use of phenobarbitone in these cases. Combination of phenobarbitone with KBr may be considered. Carbamazepine is contraindicated in cases of renal and hepatic impairment and in patients with cardiovascular or haematological disorders.

The use of carbamazepine has been recommended in dogs for cases of tail-chasing or spinning which are attributable to limbic epilepsy, and in cats for cases of spontaneous aggression (Table 6.7).

Central nervous system (CNS) stimulants

Clinical use of CNS stimulants is limited to the diagnosis and treatment of hyperkinesis, which is a rare condition in companion animals. The diagnostic role of these substances stems from the paradoxical decrease in heart rate, respiratory rate and activity level which occurs following their administration to individuals suffering from hyperkinesis. (The response to such therapy in non-affected individuals would be a significant increase in all of these parameters). Treatment with CNS stimulants may also be indicated in cases of narcolepsy, but this is also a rare condition in companion animals and would be most likely to be diagnosed after specialist intervention (Table 6.8).

Hormonal preparations

While the use of progestogens and anti-androgens may have decreased in recent years for the reasons outlined later in this section, one product with hormonal activity which is proving to be beneficial to the field of behavioural medicine is cabergoline. This drug is a dopamine-2-receptor agonist which has antiprolactin effects and is recommended for the treatment of pseudopregnancy in bitches. This condition does not only present with a set of physical symptoms but may also result in purely behavioural changes, such as aggression toward family members or other household pets and therefore cabergoline has become an important drug in behavioural prac-

tice. The onset of aggressive behaviour in bitches post spaying may in some cases be attributable to elevated prolactin levels following surgery and treatment with cabergoline can be dramatically effective in these cases. The literature also suggests that cabergoline may be of some benefit in the treatment of psychotic behaviour and reward-deficiency syndromes; therefore, its applications in the field of behavioural medicine may be wider than first thought (Table 6.9).

Progestogens were among the first drugs to include any mention of behavioural disorders in their list of indications but their effects in these situations were non-specific and, while much was written about their hormonal effects, their tranquillizing effects through central steroid receptors were largely overlooked. However, it is likely that these central calming effects were primarily responsible for their apparent success and the non-specific nature of their action, combined with the potential for extensive and frequent side-effects, has led to their being replaced with more specific psychoactive medications. Treatment with progestogens as a first-line therapy in behavioural medicine is no longer recommended.

Anti-androgens do continue to be used in order to chemically mimic castration when owners are considering surgery as a treatment option. The drug most commonly used is delmadinone acetate and dose rates are in line with data sheet recommendations. While its use may be beneficial, it is important for owners to appreciate that delmadinone does give some central calming effect in addition to its direct hormonal action and therefore it does not entirely mimic the surgical process. Cases in which delmadinone resulted in a significant alteration in the behavioural signs but surgery did not maintain those benefits have, therefore, been reported.

Table 6.8   CNS stimulants

Indications:	Dose:	Contraindications and special notes
Diagnosis and treatment of hyperkinesis.	DEXTROAMPHETAMINE Dog: 0.2–1.3 mg/kg po as a diagnostic tool – heart rate, respiratory rate and activity level to be monitored every 30 minutes for 1–2 hours following administration METHYLPHENIDATE 2–4 mg/kg q 8–12 hours as a therapeutic dose	Hyperkinesis and narcolepsy are both rare conditions. The use of CNS stimulants is therefore extremely limited.

Table 6.9   Dopamine 2 receptor agonists

Indications:	Dose:	Contraindications and special notes
Treatment of behavioural consequences of pseudopregnancy and behavioural changes post spaying in bitches.	CABERGOLINE Dog: 5 mg/kg q 24 hours for 5–14 days	Although the data sheet recommendation is for 5 days of therapy with cabergoline, clinical experience suggests that courses of up to 14 days may be necessary in cases of maternal aggression or other behavioural problems relating to persistently high prolactin levels.

Antihistamines

Although the primary indications of this drug class are not behavioural, they are nonetheless considered to be useful in the management of mild anxiety associated with car travel, as well as inappropriate night time activity and anxiety conditions in which pruritus plays a role. In these situations their sedative CNS side-effects are being exploited for their behavioural benefit. Antihistamines are contraindicated in animals suffering from glaucoma, urinary retention or hyperthyroidism and owners need to be warned of possible anticholinergic side-effects such as dry mouth or constipation. Cyproheptadine is an antihistamine with significant serotoninergic antagonist activity and has been advocated as an appetite stimulant in both cats and dogs (Table 6.10).

Alpha–adrenoreceptor stimulants

These drugs do not have a direct behavioural indication but phenylpropanolamine is commonly used in the treatment of sphincter mechanism incompetence in bitches and can therefore form part of the therapeutic approach to house-soiling in these cases. In addition, there are reports in the literature of its use in cases of submissive or excitement-related urine leaking. Increased aggression is a possible side-effect of its use and owners need to be informed of this risk before treatment commences (Table 6.11).

Alpha–adrenoreceptor antagonists

Nicergoline is advocated as a treatment for age-related behaviour changes such as sleep disorders, diminished vigour and fatigue. It acts as a cerebral vasodilator, thereby increasing blood flow to the brain and assisting in reversal of chronic hypoxia, which is implicated in the aetiology of these behaviour changes. In addition, it is reported to act as a cognitive enhancer by reversing the vasoconstrictive effect of cerebral catecholamines, to exert neuroprotective action on neural cells and to have both serotonergic and dopaminergic action. Concurrent use of other vasodilators may cause hypotension and nicergoline should not be administered within 24 hours of using alpha 2 agonists such as xylazine or metetomidine (Table 6.12).

Xanthine derivatives

Propentofylline is licensed for the treatment of canine age-related behaviour changes such as dullness and lethargy. In addition to improving cerebral blood flow through vasodilation, xanthine derivatives also improve cerebral metabolism through neuroprotective functions. Other important functions of propentofylline are its action as a glial cell modifier and its role in increasing levels of adenosine. In long-standing cases of canine cognitive decline it has been reported that the effects of single-drug therapy may not be sustained and that such cases may respond better to combination therapy with selegiline and propentofylline (Table 6.13).

Table 6.11   Alpha-adrenoreceptor stimulants

Indications:	Dose:	Contraindications and special notes
Treatment of sphincter mechanism incompetence and resulting issues of house soiling.	PHENYLPROPANOLAMINE **Dog:** 1.1–4.4 mg/kg q 8–12 hours **Cat:** 1.0–1.5 mg/kg q 12 hours	Owners need to be informed of the risk of aggression as a side-effect of treatment.

Table 6.10   Antihistamines

Indications:	Dose:	Contraindications and special notes
Treatment of mild anxiety associated with car travel, night time activity and excessive vocalisation. Indicated for mild anxiety conditions with an element of pruritus.	CHLORPHENIRAMINE **Dog:** 220 micrograms/kg q 8 hours (Max 1 mg/kg in 24 hours) **Cat:** 1–2 mg/kg q 8–12 hours DIPHENHYDRAMINE **Dog and cat:** 2–4 mg/kg q 8–12 hours CYPROHEPTADINE **Dog and cat:** 0.1–0.5 mg/kg q 8–12 hours	Not to be used in patients suffering from glaucoma, urinary retention or hyperthyroidism.

Table 6.12   Alpha-adrenoreceptor antagonists

Indications:	Dose:	Contraindications and special notes
Treatment of age-related behaviour changes in dogs.	NICERGOLINE **Dog:** 250–500 µg/kg q 24 hours administered in the morning	Concurrent use of other vasodilators can cause hypotension. Do not administer within 24 hours of using alpha 2 agonists.

Table 6.13   Xanthine derivatives

Indications:	Dose:	Contraindications and special notes
Treatment of age-related behaviour changes in dogs.	PROPENTOFYLLINE Dog: 2.5–5 mg/kg q 12 hours	In advanced or long-standing cases of canine cognitive dysfunction combination therapy with selegiline is recommended.

Pheromonotherapy (as an adjunct to behavioural therapy)

One major development in therapeutic approaches to behavioural disorders in recent years has been increasing interest in the application of so-called pheromonotherapy into the field of companion animal behaviour therapy and there are now three versions of commercial 'pheromones' available for use in veterinary practice in the UK. Two fractions (F3 or Feline Facial Pheromone Analogue – FFP and F4) are used in the cat for the management of a range of behaviour problems and there is also one canine pheromone now available (Dog Appeasing Pheromone – DAP®). Depending on the formulation, pheromones have the potential to be applied to physical objects in the environment, aerially through diffusion or directly as a spray application onto the animal or onto human hands.

Feliway®

Feliway® (CEVA Animal Health) is known as the 'familiarisation pheromone' and it is believed to provide a feeling of security for cats in unfamiliar or stressful situations. It is a synthetic analogue of the F3 fraction of the so-called 'feline facial pheromone'. Its applications reflect this belief, although the exact mode of action is as yet unclear. Feliway® is indicated for the management of indoor urine spraying, inappropriate scratching behaviour, problems during transportation and behavioural changes associated with being confined in a cattery or veterinary hospital situation. In addition, reports from those working in the field of companion animal behaviour have shown that Feliway® can be beneficial in cases of inter-cat tension in the household and in a range of feline behavioural signs which accompany high levels of unsolved stress for the cat, such as overgrooming. Within a veterinary context it can be beneficial in the consulting room environment and also in the area used for pre-surgical preparation and anaesthesia induction.

Feliway® is an environmental product and is available both as a diffuser and as a spray. The spray needs to be applied 30 minutes before cats are allowed access to treated areas because the evaporation of the alcohol carrier can be disturbing for some cats.

Felifriend®

Felifriend® (CEVA Animal Health) is a synthetic analogue of the F4 fraction of the 'feline facial' pheromone and is believed to assist in the development of an atmosphere of confidence between cats and unfamiliar people. Felifriend® is applied to the palms of each hand and is rubbed over the hands and wrists of the handler. It is marketed specifically for use in the veterinary consulting room where it is believed to reduce the cat's anxiety. It has been advocated for use with particularly fractious cats during consultation and at other times of restraint. In studies, the use of Felifriend® has significantly reduced the major signs of aggression during consultations, including attempts to bite and scratch the handler. In France, Felifriend® is also marketed for use in cases of aggression between cats in the same household and in these cases it is applied to the neck and flank region of each cat. In some cases Felifriend® has been found to induce what appears to be a panic reaction; it is suggested that this is most likely to occur when the cat is faced with a human or feline who is already strongly associated with hostility and therefore the visual signal of threat is in direct contradiction to the appeasing scent signal. The best results are obtained when the person or cat is totally unknown or where inter-cat aggression is in its early stages.

Dog Appeasing Pheromone

A recent addition to the commercially available pheromone products has been Dog Appeasing Pheromone or DAP®. This product is available in the UK as a diffuser application and one bottle is recommended to last for a period of 1 month. Refills can be purchased and applied to the original diffuser device. A DAP® spray is also available.

The product is based on a synthetic analogue of a scent signal which emanates from the inter-mammary sulcus of the lactating bitch. At this stage of puppy development the scent appears to be important in promoting calm and secure behaviour and in establishing a bond with the mother. The anxiety-reducing properties of this substance affect the adult dog's behaviour, and the applications of DAP® are varied. It has been specifically advocated in a prophylactic role for assisting young puppies in settling into their new homes and for a wide range of situations that generate fear and distress reactions, such as separation from the owner. It has also been found to be extremely effective as part of the approach to fear-related behaviours in dogs including sound sensitivity and fear of noises, such as fireworks and thunder. In such cases DAP® is recommended as an adjunct to a specially designed desensitisation and counterconditioning programme.

Chapter 7

Geriatric behavioural issues

INTRODUCTION

The rate of ageing varies with breed such that in the larger dog breeds, individuals may be considered to be geriatric at as young as 7 years of age. The corollary of this is that dogs physically age at around 1 year for every two calendar months. During the last third of the life span there is increased risk of serious or debilitating degenerative disease. Similarly, accelerated ageing is seen in cats and the combined effect is that, from the owner's perspective, a pet's health appears to decline very suddenly and rapidly.

Degenerative disease processes have a better prognosis if they are diagnosed and treated at the earliest possible stage. Even a thorough annual physical examination cannot accomplish this and so owners need to be made aware of all warning signs of changes in health and encouraged to seek help quickly.

INCIDENCE OF BEHAVIOURAL PROBLEMS

Behavioural problems are generally less common within the elderly dog and cat populations. The incidence of individual problem types within this population is also different (Table 7.1).

There is a combination of reasons for these differences:

- Many behavioural problems have a peak incidence that is before 3 to 4 years of age.
- These early problems will either be resolved, or the owner has adapted to them by the time the dog or cat has aged.
- The more seriously affected dogs and cats have been euthanised before they reach old age.

However, there are other reasons for an under-presentation of behaviour problems in older dogs:

- Owners believe that the problems they see are an untreatable, normal part of the ageing process.
- Owners are fearful of mentioning problems that may be seen as serious and a potential indication for euthanasia.

Table 7.1 Incidence of behavioural problems in the geriatric population

Increased incidence	Fear and anxiety-related:
	• 'Stereotypy/compulsive'
	• Separation-related
	• Destructiveness
	• Phobia
	Vocalisation
	House soiling
	Sleep disturbance
Decreased incidence	Aggression
	Over activity

Thus behavioural problems may be under-presented in the older dog and cat populations (Table 7.2).

MEDICAL ISSUES

The latter third of life is a peak risk period for many of the medical disorders that we know are implicated in problem behaviour. Many of these diseases are of a degenerative type and an individual geriatric dog or cat may have a number of concurrent diseases and debilities. The relationship between common clinical signs, associated medical causes and behavioural signs is set out in Table 7.3.

There are a number of reasons why this is important:

- Pain or debilitation-related irritability and self-defensiveness might cause the animal to lash out with a scratch, snap or bite in situations where it would otherwise give a warning or move away.
- Animals that have impaired senses, physical debilitation or suffer pain may not be able to mount a proper escape or avoidance reaction in situations where they are frightened. If they are not able to anticipate and avoid a situation then they may become more fearful or aggressive.
- If there is competition or a hierarchical dispute between dogs in a household, then the sensory or physically impaired dog may be injured because it is not able to react appropriately.
- The welfare of the aged animal is a concern because the programme of behavioural modification may cause further pain and stress.

Table 7.2 Behavioural problems and their causes in the geriatric dog and cat

Behaviour	Motivation/explanation
Aggression	Resource control (e.g., secondary to metabolic disease)
	Increased fear
	Poor communication with, or awareness of conspecifics (leading to status conflict in dogs, or reduced avoidance in cats and dogs)
Excess vocalisation	Loss of reassuring presence of a familiar person
	Insecurity in environment
	Increased fearful reaction to stimuli (e.g., loud or unfamiliar noises)
Destructiveness	Escape from fear-eliciting stimuli
	Attempt to reunite with owner (dog)
	Self-appeasement chewing
Waking at night (often combined with vocalisation and increased activity)	Disorientation upon waking:
	• cognitive or sensory impairment
	Day–night reversal of sleep pattern due to lack of day time stimulation/activity
Stereotypic/compulsive behaviour	Self-mutilation, pacing/circling
	• anxiety/stress (oral displacement/self-appeasement)
	• self-appeasement during pain
	• confusion, cognitive impairment
Noise phobias	Increased fearfulness/anxiety
	Cognitive impairment
	Sensory impairment
	Debilitation of avoidance/coping strategies
Separation-related	Loss of reassuring presence of owner (e.g., cognitively impaired dog)
	Loss of owner influence over behaviour

Table 7.3 Relationship between clinical signs, potential medical causes and behavioural signs

Clinical sign	Potential medical causes	Behavioural signs

Polyuria/Polydipsia	Renal disease
	Hepatic disease
	Diabetes insipidus
	Metabolic disease:
	   ● Cushing's syndrome
	   ● Diabetes mellitus
		House-soiling (increased frequency and urgency of urination)
		Increased competition for food bowl

Pain	Musculoskeletal
	Dental
	Abdominal:
	   ● Pancreatitis
	   ● Faecal impaction
	Anal gland impaction
		Increased aggressiveness
		Irritability
		Loss of mobility
		Loss of play and interaction
		Increased anxiety and fear
		Sleep disturbance

Sensory loss	Blindness Deafness Proprioceptive loss Loss of olfaction	Reduced ability to navigate environment Hypersensitivity to unimpaired sensory modalities Impaired communication Impaired avoidance behaviour

Exercise intolerance	Cellular hypoxia:
	   ● Cardiovascular disease
	   ● Anaemia
	   ● Respiratory disease
	Obesity
	Disuse atrophy of skeletal muscle
		Impaired avoidance behaviour
		Worsening phobia
		Aggression (self-defence)
		Irritability
		Frustration
		Inability to carry out normal behaviour

Polyphagia	Metabolic disease:
	   ● Cushing's syndrome
	   ● Diabetes mellitus
	   ● Hyperthyroidism (cat)
		Increased competition for resources
		Food guarding
		Food stealing
		Aggression around food

Problems of urinary outflow control	Prostatic disease (obstruction) Urinary incontinence	House-soiling
Dullness/Impaired cognition	Hypothyroidism Reduced cerebral oxygenation (cardiac/pulmonary/vascular disease)	Confusion Anxiety Loss of interaction and communication

● Cognitively impaired animals are likely to be more anxious or fearful and less able to cope with novel experiences. They may react abruptly, without warning and with little self-control or social inhibition (learned response to the social constraints of the group).

The effect is that new behavioural problems may develop in old age, or problems that were thought resolved or tolerable become more severe and unmanageable.

Unfortunately, there is a tendency for mild clinical signs to be disregarded as an inevitable part of ageing.

The prevalence of this attitude is borne out in studies of patterns of investigation of clinical signs in young and aged dogs. It has been shown that clinicians offer completely different services to the two age groups. For example, a lame young dog was several times more likely to be radi-ographed than an older one with matching symptoms. The older dog was more likely to be given symptomatic treatment on the assumption that it was suffering from degenerative joint disease. Once treated, older dogs were offered far fewer treatment reviews and changes of medication. Owners more frequently accepted symptomatic management in place of investigation. This is in direct contradiction to known data on incidence of serious disease in the two populations, and highlights the obvious need to continually review efficacy of treatment.

All medical problems should be resolved or managed as effectively as possible before a behavioural assessment is carried out:

● Full clinical examination
● Comprehensive haematology and biochemistry

- Complete review of the effectiveness of current medical treatments
- Assessment of effectiveness of current pain management

If anything, it should be assumed that the elderly dog has medical issues that will affect its behaviour unless it is proven to the contrary.

MANAGEMENT OF AGEING DOGS AND CATS

Sensory loss and debilitation are common in the elderly population and adaptations need to be made if they are to be supported. As mentioned later in this chapter, debilitated animals that become inactive are likely to become progressively less healthy. If given appropriate stimulation and interaction these animals can enjoy a comparatively good quality of life.

Sensory loss, such as blindness or deafness, are common in the geriatric dog or cat and owners can do a great deal to make these pets' lives easier. Animals can be provided with additional environmental cues that help them to find their way around and get to resources and resting places. This reduces stress and avoids complications such as dehydration. Elderly pets with mobility problems, and those with painful conditions such as osteoarthritis, may show a significant improvement in well-being if given easy access to resources close to where they spend time during the day (Fig. 7.1, Table 7.4).

Exercise patterns may need to change if an older dog is unable to cope with long walks. It has to be remembered that dogs are highly social and benefit from mental stimulation. For the older dog, walks should be made shorter but more frequent and more stimulating. The dog should be taken regularly to a park where it can spend time with other dogs, or to new places which it can investigate.

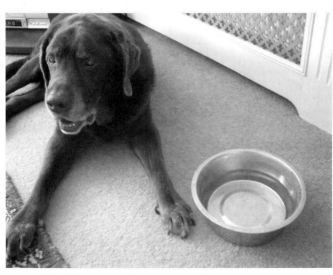

Figure 7.1   It is important to provide geriatric dogs with easy access to resources such as fresh water.

Table 7.4   Coping with sensory loss

Loss of vision	Provide extra cues that enable the pet to navigate the environment: ● Tactile: textured rugs in the middle of corridors and the centre of rooms to guide the dog away from furniture. ● Audible: leave radios playing different stations in different rooms. Place them at floor level so that the dog can 'hear' where furniture is positioned (objects block sound waves) or place them next to specific resource such as food and water bowls. ● Odor: use room fragrancers to identify different rooms. Perhaps use an odour such as lavender oil to identify the dog's bed. Avoid making significant changes in room or garden layout so that the pet is not confused. Announce all interactions by calling the pet to avoid startling and frightening it. For dogs, all walks should be on an extending leash.
Hearing loss	Try to make eye contact before interactions to avoid startling the pet. Condition the pet to anticipate interaction and reward (food treat) when touched on a particular part of the body away from the head. Train recall, sit and other signals using hand signals. Off-leash control may be improved using a remote-activated vibrating collar (not a gas or shock collar). The dog is trained to look for the owner when the vibration is felt, which then makes other commands such as recall easier.

Minimal load exercise, such as swimming, is an excellent way to maintain general fitness and muscle mass without damaging already painful joints. If other dogs are present, swimming may be an ideal opportunity to enjoy much less restricted play.

Elderly cats may derive pleasure from brief games or watching other animals play.

Obesity is a major problem in elderly dogs and some cats and owners should be encouraged to feed older animals on a nutrient-rich low calorie diet to avoid weight gain as the animal becomes less active. Activity feeding, such as the use of an activity ball or scattering food on the garden for a dog to find, or the use of small activity balls for cats, are excellent ways to increase an individual's energy expenditure and avoid weight gain (Fig. 7.2).

Managing the care of older pets

Most practices will have a large cohort of older dogs and cats that will at some time need 'geriatric care'. As mentioned previously, these pets may start to become ill and

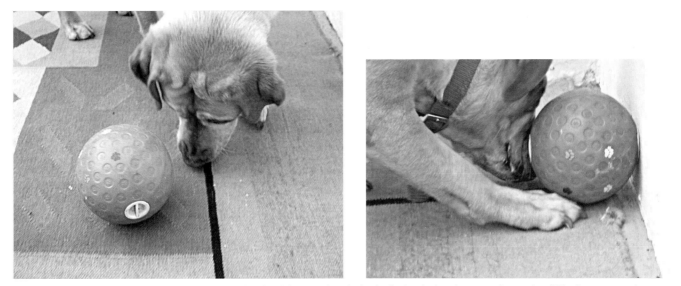

Figure 7.2   Activity feeders provide geriatric animals with mental and physical stimulation, but must be not be difficult to use or they may cause stress and anxiety.

enter a state of decline between the conventional annual health checks. Behavioural assessment is, in any case, often missed out of annual checks on the grounds of time and complexity (Box 7.1).

Box 7.1   Suggested methods for improving care for impending geriatric cases

- Regular planned reviews of pain control and disease management.
- 6-monthly (or more frequent) nurse appointments to follow through a checklist of behavioural and general health indicators.
- Regular weighing (good indicator of reducing activity).
- Provide owners with a basic questionnaire on behaviour and general health, to be completed in advance of all health checks.

COGNITIVE IMPAIRMENT

The signs of cognitive impairment will often precede other organic signs of ageing and are a good indicator of general health. Thus, behavioural change may be the first indicator of the need to intervene more widely in the health of the geriatric dog. Owners should be made aware of the mildest signs of this condition so that they bring affected dogs for treatment at the earliest possible stage. It is vital that the signs of cognitive impairment are not taken for natural signs of old age.

Cognitive impairment in cats often goes entirely unnoticed because the major part of the cat's activity pattern occurs outside the home. Reductions in hunting, territorial activity and other outdoor activity are often missed. Owners merely report that the cat spends more time at home or asleep. There may be increases in vocalisation, anxiety and dependence.

Cognitive impairment is a serious problem, indeed it is a life-threatening disease for many elderly dogs. Owners are not aware that in early cases the signs of impairment are treatable or temporarily reversible, so they may not bring these cases to the clinic until they have progressed too far. Loss of activity and normal interaction with the owner impairs the human–animal bond so that when the dog begins to disturb the owner's sleep, bark incessantly or soil in the house, it is more likely that owners will bring the animal to the clinic for euthanasia.

So, for the sake of the pet's health and welfare, we need to encourage owners to discuss subtle changes in the behaviour of their ageing pet.

Certain forms of human and animal cognitive dementia share similarities and it is worth comparing them. Human age-related dementia is subdivided into numerous categories. The three commonest forms are:

- Pseudodementia
- Vascular dementia
- Dementia of the Alzheimer type (DAT)

PSEUDODEMENTIA

Pseudodementia is a type of depression seen in elderly human patients. Signs are typical of other forms of depression but this condition is often confused with true dementia because of the complicating effects of the specific forms of debilitation that accompany old age. There is a general reduction in activity and social interaction, and a loss of interest in occupations the individual formerly found pleasurable. There may be memory loss, anxiety, and other complications that follow from depression.

Pseudodementia generally arises out of debilitations that interfere with the individual's ability to carry out normal activities. For example, the degradation of vision, hearing or mobility. Without the mental stimulation of regular communication, activity and involvement with the environment, the individual becomes withdrawn, frustrated and anxious.

In man it has been shown that pseudodementia is entirely reversible and does not appear to be associated with any histopathological changes. However, the condition may be made worse by the onset of the gradual depletion of neurotransmitter function that occurs with age.

There is no recognised equivalent diagnosis to pseudodementia in the dog or cat, but the factors that create pseudodementia in man are present in the canine and feline populations too and there is every reason to think that many elderly animals suffer from an analogous condition. To recognise the potential for pseudodementia is important because it contributes to a general decline in physical and mental health. For example, in man pseudodementia is a risk factor for developing other more serious forms of dementia. Individuals that become depressed as a result of debilitation will suffer a more rapid decline in fitness and general health.

Human sufferers of pseudodementia respond very rapidly to basic rehabilitation; better pain management, treatment of debilitating disease and the provision of stimulating activities that are within the capabilities of the individual. Precisely the same approach should be used in older dogs and cats that have no specific cognitive impairments but are generally depressed in mood.

VASCULAR DEMENTIA

Vascular dementia and dementia of the Alzheimer type (DAT) are the commonest forms of dementia in man. Vascular dementia results from poor oxygenation of the brain due to circulatory impairment. There are probably numerous types of this condition, resulting from different patterns of cerebrovascular obstruction, including infarcts and emboli. Risk factors in man include atherosclerosis, hypertension, cardiac arrhythmia, diabetes mellitus and hyperlipidaemia.

Some of these factors are also common in the canine and feline population and cases of dementia relating to a primary cerebrovascular defect are probably also common.

To identify and resolve treatable causes of vascular dementia is important because these animals will only obtain limited benefit from drug and dietary treatments intended for Alzheimer type dementia. Drugs such as propentofylline are being licensed for the treatment of human vascular dementia and also for the treatment of cognitive decline in the dog. However, the general success of such drugs in treating canine dementia is not an indication that canine patients share identical pathology with human vascular dementia sufferers.

DEMENTIA ALZHEIMER TYPE (DAT)

Dementia of the Alzheimer type is the commonest form of dementia in man. The pathology and pathophysiology are relatively well-described and broadly similar to that seen in cognitive dementia in dogs. A simplified description of the changes seen in both dog and man are listed below:

- Mitochondrial metabolism becomes defective producing more metabolic waste (free radicals) per unit of energy.
- Antioxidant mechanisms that normally defend tissues against oxidative damage are overwhelmed by the excess production of free radicals.
- Repair processes are ineffective because there is insufficient energy production to fuel both maintenance and repair.
- The oxidation of lipid and protein components leads to cellular damage and increased production of beta-amyloid.
- Beta-amyloid and lipid peroxides are themselves neurotoxic and so a spiral of cellular damage begins.
- Histologically, there is deposition of beta-amyloid in microscopic plaques, beginning in the frontal cortex and sweeping rearwards throughout the cerebrum, leading to a characteristic progression of symptoms.
- Beta-amyloid is also deposited in vital structures such as the hippocampus (responsible for short-term memory formation).
- The situation is further complicated by the fact that beta-amyloid provokes an inflammatory response which further interferes with local nerve function; and the histological changes extend to damage to the microcirculation of the brain so that oxygenation of tissues is reduced.
- A vicious cycle of degeneration and increasing beta-amyloid deposition will develop.
- There is also accompanying reduction in neurotransmitter production and recycling.

The severity of dementia in both dog and man correlates very strongly with the quantity of beta-amyloid present in the brain. It is probable that a similar process is present in the cat.

This process of degeneration can be divided into two phases. During the first (initiation) phase there is a general impairment of neurological functioning due to neurotransmitter depletion, cellular metabolic disturbance and oxidation, but the amount of beta-amyloid is quite low. In the second phase, significant quantities of beta-amyloid have been deposited. The effects of oxidation and toxicity of oxidised cellular components creates a spiral of damage that is more rapid and irreversible.

Beta-amyloid and tau protein are seen in the plaques of feline, canine and human patients, but the organisation and distribution are different. In man, the beta-amyloid plaques are quite large and focal. Tau protein forms 'tangles' that are a microscopically visible component of each plaque. In the dog, the beta-amyloid plaques are smaller and more diffusely distributed within the brain. Tau protein is chemically detectable in the plaques but does not form large tangles. Cats also have large and focal plaques which otherwise biochemically resemble those in the dog. Larger plaques are associated with more severe and permanent local neurological impairment.

These histologically observed differences in pathology appear to be important for the differing progression and progress of the disease in the three species. In man, the damage caused is apparently permanent and irreparable; no treatments have as yet significantly delayed or reversed any signs of human DAT. In dogs, the outlook is more positive. Behavioural signs of dementia are often temporarily reversible and the progress of the disease can be dramatically slowed down. In humans, no matter how aggressively it is treated, this disease is the primary life-threatening condition. Dogs have a much better prognosis because, if treated at a sufficiently early stage, the progression of the condition can be slowed to a point that other medical disorders are likely to replace dementia as the life-limiting condition. The outlook for feline patients is uncertain, but the size of plaques and general lateness of diagnosis mean that the prognosis is less good than for the dog.

It may be that the more diffuse beta-amyloid in the canine patient causes less severe damage and allows for more gradual remodelling so that function is taken up by other nervous tissue. Alternatively, the different role of tau protein in human beta-amyloid plaques may be relevant. Certainly, the functional demands on the canine brain are substantially less than those on the human so the dog is able to appear relatively normal, even when severe impairments are present.

COGNITIVE DEMENTIA IN THE DOG AND CAT (ALZHEIMER–LIKE)

DIAGNOSIS

This form of dementia closely mirrors DAT in terms of clinical effects and pathology (see above). Early diagnosis is critical. To treat these cases effectively, we must intervene during the earliest stages of the disease when damage is less critical; for example, during the first phase of impairment. Behavioural changes in early dementia are quite subtle and easily confused with depression and the effects of illness. Many owners write them off as 'just old age'.

In the early stages of dementia we might typically see quite nondescript signs that are often hard to attribute to any specific cause:

- lethargy and depression
- reduced activity
- reduced social interaction
- loss of play
- mild disturbance of sleep pattern
- mild increases in fear and anxiety.

These changes are linked to the initiation phase of the condition, so it is particularly important to catch cases at this stage. There will be mild cognitive impairment and these dogs can be differentiated from ones with debilitation and depression by the lack of response to improved medical management and environmental stimulation.

As the disorder progresses, more severe signs emerge that are linked to five underlying degenerative processes:

1. Generalised and localised cortical impairment (frontal cortex, motor cortex, etc):
   - changes of 'personality'
   - confusion and failure to interpret sensory information correctly (staring into space or at inanimate objects)
2. Loss of learned behaviours:
   - house-training
   - control commands
   - social inhibition (ignorance of the restraining influence of the presence of other individuals, including the owner)
   - food snatching and stealing in front of the owner
   - elimination in front of owner
3. Changes in emotionality:
   - worsening of existing fear and phobia problems
   - increased anxiety
   - depression
   - irritability
4. Impaired ability to form new short-term memory:
   - repetition of behaviour (e.g., requests for attention, food, or to go outside)
   - difficulty acquiring new learning (e.g., being house-trained again)
5. Specific neurological impairments:
   - loss of proprioception
   - sensory impairment (central blindness, central deafness)

The mixture of symptoms seen in any individual case is quite unique. A large proportion of the animal's consistent pattern of responses that we might call 'personality' is learned during life. In particular, this includes patterns of social inhibition in which the animal learns to suppress highly motivated behaviour according to the social context.

For example, many young dogs will try to snatch food from the plate of a person or another animal, but they rapidly learn that this is unacceptable. Likewise, an attention-seeking dog learns not to pester its owner. Dogs with dementia lose these inhibitions and may return to acting purely on current motivation. Punishment, including ignoring behaviour, has little or no effect other than to distress the animal and risk conflict with it.

Despite the fact that a decline in interaction is often cited as an indication of dementia, this is not always the case. In some individuals the level of attention-seeking increases. There are many reasons for this; for example, if the animal's level of anxiety forces it to demand more reassurance from its owner or because it still feels hungry and cannot remember when it last asked for food. So it is best to remember the underlying factors in dementia-related behavioural change and then to use them to interpret the animal's current behaviour.

As the condition progresses further, there is an accumulation of damage in specific areas leading to discrete neurological signs such as ataxia, central blindness or deafness. These sensory losses are often confused with actual primary sensory loss, especially in dogs with already limited vision. Usually an examination will reveal that the animal's actual hearing or vision loss is not enough to account for the overall sensory impairment. In these cases, it is damage to the CNS which is leading to the loss of functional vision or hearing because the animal is not able to process and interpret the sensory information it is getting. Even at this advanced stage there is some value in treatment.

It is relatively easy to pick up moderately severe cases, but early and severe ones are more difficult. The former because owners may assume that what they are seeing is the effect of normal ageing, the latter because the more obvious signs of cognitive dementia are obscured by severe neurological signs.

High-risk periods for the geriatric pet

Certain events are known to place additional stress on patients and represent a unique risk to the cognitively impaired pet (Table 7.5).

Preparations can be made for these events so that their impact is minimised. For example, using dietary modification and the administration of psychoactive, antioxidant or neuroprotective drugs in advance of planned events, such as general anaesthesia. Pre-operative blood screening, together with continuous intra-operative and recovery blood pressure and oximetry measurement, are essential for proper anaesthetic management.

Wherever possible perioperative pain relief should be used to reduce the uncomfortable after-effects of prolonged recumbency, and reversible or short-acting sedatives and induction agents should be used so that anaesthetic duration is minimised. The animal should be returned to a familiar environment as soon as safely possible after recovery.

In the dog, Dog Appeasing Pheromone (DAP®) can be used to aid familiarisation with new environments. For example, if a DAP® diffuser is installed in the dog's home a few days prior to a change of environment, then the new environment will seem more familiar and less threatening if a DAP® is installed there too. This effect can be used to reduce stress for older animals that are to be hospitalised or come to the clinic for procedures.

Table 7.5 Veterinary procedures and environments

	Event	Effect
Veterinary procedures	Anaesthesia/sedation Surgery Medication Examination	Hypoxia, hypovolaemia, low blood pressure, after-effects of drugs Blood loss e.g., steroids, tranquillisers Emotional and physical stress, fear, anxiety
Change to a new environment	Hospitalization Kennelling House move	Loss of familiar cues that enable animal to comprehend environment Emotional stress
Alterations to current environment	New pets Children Change of owner routine	Changes in status (dog), competition for resources (food, attention) Loss of owner attention, unfamiliar noises/activities Loss of reassuring presence of owner

TREATMENT

Treatment should have several aims:

- Delay progression of disease (where possible).
- Return mental function to a level at which normal behaviour may be re-established.
- Retrain lost behaviour.
- Re-establish relationships with people and other animals in the house so that social support helps to maintain improvement

The treatable underlying mechanisms of cognitive dementia are:

- depletion of neurotransmitter function
- localised inflammation around beta-amyloid plaques
- mitochondrial inefficiency (producing more free radicals per unit of useable energy)
- depletion of cytochemicals needed for cell repair
- ongoing oxidative damage.

There are several approaches to correcting these faults which may be used in combination with each other.

Dietary modification

There is considerable evidence that dietary supplementation can be used to improve mitochondrial metabolic function and assist oxygen free-radical scavenging mechanisms.

Trials also suggest that these supplements are equally effective in vivo, improving neuronal metabolic function and boosting CNS antioxidant reserve. Supplements with demonstrable efficacy include vitamin E, n-acetyl-l-carnitine and alpha-lipoic acid which have been trialled in a number of species, but most specialist diets also include a range of other antioxidant chemicals and additives.

The diet should also include increased levels of cellular repair materials such as essential fatty acids. Low protein, high carbohydrate diets made with high-quality protein and vitamin B supplementation can be used to increase the levels of the neurotransmitter serotonin (5-HT), which may be useful in dogs that are suffering from chronic anxiety.

Of course, such diets must also be compatible with whatever medical problems the animal is also experiencing, but most senior and disease specific diets can be modified easily and safely to give benefits to the cognitively impaired animal.

Dietary modification of this kind should be the mainstay therapy to delay progression of dementia and should be instituted in dogs with the earliest signs of dementia. Owners can expect to see improvements within 4 to 6 weeks of dietary change.

Dietary modification is also potentially useful for senile cats, but early intervention is even more important.

Drug therapy

In behavioural medicine, psychoactive drugs are primarily used to correct neurotransmitter abnormalities, but some of these drugs have specific properties that may be useful for the cognitively impaired dog or cat. Drugs such as propentofylline and nicergoline have specific effects on cerebral circulation in the dog.

Drugs should be carefully selected to complement dietary modification in line with anticipated neurotransmitter problems or cerebral oxygenation/perfusion problems.

Where cerebral oxygenation is an issue, all efforts should be made to correct any cardiovascular or pulmonary problems that may be the root cause.

Table 7.6   Drug therapy: effects and drug types

Effect	Drug types
Improve cerebral circulation	Propentofylline
	Nicergoline
Antioxidant effects	Selegiline
	Propentofylline
	Nicergoline
Improve neurotransmitter function	
Dopamine	Selegiline
Serotonin	Clomipramine
Neuroprotective effects	Selegiline
	Propentofylline (cholinergic neurons)

Herbal drugs such as valerian, St. John's Wort and skullcap should be avoided, especially in the cat, because their safety and effects on cognition are unquantified. Many of these drugs are general CNS depressants with sedative properties, which makes them unsuitable for treating dogs with cognitive dementia. Some, like St John's Wort, have effects on neurotransmitters and may interact with conventional serotonergic (clomipramine) or dopaminergic (selegiline) drugs to produce adverse effects.

The choice of drug should depend partly on the anticipated pathology or pathophysiology and partly on the behavioural signs of the condition being treated.

The dopaminergic drug selegiline is useful for cases where there is behavioural inhibition and impaired learning because this drug increases exploratory behaviour and the intensity of the experience of reinforcement. In particular, this assists with the retraining of learned behaviours. Selegiline is also useful for cognitively impaired dogs that have fear-related problems, especially if fearfulness has increased as a result of cognitive changes.

Serotonergic drugs such as clomipramine and fluoxetine are useful for animals that suffer from chronic anxiety, attachment problems and sleep disturbance. They should not be used in combination with dopaminergic drugs such as selegiline. When switching between serotonin re-uptake inhibitor and monoamine oxidase inhibitor drugs, there must be a **minimum** 14 day washout period, when neither drug is given, to prevent the occurrence of potentially fatal serotonin syndrome (Table 7.6).

It is important to remember that while these drugs may be used in the cat, they are not licensed for this species and dose rates must be checked with current references.

Changes in behaviour may be slow with psychoactive drug treatment, with a partial response seen after 4 to 6 weeks and sometimes waiting until 8 to 10 weeks for a truly significant response.

Short-term drug treatments may be used to deal with problems of sleep disturbance which can be very difficult for owners to cope with. Dogs with cognitive dementia will often find it hard to get to sleep or may wake up at a specific time in the night. Chronic anxiety is linked to waking in the first third of the sleep period. In other cases, the dog wakes an hour or two before the owner is up, which creates insecurity and anxiety. The aim, if using short term sedatives, is to help the dog to sleep through the periods when it might awake and cause a disturbance but leave it fully awake during the day so that the owner can exercise it more and try to return the animal's pattern of activity to normal. The choice of drug should be appropriate to the type of sleep disturbance, with short-acting drugs being suitable for early night-time wakefulness. Strongly sedative drugs, such as acepromazine, should be avoided where possible because they produce hangover effects that affect cognition during the daytime.

Benzodiazepine drugs such as diazepam may produce a short-term sedative effect, but they too should be avoided because the memory impairment they produce will interfere with retraining and may exacerbate some of the behavioural problems. Benzodiazepines are toxic when given orally to cats. Caution should be exercised over the prescribing of benzodiazepines due to their abuse potential in the human population.

Sedative antihistamines such as trimeprazine tartrate (Vallergan®) are often very useful because they produce short-term sedation without any after-effects. This drug works well in combination with behavioural therapy to alter sleep patterns. In most cases, sedation should be needed for only 1 to 2 weeks if other behavioural therapy is used to alter the sleep pattern.

Behavioural therapy

This can be divided into three components:

1. Making the environment more accessible to the geriatric pet.
2. Retraining the behaviours that the animal has lost through cognitive impairment.
3. Providing environmental enrichment to stimulate and maintain mental processes and to improve quality of life.

Environmental modification to improve accessibility

The two main problems for these dogs are locating, and then getting to, the resources they need. Pain or frustration experienced when using stairs or climbing onto furniture, for example, can make dogs irritable and aggressive. Many older dogs with back problems will object to being removed from furniture simply due to back pain. Not being able to find or comfortably visit a water bowl is a potential cause of mild dehydration, especially for any animal fed on a dried diet.

Certain simple changes will make resources more useable for the less mobile pet and help to reduce competition with other animals in a multi-pet household:

- Additional water bowls close to resting areas.
- Additional resting sites.
- Steps/ramps to get on and off furniture (if desired).

Pets with defective vision may need to be given extra cues that enable them to navigate the home:

- Carpets and rugs to give a tactile identification of central floor spaces and corridors so that the animal can move about confidently without bumping into things.
- Quiet radios placed at the animal's level in different rooms close to resources so that the animal can use sound to locate them.
- Different scents to identify specific rooms so that the pet can locate them.

These changes also benefit anxious or confused pets by giving them additional navigation cues. Confused animals also benefit from having properly designed bed areas, with a well-padded wrap-around basket, nearby night-light and a piece of the owner's recently worn clothing to aid famil-

> ### Box 7.2 Immediate action: sleep disturbance due to cognitive dementia
>
> *Make the resting place more comfortable and familiar:*
>
> - Install a night-light next to the resting place.
> - Add a piece of the owner's unwashed clothing.
> - Make it well-padded with high sides so that the dog can get comfortable and feels safe.
> - Install a DAP diffuser next to it.
> - Keep windows closed to avoid ingress of sound.
> - Use heavy curtains to stop the early morning light waking the dog up.
>
> *Increase daytime activity levels:*
>
> - Short walks and lots of play throughout the day.
> - Activity feeding.
> - Wake the dog regularly the during day; don't allow it to sleep all the time.
>
> *Use a short-term sedative to improve sleep:*
>
> - Trimeprazine tartrate (Vallergan).
> - Small amounts of sedative lavender oil on the dog's bedding.

iarity. Large dogs may benefit from a raised bed that is easier to get in and out of (Box 7.2).

Retraining behaviour

Some behaviour, such as house-training, may be completely lost, but in many cases there is a residue of original learning that simply needs to be reactivated.

It is essential to avoid using positive punishment to retrain new behaviour because this will simply cause fear and stress. Cues and reinforcement need to be clear and intelligible to the animal. Conditioned secondary reinforcers are useful because they may be tailored to the individual animal's perceptual abilities. For example, although clicker training is often very valuable, touch or light flashes may be used as alternative conditioned reinforcers once associated with a suitably motivating reward (e.g., food).

It may also be necessary to retrain the animal to reduce its attention-seeking behaviour once it is not showing signs of anxiety or confusion and will not suffer distress at being ignored.

Environmental enrichment

There is no point in giving medication and a specialist diet in order to improve cognitive ability if we do nothing to stimulate the animal. Indeed, a mentally functional animal with nothing to do is a potential welfare problem.

There are some simple things that can be used to exercise the animal's mental abilities, none of which require a lot of effort from the owner:

Activity feeding This can be as simple as scattering dried food for the pet to find, but can include homemade or manufactured feeders (Havaball®, activity ball, Buster Cube®, miniature activity balls for cats). It is best to start with very simple and undemanding exercises that replace only a small proportion of the animal's daily food intake and then to increase the range and complexity of feeders and food-finding opportunities as the pet seems able to cope.

Exposure to stimulating environments Debilitated dogs may not be able to walk far but they should still be taken daily to interesting places so that they can sniff around and meet other dogs and people (if this is something they have previously enjoyed). Even a couple of short (5–10 minute) periods are beneficial to an otherwise housebound dog.

Low or zero-load exercise, such as swimming, is a good way to improve strength and stamina in older dogs that have become sedentary and unfit. It is also a good opportunity for fitter animals to enjoy more vigorous play and social contact with less risk of pain.

Play Owners should make a list of the games that the animal used to enjoy when it was younger. Some of these may be beyond its abilities but others may be safely adapted to suit an older animal. It is also good to create new games based on reliable motivators like food. For example, teaching a dog to play a food-finding game on command.

Social contact Geriatric and cognitively impaired pets often become socially isolated because they become less demanding. Owners should be encouraged to interact with their pet more often, but less often *on-demand* from the pet. This may include invitations to play or have contact. For dogs, this should also involve group play and contact with other dogs that the animal has previously got on well with.

PROGNOSIS

Cognitive dementia is always progressive. It has been shown that dogs with one major sign of dementia will progress to have at least one further sign within 12 to 18 months. The course of the disease is very variable and in some cases dogs will show severe signs within only a few months.

However, the animal's current level of disease is composed of both reversible and irreversible brain changes:

1. Reversible/treatable:
   - inflammatory responses around beta-amyloid plaques
   - neurotransmitter system deficits
   - mitochondrial metabolic defects
   - oxidative damage
2. Irreversible:
   - cellular death
   - deposition of beta-amyloid plaques

So, in fact, many of the processes underlying dementia in dogs are treatable, although a combination of approaches is needed in many cases. In any given individual, it is hard to assess whether signs are (temporarily) reversible or not, so it is difficult to prognosticate.

Table 7.7 contains some guidelines; however, these are only approximate.

Table 7.7 Prognosis

Prognosis	Signs (at time of presentation)	Benefit of treatment
Good	Only minor signs of short duration (<6 months)	Appropriate therapy may return almost all of normal function (temporarily). Dementia may not be life-span limiting condition.
Moderate	1 to 2 major signs	Therapy may delay onset of further signs and may return current functioning to 'normal' temporarily. In older dogs dementia may not be life-span limiting.
Guarded	3+ major signs with significant progression over <6 months	Therapy may delay progression but may not return all function to normal, even temporarily.
Guarded–poor	Major signs with one or more neurological deficit	Therapy may delay progression but functioning will probably not return to normal, even temporarily.

ADVICE SHEETS THAT MAY BE RELEVANT TO THIS CHAPTER

In Appendix 2:

2. Jumping up
3. Reward and punishment
5. Reducing possessiveness through play
8. Play and calm signals
9. The 'come away' command
11. Attention-seeking and the 'no' signal
12. Click-touch training
16. Environmental enrichment for dogs
17. Using food rewards for training
18. Food for work
19. Introducing the clicker

In Appendix 3:

1. Improving the outdoor environment for cats
2. Improving the indoor environment for cats

PART 3

Canine behavioural problems

PART CONTENTS

Chapter 8

Canine fear, anxiety and phobia-related disorders

INTRODUCTION

Many behavioural problems have fear or anxiety as a normal underlying emotional motivation. Some of these conditions have outward signs of aggression, so there is something of a crossover between the information in this chapter and the one on aggression.

UNDERLYING CONCEPTS IN FEAR AND ANXIETY DISORDERS

Fear

Fear is the apprehension of a stimulus, object or event. The most important thing to remember about fear is that it is a highly adaptive response, which is essential for survival. When animals respond to stimuli in their environment, there is a complex range of potential reactions and the selection of a response that is both specific to the stimulus encountered and to the situation or context in which it is found will depend on two very important factors. First, there is a genetic influence on behaviour, which influences the species and breed-specific behavioural responses that have become established over generations. Secondly, there is an individual aspect of behaviour which has been established through the process of learning and which reflects not only the animal's innate response to specific stimuli but also its experience.

The key feature of fear is that the behaviour is directional, related to the location of the stimulus. The object of fear will always initially be the focus of the dog's attention (Box 8.1).

The animal's aim is to reduce the sensation of fear either by repelling, escaping from or evading the source of the fear. If this is not possible, then the animal will freeze and wait for an opportunity to engage another response, or engage in displacement activity that is a form of self-appeasement or self-distraction.

The most significant patterns of behaviour for fearful animals are therefore the four Fs:

- Fight
- Flight
- Freeze
- Fiddle about (displacement or self-appeasement behaviour)

The choice of whether to fight, flee, freeze or self-appease depends upon the situation but the tendency to choose one over another also varies significantly with breed and species. Cats are inclined to engage in escape as the primary response to fear or threat, which is why they object so strongly to restraint and entrapment. If this escape response is frustrated in any way, then the cat is quite likely to shift to overt aggressiveness in an attempt to re-establish a means of escape.

Breed variation among dogs is also considerable. Certain types of dogs have been deliberately bred to behave in a particular way when faced with threat or frustration. Experimentally, puppies have been raised in relative isolation and then exposed to a range of novel stimuli such as furniture or people. Their behavioural response to the novel stimuli has then been studied. Some breeds, such as beagles, would immediately freeze almost to the point of catatonia. Others, like certain small terriers, would show the opposite by barking and running around the novel stimulus. We know that all the groups were experiencing fear but their reactions were entirely different.

To some extent we capitalise on the freezing behaviour. Most dogs, for example, will freeze when put on an examination table. Unfortunately, some dogs are seen as obstruc-

tive when they become aggressive and self-defensive instead of freezing. They tend to get labelled as 'dominant' when, in fact, they are merely expressing a breed-specific response to fear that is incompatible with what *we* want them to do.

Another feature of the behaviour of frightened animals is the 'fear-potentiated startle response'. Put simply, the fearful animal is very easily startled by small noises or movements. So another indicator of fear is the extreme jumpiness that the animal displays. This makes the fearful animal a volatile individual.

Approach–avoidance conflict

An animal may be both drawn to investigate something and apprehensive of approaching it. This conflict is critical in understanding how we treat fears and phobias of all kinds.

In Figure 8.1 there are two lines drawn. One indicates the tendency to approach and the other the tendency to avoid. At longer distances, the tendency to want to approach is greater than that to avoid and the animal will move closer. The tendency to avoid increases as the animal approaches until it becomes great enough to stop the animal going further. So the animal will *voluntarily* approach only as close as the crossover point; closer than this will produce feelings of fear which the animal will not choose to experience. At this distance the animal will stop and oscillate about that point, sometimes going a little closer and a moment later moving further away. There is hesitancy and anxiety.

If the object does not move or make any noise then apprehension will gradually decrease, with a lowering of the avoidance line. The dog tentatively approaches closer to the object until it is sure that there is no threat. Finally, it will lose its apprehension and ignore the object. If the dog were forced to go closer than it would approach voluntarily, then we would expect it to experience profound fear.

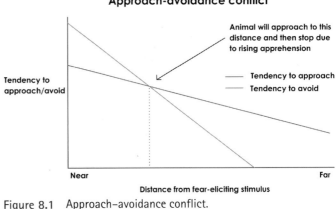

Approach-avoidance conflict

Animal will approach to this distance and then stop due to rising apprehension

Tendency to approach/avoid

— Tendency to approach
— Tendency to avoid

Near   Far

Distance from fear-eliciting stimulus

Figure 8.1 Approach–avoidance conflict.
(J. Gray, Psychology of Fear and Stress, Cambridge University Press, Cambridge, 1979)

Understanding approach-avoidance conflicts enables us to make some useful predictions about behaviour:

- At distances further than the crossover point, the dog attends to the stimulus but is not apprehensive of it. It still desires to move closer.
- At distances closer than the crossover point, the dog experiences fear.
- Two dogs that approach to the same distance may be experiencing completely different levels of fearfulness. One may only be lured close by the presence of food whilst, in fact, being quite terrified.
- The height of the avoidance line will vary dynamically with the potential threat from the object or person. Sudden movements or sounds will make the avoidance line go higher and the degree to which this happens depends upon the individual dog's response to these changes.

Since fear potentiates the startle response and may recruit aggressive behaviour, we must be wary of the fact that a dog that comes close may also become very fearful and likely to react very suddenly. For example, it would be unwise to lure a fearful dog too near using food or some other reward because this brings the animal within attacking distance at a time when its responses are most likely to be sudden, rapid and violent. Also, if the dog is being restrained on a leash, there is a risk of redirected aggression if the dog has shown this kind of behaviour in the past.

We know that, beyond the crossover point, the dog is not experiencing fear; so regular and repeated exposure beyond that distance would enable the dog to habituate to the presence of the stimulus. Gradually, apprehension would decrease and the dog would voluntarily go closer. This does not risk flooding the dog with fearful experiences and does not place anyone at risk. It also minimises the chance of aversive experiences during training. We can see that a relatively static and unvarying stimulus is easier to adapt to than a moving and changing one that produces wild fluctuations in the height of the avoidance line.

Information from the approach–avoidance model can be applied to fears or phobias of noises as well as objects or individuals. Instead of varying distance, sound intensity might be varied.

Anxiety

Anxiety can be defined as the apprehensive anticipation of threat.

The function of anxiety is to broaden the animal's attention so that it is prepared to react to any threat. It is most likely in unfamiliar situations or where the animal has had aversive experiences.

The key difference between anxiety and fear is in the word 'anticipation'. For the anxious animal no threat is present and anxiety is under the control of stimuli that are not a main object of attention. These are contextual cues relating to features of the environment the animal is in (enclosed or open space, presence or absence of trees, odours, etc.).

The dog often responds to a series of these stimuli, which results in increasing anxiety: for example, a series of actions performed by the owner as he or she prepares to leave the house or in response to changing weather conditions that might predict a storm (wind, change of temperature, clouds overhead, rain, etc.).

The intensity of anxiety experienced depends upon the level of arousal and the nature of the threat or danger that is anticipated. For some dogs with firework or thunder phobias, the potential threat they anticipate is so severe that they will respond anxiously to all sorts of very subtle contextual cues, such as approaching darkness or smoky odours in the atmosphere. These dogs may show signs of chronic anxiety throughout an entire season.

Since there is no focus for the emotional state and the dog is actually in a state of readiness for a threat, a number of anxious behaviours are shown in Box 8.2.

Chronic anxiety also produces pervasive effects on behaviour, leading to disturbance of sleep and chronic fatigue. Animals that have been anxious during a walk will be abnormally tired when they get home to an environment that feels safe.

Anxious animals may show hesitancy and this is important when considering medication. Anxiety may be the reason for aggressive behaviour or it may be the only thing that inhibits the dog from completing an aggressive attack. Drugs that cause disinhibition of anxious hesitancy can therefore increase the chances of an aggressive attack. This problem is most frequently encountered with benzodiazepines (diazepam) and tricyclic antidepressants (amitriptyline, clomipramine), and phenothiazines such as acepromazine.

Being anxious is exceptionally unpleasant and animals will seek any opportunity to reduce their arousal and anxiety. We can therefore treat anxiety with medication, but we can also teach the animal to carry out behaviours that reduce anxiety or selectively reinforce non-anxious behaviours.

PHYSIOLOGICAL AND NEUROCHEMICAL MECHANISMS UNDERLYING FEAR AND ANXIETY

In order to understand the physiology of fear, it is necessary to look to one small area of the brain where the control

---

Box 8.2   Typical behavioural signs of anxiety

- Arousal (including increased heart and respiratory rate)
- Hypervigilance/scanning
- Hesitation in completing a behavioural sequence
- Loss of selective attention
- Restlessness
- Increased locomotor activity
- Increased heart rate and respiratory rate (e.g., panting)

centre for this important survival mechanism is located – the amygdala. This structure is involved in the generation of the signs and symptoms of fear, anxiety and phobia and, in its role of mediating fear responses, the central nucleus of the amygdala makes connections to other important areas of the central nervous system (CNS), such as the hypothalamus, the dorsal motor nucleus of the vagus, the parabrachial nucleus, the locus coeruleus and the paraventricular nucleus.

There are a number of responses involved in the fear reaction including autonomic, neuroendocrine and muscular responses. The autonomic response is associated with increased activity of the sympathetic nervous system, resulting in a flight or fight response. This involves various reactions that prepare the body for action, such as increased arousal and agitation, peripheral vasoconstriction and secretion of thick viscous saliva from the submandibular salivary glands. At the same time, there is a decrease in parasympathetic activity.

The amygdala is involved in the control of these autonomic responses, both directly through the dorsal motor nucleus of the vagus and indirectly through the lateral hypothalamus. The orbitofrontal cortex is involved with the behavioural response that is associated with the emotion of fear and is believed to initiate autonomic responses to conditioned stimuli acting as either reinforcers or punishers.

The medulla of the adrenal gland is involved in the fear response through the release of epinephrine (adrenaline), norepinephrine (noradrenaline) and dopamine and contributes to the preparation of the body for action by increasing the heart rate and blood glucose levels. Epinephrine release is also believed to increase cognitive function and assist the animal in clear thinking, which increases its success in escaping from the perceived threat.

Hypothalamic control of the release of corticosteroids from the adrenal cortex is another feature of the fear response but is not unique to fearful reactions and is seen in association with other emotional responses, including those of a positive nature. The stress response is basically a mechanism for generating arousal to prepare the individual for defence or activity and the aim of the system is to return an individual to within its normal homeostatic parameters.

Cortisol receptors are widely distributed throughout the body and, as a result, the effects of cortisol release are wide-ranging. Amongst the most readily recognised effects are those relating to glucose metabolism. Through the action of cortisol, blood glucose levels are increased to provide a supply of energy for muscular activity. In addition, cortisol has a direct effect on the brain and is believed to increase arousal in the CNS through the hindbrain and locus coeruleus pathways. The sex hormones are also affected by cortisol and there is a decrease in the sensitivity of gonads to lutropin (luteinising hormone) and a resulting decrease in libido and fertility in animals exhibiting a stress response.

Cortisol release is controlled by a negative feedback system involving the hypothalamus, anterior pituitary and adrenal gland and, while the short-term effects of cortisol are adaptive, in a stress response prolonged release of high levels can have wide ranging negative effects on the body.

The neurotransmitters associated with fear and stress

There are four neurotransmitter systems that are of interest when studying the physiology of the fear response and an understanding of their involvement in the process can be helpful when considering the use of pharmacological intervention in clinical cases.

Noradrenergic system

Norepinephrine is an important neurotransmitter within the CNS and mediates a range of behavioural and physiological reactions associated with the emotional response of fear.

The noradrenergic neurons projecting from the locus coeruleus are of particular interest in this context, along with their connections to limbic and cortical regions, since the locus coeruleus plays a central role in the efferent pathways of the fear response. Norepinephrine is also released from the hypothalamus and frontal cortex.

Increases in noradrenergic transmission are associated with increased arousal, awareness, vigilance and signal detection in a state of fear, and also with control of the facial expressions of fear through the trigeminal and motor nuclei.

Activation of the beta-adrenergic system affects long-term memory of negative events through plastic changes in central adrenergic mechanisms and this enhancement of memory is obviously adaptive for the animal. The most important site of catecholaminergic activity in relation to memory-enhancing action is believed to be the amygdala.

Serotonergic system

The role of serotonin is not clearly defined but it is believed to be important in the mediation of anxiety, with an increase in serotonin release being associated with stress and anxiety. It is the serotonergic system located in the dorsal raphe nuclei that is of particular interest in this context, through inhibition of adaptive and social attachment behaviour. Adequate serotonin release is believed to be instrumental in some fear responses but there is no firm evidence for a link between the release of serotonin and the display of anxiety-related behavioural responses.

Some research has illustrated differences in the anxiety-related serotonergic activity of individuals with different rearing environments and it is believed that the role of serotonin is related to the responsiveness of the serotonergic system, which in turn is affected by prior experience.

Dopaminergic system

Dopamine release occurs primarily in the prefrontal cortex and amygdala, and certain populations of dopamine neurons are selectively activated during the stress response. Histochemical studies have shown that the neurons of the lower brain stem, where the reticular activating system is located, contain norepinephrine and dopamine and that these neurons have widespread synaptic connections with the limbic system in which the amygdala is situated. The limbic system is a phylogenetically ancient part of the brain that governs a range of emotional functions.

GABA-ergic system

GABA (γ-aminobutyric acid)-mediated neurotransmission is known to be affected by stress and the effects of this inhibitory neurotransmitter on the tone of the serotonergic and noradrenergic systems is believed to be significant in this regard. The influence on the serotonergic system is believed to be instrumental in the anxiolytic effects of GABA and hence of GABA agonists.

SUMMARY OF TREATMENT METHODS

Preventing the development of fear and anxiety

Fear, and the anxiety that arises out of it, develops in order to protect the individual from potential harm and it results from a learning process in which an individual associates certain stimuli with unpleasant outcomes, either in terms of emotional response or physical experience.

It therefore follows that the development of fear within an individual will depend to a large extent on its experience. The acceptance of stimuli as 'normal' (and therefore non-threatening) arises from early experience, and fear is most likely to develop in reaction to stimuli that are not encountered during the early stages of life. This explains the importance of the so-called sensitive period in puppies and highlights the need for novelty and complexity within the environment at this stage of development.

However, fear responses can be triggered at any stage of development and, while prevention measures can be targeted toward very young puppies, they should also be applied to older animals when encountering new or potentially challenging environments and events.

We may take advantage of latent inhibition to protect individuals from developing negative associations with events or contexts. This can be done by deliberately organising a number of highly positive experiences that will then block the acquisition of negative learning. Hence, we encourage dogs to visit the veterinary practice regularly on a 'social' basis so that they may be given food treats, pleasurable contact with people and play. This can help to decrease the negative reaction to that environment even when the animal finally has to endure an unpleasant procedure such as vaccination.

Desensitisation and counterconditioning

Desensitisation is used to reduce fearful and phobic reactions to stimuli. After a large number of neutral presentations of the stimulus, it ceases to produce a significant emotional effect.

Counterconditioning is used to create a new and positive emotional response with the desensitised stimulus (Fig. 8.2). After being counterconditioned, the same stimulus is paired with events that produce an unconditional positive emotional response that conflicts with fear. Typical examples are food and play.

The ultimate result is that, every time the stimulus is experienced, there is an emotional swing toward a relaxed

Figure 8.2 In counterconditioning, the aim is for the previously fear-eliciting stimulus to come to evoke a pleasurable emotional state.

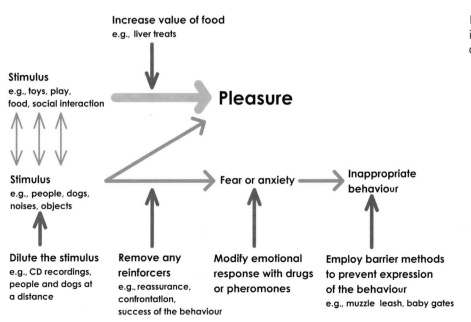

and happy emotional state that is in direct conflict with the fear that was previously present. This has a blocking effect that reduces the chance of resensitisation and generalisation. Desensitisation and counterconditioning therefore work in concert to reduce and replace the conditioned emotional response of fear and can be used to treat any fear or phobia problem. Where there are fears or phobias of multiple stimuli, it is best to treat each one separately and divide any complex stimulus into several more easily treated individual components. For example, the visual and audible stimuli associated with traffic or the different noises experienced during a storm or firework event.

If the unconditional appetitive stimulus is insufficiently significant to the dog, then fear may continue to be elicited because this emotional state takes priority. To prevent the continued expression of undesirable behaviour and emotional states during training, the fear-eliciting stimulus may need to be diluted, and any reinforcers for the fearful or anxious behaviour must be removed. Alternatively drugs may be used to modulate emotional states (see Fig. 8.2).

Practical aspects of desensitisation

First, the precise desensitisation stimulus must be identified and differentiated from other stimuli that may also evoke a response. Next, a way must be found to reduce the intensity of this stimulus to below the threshold that produces an emotional response.

Ways of reducing the impact of the stimulus might include:

- reducing sound intensity
- producing smaller versions of the stimulus
- presenting the stimulus in a different way or in an unusual context
- placing the object of fear further away
- partially obscuring vision of the object using a fence or a screen.

For desensitisation to be effective and non-stressful for the dog, the stimulus must be minimally salient; the dog should initially notice that the object or sound is present but must not show signs of fear or anxiety.

The dog is exposed to the attenuated stimulus for short periods of 5 to 10 minutes several times each day until it barely notices when the stimulus is presented. At this point, the level of the stimulus is increased to the minimally salient level again and the process is repeated; that is, the sound volume is turned up, or the test object is replaced with a bigger version, or the object is brought slightly closer.

This cycle is repeated until the dog can tolerate the full stimulus without reacting emotionally. At this point the dog is desensitised, but this process is easily reversed. A sensitising or intensely fear-eliciting experience with the stimulus may cause the dog to revert to fearful or phobic response. The training is carried out in a number of different contexts, including those most relevant to the fear or phobia. In reality, it is often very difficult to progress smoothly from fake or attenuated stimuli to real ones and ingenuity may be required.

Practical aspects of counterconditioning

Before beginning counterconditioning, there must be minimal reaction to the stimulus at the intensities at which it will be presented during training. If the emotional response to the stimulus is anywhere near as great as the emotional response to the unconditioned stimulus we are trying to associate with it, then the response will be negligible. If the emotional response to the fearful stimulus is actually greater, then we may condition aversion to the other unconditioned stimulus (Table 8.1).

The timing between the stimuli is critical. We want the previously fearful or phobic stimulus to predict and coincide with the positive unconditioned stimulus so that, when it is heard in the future, the animal is anticipating a pleasant rather than aversive event.

As with desensitisation, the intensity of the previously fearful or phobic stimulus should be low to begin with and then gradually raised over a number of training sessions.

Two variations on counterconditioning may be:

1. With a long continuous stream of stimuli.
2. With individual separate stimuli.

With the first type, the animal is presented with a long stream of closely-spaced stimuli, all of the same intensity. This might be a continuous recording of the noises of which the animal is frightened. The playback system would be switched on and, as soon as the sounds start, the owner would put the dog's food on the floor or start a game. The sounds would be stopped when the dog comes to the end of the meal or the game stops. This method of counterconditioning may be used with the same recorded sounds as were used for desensitisation.

The second type is used to associate a single noise or presentation of the previously phobic stimulus with a

Table 8.1 Effect of relative emotional impact on counterconditioning

Relative evocative strength of previously fear evoking (*FE*) and emotionally positive counterconditioning stimuli (*CC*)	Result
FE > CC	Dog learns to fear the stimuli associated with the counterconditioning event
FE = CC	Little or no response to training
FE < CC	Effective counterconditioning takes place

short burst of reward. For example, a single quiet banging noise is played and, as soon as it is heard, a food treat is given to the dog or a brief game starts. A dog might be engaged in play every time it sees another dog or person that it previously feared. Through repetition, the dog learns to anticipate a positive outcome when it hears unexpected single noises or sees the thing of which it was fearful.

Instrumental conditioning

When fearful or anxious, dogs may be unsure how to cope with a situation. This can result in bolting behaviour or prolonged stress. If the dog discovers that aggressive behaviour, such as barking, growling or snapping at fear-eliciting stimuli has the effect of driving them away, then there is a danger that its strategy may shift from avoidance to offensive aggression. During development, animals usually learn to orientate away from fearful things and toward their mother or another suitable protector. This response changes with maturity and increased self-reliance and, in some cases, it never properly develops because the dog is not given suitable cues that support it. However, this strategy of looking away from fear-eliciting stimuli can be trained using a 'come away command'. Details of this training are included in a handout in Appendix 2. Essentially, the dog is rewarded for moving back to the owner when commanded to do so in a range of normal and then mildly fear-eliciting situations.

Exclusion of medical differentials

It is essential when investigating a potential fear or phobia case to rule out the medical differentials for the behavioural symptoms that are being exhibited (Table 8.2). This is especially important when the use of psychoactive medication is being considered. Some of the differentials can be excluded on clinical examination and medical history but

Table 8.2 Medical differentials for phobia cases

Medical conditions affecting sensory perception	Medical conditions affecting cognition
Partial deafness, e.g., in upper range	Seizures
	Brain tumours
Touch hypersensitivity (hyperaesthesia)	Dementia
	Hepatic disorders
Blindness	Thyroid disease
Dementia	Cushing's disease
Old age changes (non-dementia)	Addison's disease
	Iatrogenic – acute or high level
Pain foci	chronic use of steroid medication

others will involve a combination of these approaches and the use of further diagnostic tests.

Once the medical differentials have been excluded, the choice of medication for the phobia will depend on whether a short or long-term approach is appropriate.

General treatment of specific fears

The general approach is the same in all cases. All stimuli and events that evoke fear must be identified and means found of presenting them in a controlled manner as part of desensitisation. All other uncontrolled exposure to the stimuli should be avoided. Punishment is inappropriate in cases of fear because the animal may associate this additional aversive event with the one that it is already facing. The result is that fear increases in the future. Training routines may have to be developed to deal with the specific nature of the fear, and care must be taken not to place people, animals, and property at risk with potentially aggressive dogs.

FEAR OF ANIMATE OBJECTS (PEOPLE AND OTHER ANIMALS)

Dogs with a fear of people may vary in the range of their fear from those with a selective fear of people with a certain type or appearance (based on gender, size, age, and appearance), to those with a general fear of any unfamiliar person, regardless of type. The same is true of fear of other animals. The movement of the person or animal constantly changes the dog's willingness to approach and the dog cannot naturally approach closer in the way that it would with an inanimate object as its approach–avoidance conflict gradually subsides.

DIAGNOSIS

Typical signs of fear are seen, as described earlier, with approach–avoidance conflict. There is a variation in type of response from passive and avoidant to overtly aggressive. Immature fearful dogs often adopt an avoidant pattern of behaviour: retreating, running away or hiding. As the dog reaches maturity, this same fear give rise to more overtly aggressive behaviour as it attempts to defend itself. There is therefore a vital window of opportunity to treat fearful young dogs before they start to develop self-defensive aggression.

It is quite common for fear-related problems to be misinterpreted as stubbornness when a dog refuses to obey commands because it is being coerced to carry out behaviour that will increase its fear. This situation typically occurs during veterinary consultations or grooming and may finally drive the dog to become aggressive. It is therefore important to recognise signs of fear (Fig. 8.3).

Good history-taking is vital in order to find out about specific incidents or attacks which may have caused an

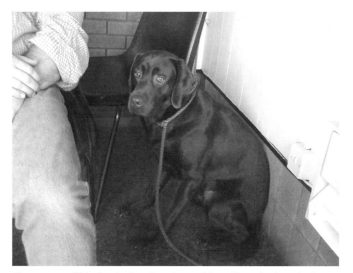

Figure 8.3   This dog is showing signs of fear. Note the hunched body posture against the wall, the slightly lowered head position, facial tension and appearance of the eyes.

increase in fear. Likewise, we need to know about any experience that has occurred in sensitising contexts, such as exposure to dogs or in a noisy or stressful context (town centre, training class).

TREATMENT

Apart for treating the condition, the main aim is to make sure that the situation does not progress to aggression and that people are not placed at risk (Box 8.3). It is particularly important, for example, not to use rewards to lure dogs closer to people and animals because this will intensify fear and create risk of stress to the dog or provocation of an attack.

It is also vital to avoid any kind of punishment when treating fearful dogs. Punishment merely intensifies the negative emotional experience of an already stressed animal and will probably make the dog more fearful, and potentially aggressive, in the future.

Dogs with fear-related problems do not benefit from being coerced into 'facing up to' the things they fear. This may make the problem much worse.

As with any other form of aggression, the key is to identify the precise stimuli or stimulus elements that evoke fear. In the case of a poorly socialised dog, it may be any aspect of human appearance that the dog did not encounter and learn to accept as a puppy (people wearing beards, glasses, hats, etc.). Often there are specific details of appearance that the dog will respond to and some things are, by their nature, more frightening. Very tall people wearing dark clothes look larger and more menacing. Large black dogs tend to evoke more fear.

Once all fear-evoking stimuli have been identified, they should be listed in order of the level of fear they evoke. The dog is desensitized and counterconditioned to each stimu-

lus in turn, starting with people of whom the dog is least fearful, presented in the most nonthreatening way; typically seated and ignoring the dog. As the dog comes to tolerate the seated person, it would then be conditioned to ignore the person as they move slowly around and begin to interact with it. This process would then be applied to a wide range of people with different appearances, but it is also easy to reuse the same people, modifying their appearance with fake beards, moustaches, hats, coats and other apparel so that the most use is made of the 'stooges' that can be employed.

Counterconditioning is carried out with stimuli that have already been desensitised or already evoke minimal fear. In counterconditioning, the appearance of the stimulus is immediately followed by the presentation of some activity that the dog is known to find unconditionally enjoyable, such as eating food or playing a game. For example, each time the stimulus is encountered, at a distance at which the dog is not fearful, the owner gets out a toy or places some food treats on the ground for the dog to eat. Over a number of repetitions the dog will show signs of positive anticipation of food or play whenever the previously fear-eliciting stimulus is encountered. The distance for the stimulus at presentation is gradually decreased over a number of exercises.

Initial counterconditioning can be followed with an instrumental procedure such as the 'come away command'. During a number of training sessions, the dog is trained to come away from a range of different non-fearful stimuli when it is on a walk. The dog is rewarded for following the owner away and sitting down for a treat. The dog is then trained to perform the same 'come away' from mildly fear-eliciting stimuli or counterconditioned stimuli. Once a dog has learned to associate distant or mildly fearful stimuli with a positive experience, such as play or feeding, then the dog can be commanded to come away and sit when that stimulus appears and comes closer. This enables the owner to lead the dog out of a potentially troublesome situation. The dog is then repeatedly rewarded throughout the period that it stays sitting and does not attempt to run away or show aggression to the person or dog that passes by at a distance. This offers a good intermediate method of management of the dog in real situations in which the owner needs to gain control of the dog as a potentially frightening situation develops.

Dog appeasing pheromone (DAP®) is theorised to increase the sense of familiarity of situations and also reduces anxiety. This might prove useful in the treatment of fear of people introduced into the home (Box 8.4).

Drug therapy

Psychoactive drugs may be used to assist progress in behavioural therapy. The choice of drug type depends upon whether the predominant emotional state is fear or anxiety and whether altering this emotional state will improve treatment success or not.

Anxiolytic drugs

Anxiety is a component of fear-related problems in two ways. First, the animal may anxiously anticipate the arrival or actions of the fear-eliciting individual. This anxiety may be chronic and immensely unpleasant for the dog. It may try to reduce its experience of anxiety by using an aggressive display or attack to repel the potential threat. Secondly, anxiety may have an inhibitory effect on the dog's actions; to attack the source of threat requires approaching until close, which carries a risk. If the dog is uncertain of the outcome of an aggressive attack, it may be hesitant to carry one out. So anxiety can be either the emotional motivation for an attack or the only thing that prevents one.

Before using an anxiolytic drug, it is essential to assess the precise role of anxiety in an individual case. If a dog approaches the subject of its fear and hesitantly lunges forward to snap at it, then using an anxiolytic drug might disinhibit the dog and allow it to complete the aggressive manoeuvre. If the dog paces, pants and wanders restlessly but never approaches the object of its fear and always shows signs of avoidance, then an anxiolytic drug might be beneficial.

However, there are many different classes of drug with different anxiolytic effects. Not all will be suitable for the treatment of behavioural problems.

The commonest groups are the benzodiazepines (diazepam, alprazolam), SRI (clomipramine), SSRI (fluoxetine, sertraline), and phenothiazine drugs (acepromazine). Each of these drugs has subtly different effects on different aspects of anxiety. Benzodiazepines have the widest range of effects, significantly reducing anxiety in all situations and all animal models of anxiety. These drugs are unsuitable for use in cases where there is fear or aggression because they produce powerful disinhibition and make dogs dangerous and unpredictable. They also block short-term memory formation which interferes with any kind of behavioural therapy.

SRI and SSRI drugs produce less serious disinhibition of aggression than benzodiazepines, but they still carry a risk and should only be used after thorough assessment. Phenothiazine drugs, like acepromazine, are often used as sedatives, but are unsuitable for treating dogs with fear-related problems. They can produce disinhibition but do not provide any useful therapeutic anxiolysis.

Drugs that reduce apprehension

Selegiline has proved highly effective for the treatment of specific fears. Selegiline increases confidence and exploratory behaviour whilst reducing apprehension. The improvement in confidence is unstable during the first 6 to 8 weeks of induction and care must be taken not to allow the dog to get into situations with which it is unable to cope during this period.

Selegiline increases the intensity of rewarding experiences which can be an advantage when carrying out counter-conditioning based therapies. It can also alter hierarchical relationships between the patient and other dogs or people within the home. Caution should be exercised when giving this drug to low-ranking individuals in multi-dog households because it may give them confidence to challenge what was a functioning and harmonious hierarchy. It should not be used where some kind of status-based aggression problem exists between the dog and a person.

Box 8.4   Treatment: fear of animate objects (dogs, people)

- Identify objects of fear and contexts that evoke anxiety.
- Create a list of features and types of stimuli, placing them in order of the severity of response they evoke.
- Desensitise and countercondition responses to these stimuli using volunteers who can be disguised to simulate a range of different appearances (of people).
- Training should begin with the stimulus at a distance.
- Over a number of sessions it may come closer, make more and faster movement and make more noise.
- Avoid uncontrolled exposure to real stimuli.
- Use a 'come away' command to control the dog in real situations where fear-eliciting stimuli are encountered in an uncontrolled manner.
- DAP® diffuser will help if fear is of a stimulus that is encountered in the home; a DAP® collar may help if the stimulus is encountered outside.
- Psychoactive drugs may be considered for severe cases (with caution).

PROGNOSIS

A good prognosis is associated with cases that are of short duration in an otherwise well-socialised dog that has only one fear-related problem. These are typically dogs that have previously had a normal response to the now fear-eliciting stimulus, having developed fear as a result of some aversive incident. There is a better prognosis for dogs that generally can be kept away from the fear-eliciting event or stimulus but can also easily be trained with it. Dogs that had a range of fear-related problems at the time of acquisition as a puppy but who have overcome these fears and now behave normally, apart from the remaining one or two fear problems, also have a good prognosis because they have naturally become less fearful over time. Dogs with a lack of early experience during the sensitive period and a persistent pattern of fears that extends from puppyhood into adulthood, have a guarded to poor prognosis.

PHOBIA

The human psychiatric definition of phobia is 'irrational' fear that is out of proportion to the actual level of threat. Animals cannot recognise whether or not what they are experiencing is a genuine threat, so this definition is unusable in the veterinary context. However, the subconscious nature of phobia is such that even a highly rational being is unable to overcome the intense experiences that it produces.

It is better to focus on the functional and observable features of phobic fear that differentiate it from normal adaptive fear. As mentioned previously, normal fear is a healthy control that protects us from danger and it is largely proportional to the risk of harm. The effect of phobia is to limit normal behaviour (Box 8.5).

A person who has a normal fear of traffic would avoid walking across the road unless it was clear. One with a phobia of cars would not go near a road if there was any chance of a car appearing and would refuse to get into a car or go anywhere near one. They might not even be able to look at a picture of a car or watch a film with a car chase in it. Thus, fear protects and phobia cripples.

Phobias may develop with any stimulus that can evoke normal fear but there are certain kinds of stimuli that are more commonly linked to phobia. In man, sound sensitivity problems are common in children under 5 years of age, but sounds phobias are very rare in adults. There is apparently a spontaneous 'cure' when the child becomes able to understand the origin of loud noises like fireworks and these children often go on to develop a fondness for firework displays. Visually-based phobias are commonest in man and include fear of animals, inanimate objects and situations such as confinement, open spaces or heights.

Sonophobia is by far the commonest phobia in dogs but other phobias do occur. Many of these develop from phobias of loud noises that have created severe sound sensitivity and generalisation (Table 8.3).

Visually-related phobias do develop without any direct connection to a sound phobic event but this may be because the dog has a poor socialisation history and is therefore suffering from a large number of other anxiety and fear-related disorders. Poorly socialised dogs often show apprehension of a lot of new objects when they first meet them and in susceptible individuals that have experienced traumatic events, this may go on to create the conditions for phobia development. The principles of treating phobias are the same, no matter what the phobic stimulus (Box 8.6).

Box 8.5   Differences between phobic and normal fear

- Phobic fear is intense and out of context so that it limits normal behaviour.
- Phobic fear is 'all or nothing'; once a certain threshold is reached the fear expressed becomes very intense and unrelated to the intensity of the stimulus. This threshold can be very low, so the animal's response seems to us to be disproportionate to the stimulus intensity.
- Unlike normal fear, phobic fear persists long after the actual threat has gone away.

Table 8.3   Sonophobia

Visually related phobia	Relationship with sonophobia	May generalise to:
Flapping cloth (flags, washing)	Association with wind as predictive cue for storms Noise of flapping in high wind may sound like a quiet bang or pop	Large birds Plastic bags blown by wind Hot air balloons Paragliders or kites Brightly coloured clothes Cloudy skies
Hot air balloons	Sudden loud noise when burner switched on	Kites or paragliders Whooshing and rumbling noises (central heating boiler) Brightly patterned fabric (including clothes)
Onset of darkness in evening	Darkening sky is predictive cue for storm Darkness precedes firework displays	Any sudden period of darkening sky Cloudy skies Large cloud passing overhead
Cars and traffic	Often begins as a sonophobia	Other fast-moving objects

DIAGNOSIS

It is important to rule out any medical disorder that contributes to fear and phobia. For practical purposes, it is useful to divide phobia development into two stages:

Stage 1: *Simple phobias* in which the animal responds phobically to a limited number of stimuli and has developed a method of predicting and coping with the phobic event. The owner may not regard this animal as having a problem.

Stage 2: *Complex phobias* in which the response has generalised and the dog has lost its means of coping because it cannot either predict or avoid exposure.

The vast majority of dogs that are suffering from phobias are in stage 1. They have learned a pattern of cues that enables them to reliably predict a phobic event and a means of escaping from it, or minimising exposure to it. They make very few errors so that, between phobic incidents, they appear to be normal. In most cases, their owners are only concerned with their behaviour at times of phobic exposure.

However, there is a general trend towards worsening phobia, either because of repeated exposure to the phobic stimulus or because of specific kinds of experience that make the phobia worse. Over time, the majority of phobic dogs will develop additional phobia-related problem behaviour that will cause their owners concern.

Phobias become more problematic due to:

- increasing sound sensitivity
- generalisation
- learning and generalisation of predictive cues
- experience of situations in which the dog was unable to predict the phobic event
- experience of situations in which the dog was unable to mount an escape or avoidance reaction.

Increasing sound sensitivity

Some dogs will become so sound sensitive that they will startle at any sudden noise. This may be due to fear-potentiated startle or generalised anxiety, and the dog is at risk of developing a range of new sound fears and phobias.

Generalisation

Any stimulus, simple or compound, has a set of recognisable properties:

- Sound: loudness, duration, and the range of frequencies the noise contains
- Person: height, hair colour or clothing
- Dog: size, markings

Generalisation is the process through which the response to one stimulus is gradually transferred to other stimuli that share some of the same properties. We see this a great deal with noises like thunder, fireworks, guns and crow-scarers because these are all obviously very similar.

However, we need to remember that the hearing and vision of animals is not entirely like our own. The frequency response of their hearing typically extends much higher than ours but misses out on the lowest frequencies that we can hear. Compared to our own vision, that of the dog has generally poorer resolution, cannot discriminate colour as accurately and is designed to pick out movement more vividly. The features of a stimulus that are salient and inclined to become generalised are not the same as those for a person.

Generalisation is most troublesome when the animal begins to react to normal everyday sounds to which it has been regularly exposed without any reaction. Audible examples include car doors slamming, cupboards closing, heavy footfalls on stairs or the sound of logs popping on a fire. It is potentially very serious when dogs gradually generalise responses to these kinds of noises.

Predictive cues

When a frightening or phobic event occurs it is essential for the individual to find ways of avoiding the same experience again. This means learning what other events predict the one of which we are frightened. These predictive cues are learned like any other piece of classical conditioning.

Predictive cues include:

- whistles and whooshes that precede a firework bang
- wind/rain/darkness before a storm
- the smell of burning in the air before fireworks.

Unfortunately these cues are likely to generalise so that the dog begins to become anxious or to mount an escape response when they hear similar noises. Typical examples of generalised predictive cues are noises like the bleep of a mobile phone or the squeak of brakes. Predictive cues and the stimuli to which they generalise are usually very common, which means that the dog experiences a larger number of phobic or fearful events.

Wherever there is evidence of generalisation to normal everyday noises, this is an indication of a severe phobia problem.

Problems arising from a loss of predictability of phobic events

In stage 1 of phobia dogs are able to predict the phobic event, leaving themselves enough time to find an escape route or somewhere to hide.

If the dog is not able to predict a phobic event, its ability to cope is undermined. A typical example is when a dog hears a single gunshot close by when on a walk in an open field. The dog has no certain means of determining whether another such event might occur. The cues are contextual ones, so the dog may seek to avoid returning to that location again. These dogs will refuse to go to certain places on walks and, if the contextual avoidance generalises, they then refuse to go to other similar places too.

If there are one or two salient cues in the environment then these may become associated with the phobic event even if they are completely unrelated; this could be an unusual noise, person, animal or object that just happened to be around at the time.

Problems arising from a loss of ability to mount an escape or avoidance reaction

A proper escape response has several components:

- Localise the origin of the phobic stimulus.
- Move away from it along a decreasing gradient of exposure.
- Seek refuge in a location where exposure is perceptibly lower.

Animals also derive a greater sense of escape if the environment they escape to is different from the one where the phobic event was experienced. Laboratory animals will slowly learn to press a bar to prevent an anticipated shock. They will learn much faster if pressing the bar alters illumination or some other property of the environment so that the context has effectively 'changed'.

There are many reasons why an escape route may fail:

- Animal is shut in a room where it cannot get to its favoured escape place.
- Owners move furniture so that corners where the dog would hide are inaccessible.
- Owners move to a home where the dog has no reliable learned escape route.
- Sounds levels are consistently high throughout the environment the dog is in so that it cannot reduce its exposure.

- Another dog in the household defends the area to which the dog needs to escape.

Dogs will do terrible damage to a home in order to find somewhere to hide or to get out of a room where sound levels are high, so they must always have access to an escape route. Escape routes are chosen on the basis of the reduced sound level in the range that the dog is most sensitive to or frightened of. Small rooms in the middle of the house, or rooms with small windows, are often preferred because sound levels are lower. Some dogs will put their head into a corner of a room where two solid walls meet because the boundary effect created will reduce sound intensity. The corner also gives the impression that the sound level ahead of the animal is lower than that behind. This can cause the dog to try to dig into a corner or at least stand there for long periods.

Rooms have a characteristic resonance related to their dimensions. If the resonance increases the sound pressure level of the noises of which the dog is scared, the dog will want to leave that room when the noise starts. Rooms with solid walls and a lightweight flat roof can function as a 'bass trap', artificially boosting low frequencies. In the UK, this is typical of the construction of kitchens and household extensions, which makes them a dangerous choice of place to confine a pet during phobic events.

The phobic stimulus may itself have properties that make the situation worse. Many sound phobias are of low-frequency sounds like bangs and rumbles. High-frequency sounds are relatively directional and the higher-frequency range is used by people and animals to localise the origin of sounds. Solid objects block or absorb them. Low-frequency sounds pass through most objects and are relatively non-directional.

This means that it can be very hard for the dog to mount a satisfactory escape response if it is in a confined area or an open space when it hears a sequence of loud noises. The sound level is the same regardless of where the animal goes and there is no sense of escape due to change of context. In this situation the animal may become disorientated and confused, entering a state of panic because it is unable to get away. These dogs are at risk of developing anxiety over 'confinement' or restriction of escape response. Such dogs often show signs that are remarkably similar to separation anxiety; they will attempt to break out every time they are confined in a particular room regardless of whether or not there is any noise event. The difference is that they are only concerned with getting out of the room or the house and have no interest in finding the owner.

In contrast to this, there are situations in which the owner has become vital to the dog's coping behaviour. Instead of running to hide somewhere, the dog seeks comfort from the owner. If the owner is not present during a phobic event, the dog may become very distressed because it is unable to find safety. Once again, these dogs may be presented with 'separation anxiety' when, in fact, they are phobic and have no problem of attachment.

MANAGEMENT OF PHOBIA

A handout detailing short-term management of phobic events is included in Appendix 2.

The key aim of management is to prevent phobia problems from worsening and to enhance the animal's ability to cope while treatment is undertaken.

General advice includes:

- Avoid any predictable phobic exposure.
- Do not take a sound-sensitive animal to places where phobic events are possible. For example, fields where there is shooting or a crow-scarer.
- Avoid close proximity to the launch sites of fireworks where dogs will hear the whistles and whooshes that can generate generalisation to other sounds.
- Do not restrict access to escape routes unless there is a very important reason to do so. Try to open up opportunities to escape.
- Do not sympathise with or get angry with a fearful or phobic dog as either will add to the emotional intensity of the situation and will increase the likelihood of future problems.
- Do not force animals to confront their fears by, for example, dragging them to places where they are reluctant to go.

Many dogs have already learned an appropriate escape response that takes them to a place in the home where the sound level is reduced and they feel safer. This is usually in a room with small windows and something sound absorbent that the dog can get inside, underneath or behind (e.g., heavy furnishings such as a bed or sofa).

Some dogs will go to such places and then come out again and search for somewhere else. This is because, although the level of sound in the first escape place is lower, it is not sufficiently reduced to enable the dog to feel any abiding sense of relief. As the phobic event continues, the dog becomes more fearful again and has to find another hiding place.

The dog can be helped by improving the quality and availability of the refuge. To determine what kind of improvements might be made, it is useful to study the precise nature of the escape place that the dog already chooses. Wooden and partition walls do not absorb low frequencies, windows transmit noise and large panes of glass may resonate. Heavy soft furnishings absorb sound. Solid walls not only block the entry of sound from outside but also create a boundary effect that reduces sound intensity close to the wall and this effect is magnified in corners.

Most dogs will therefore pick rooms with solid walls, preferring corners and the cover of heavy furnishings or fitted wardrobes. Bathrooms are also a favourite, possibly because they often have solid walls and are either in the middle of the house or have small windows so that less sound comes in.

For a dog that often hides under a bed in a spare room, modifications might include:

- putting up heavy curtains to block sound and light from outside
- keeping windows closed
- piling extra blankets and old coats onto the bed to help absorb sound
- putting on background music that helps to disguise what is going on outside
- installing a DAP® diffuser close inside the place where the dog hides.

For some dogs, a new refuge might need to be created that is more accessible and provides the basic features.

A wooden box fitted into a corner of such a room might also make a good refuge but the walls need to be thick and damped with layers of foam and blanket. The door should be made from thick overlapping blanket to block out light. This kind of refuge only works if it is placed in a position where the dog feels safe and the noise level inside is genuinely reduced in the frequency bands to which the animal is sensitive. Knocking on the outer shell of the box while your head is inside is a good way to test the shelter. If there is a dull thud it is well damped, if it booms then there is unwanted resonance.

Animals can be clicker-trained to use the refuge as a den or sleeping area. This is a very useful way to reduce the constant aggravation of a dog that wakes and paces or digs during the night. If the animal can be encouraged to sleep in such a box, there is much less likelihood of it waking when it hears noises at night (Box 8.7).

This kind of bolt-hole is only used as a means of *managing* phobia, because the aim is to teach the dog to ignore sounds and not to constantly seek the refuge. However, if the dog is elderly or suffering from cognitive problems, it may not be possible to completely desensitise and counter-condition, so a refuge may be an appropriate permanent means of management.

Box 8.7   Providing a bolt-hole for phobic dogs

Where possible choose a place to which the dog has already shown a tendency to go. The dog must be given access to this place at all times and its choice to go there never impeded. Improvements may be made to make the bolt-hole better:

- A DAP® diffuser installed close to the dog's resting place in the bolt-hole.
- Piles of blankets to hide under.
- Windows shut, heavy curtains drawn to block out light.
- Pieces of owner's clothing carrying their body odour placed in the bolt-hole.
- Background music playing to block out external noise.

An owner handout for coping with phobic events such as thunderstorms and fireworks is included in Appendix 2.

Counselling owners to respond appropriately to the animal's behaviour

Many owners either try to soothe the animal or get cross with it when it becomes fearful. Both responses are wrong because they result in increasing the intensity of the emotional experience or rewarding inappropriate behaviour. It is best to encourage owners to ignore the animal's fearful behaviour but then reward it when it shows signs of recovery. A good refuge will help with this because many owners are forced to intervene when the animal digs or damages furniture in an attempt to find relief from fear.

TREATMENT: DESENSITISATION AND COUNTERCONDITIONING

These treatments are the only ones proven to produce long-term benefits. Desensitisation must be very thorough before counterconditioning can begin and it may take several months in severe cases. If using recordings or other simulated stimuli it is important to make them as realistic as possible (Table 8.4).

Some dogs show an intense reaction even to very low-level stimuli, such as sounds played on a tape deck. For these animals the realism of the stimulus should be decreased. In the example of sound recordings of thunder or fireworks replayed through a home stereo, this might mean reducing the level of bass frequencies, switching one speaker off or muffling a speaker with a cushion. If the dog's sound sensitivity is extreme it may become a barrier to behavioural therapy and may benefit from drug therapy.

Instrumental learning

Clicker-training can be used to teach specific behaviours that can then be used in counterconditioning or anxiety reduction. For example, the dog may be trained to adopt a calm and relaxed posture on cue.

This calm state can then be produced on cue and used as part of counterconditioning. It can also be used to collapse states of anxiety by giving the animal a behavioural outlet that reduces the arousal and anxiety.

Reducing escape responses

Some dogs attempt to flee, even from very small noises, when they are not actually experiencing any fear or anxiety. This kind of avoidance response is, in a sense, like superstitious behaviour in people. The dog cannot habituate to the stimulus because it never stays around long enough to experience it.

For dogs that show this kind of fearless avoidance behaviour, it can be useful to limit their ability to escape during training. A long line may be used to slow down the escape, and then the dog is rewarded in some way for coming back

Table 8.4　Common errors when using sound recordings to treat noise phobia

Behavioural treatment has no effect: sounds are unrealistic	
Cause	Effect
Inadequate bass frequencies	Sound is not representative of the real phobic event
Speakers placed too close to each other, or recording played back in mono	Sounds are localised, which is different from real fireworks/thunder
Speakers incorrectly positioned away from window areas	Dog is aware that real external sounds normally come from window

Desensitisation or counter-conditioning makes problem worse	
Cause	Effect
Sounds on recording are widely spaced and vary greatly in volume	This is a sensitising pattern to which habituation will be impossible
Playback levels are not set correctly for each session (set too loud)	Dog shows signs of fear during training and is therefore being flooded rather than desensitised
Desensitisation or counterconditioning carried out in a closed room	Dog cannot escape if sound volume too high
Speakers placed too close to the refuge dog uses to get away from the sound (e.g., in corner)	Dog cannot hide if it becomes fearful

again before it has completed its escape. Quite quickly the dog will learn that, for this minimal sound level, an escape is not necessary, and conventional desensitisation can begin. This method must not be used if the dog is actually fearful.

It is dangerous to confine dogs during desensitisation and counterconditioning because, if levels are set wrongly, the dog may become distressed if it cannot escape.

TREATMENT: DRUG THERAPY

Drug therapy can be used as a short-term strategy to enable a patient to deal with an inevitable event or circumstance, or as a long-term treatment which assists in the application of behavioural modification techniques over a period of weeks and months. The aim in these two scenarios is very different and the drug classes that are appropriate will also differ (Box 8.8).

Short-term drug therapy

The traditional pharmacological approach to treating fears and phobias in dogs has been the administration of sedatives and tranquillisers. These drugs make the animal unreactive and remove the symptoms of fear that owners find so distressing. However, such an approach has serious implications in terms of animal welfare.

Many of these drugs sensitise dogs to auditory stimulation and block motor activity, while leaving sensory perception unaffected. The ethical considerations of such an approach cannot be ignored and the fact that their use may lead to an exacerbation of the sound phobia limits their usefulness in these cases (Table 8.5).

Neuroleptics

The most commonly used drugs from this class are the phenothiazines, of which the most frequently prescribed example is acepromazine (ACP). The drug exerts its therapeutic actions by blocking dopaminergic receptors in the brain and has been effective in the suppression of symptoms of sound phobias.

However, the action of these drugs is not selective and their therapeutic effects cannot be achieved in isolation from CNS depression. Sedation may be desirable in short-term use but many owners object to having a dog that is unable to move properly and requires constant supervision to prevent injury.

The major disadvantage of ACP is that it blocks motor responses while leaving sensory perception unaffected. Sound-sensitivity is actually increased by this drug. The dog is therefore fully aware of the fear-inducing stimulus but limited in its ability to react. This can result in worsening of the phobia over time and treatment with ACP for firework phobias can be associated with increasing severity of the phobic reaction from year to year.

The major behavioural contraindication is aggression, since ACP can lead to behavioural disinhibition. This is very dangerous where anxiety is only just suppressing aggressive behaviour.

There are medical contraindications for ACP, including epilepsy, brachycephalic breeds, history of respiratory depression, hepatic dysfunction, renal compromise and hypotension. Prior to use of ACP, all patients should receive a biochemistry screen for renal and hepatic function. Use of ACP in geriatrics (over 8 years of age) carries particular medical concerns in terms of hypotensive effects.

Beta-blockers

These drugs block beta-adrenergic receptors which are responsible for many of the autonomic symptoms of fear and anxiety, such as rapid heart rate and trembling. The most frequently prescribed example is propranolol, but other examples used in veterinary behavioural medicine include atenolol and pindolol.

These drugs reduce anxiety and decrease the somatic symptoms associated with the anxious state. Primarily, they are used as sole drug therapy for situational anxieties but have been advocated in some literature for treatment of sound phobias. They are rarely effective in severe phobic reactions. They may be useful in predictable situations of sound phobia when the drug can be given 30 minutes to 1 hour before effect is needed. The effect may be more powerful if the drug is given in combination with pheromonotherapy (DAP®).

Table 8.5   Drugs for short-term phobia therapy

Drug	Recommended dose for noise phobic dogs – these drugs should be administered as necessary (*prn*)	Maximum daily dosing routine if not used prn	Delay in onset of action
Acepromazine (POM*)	0.1–2.0 mg/kg prn	1–4 times daily	20–30 minutes (given PO)
Propranolol (POM)	0.1–3.0 mg/kg prn	tid	30 minutes
Diazepam (POM)	0.55–2.22 mg/kg prn	2–3 times daily	30 minutes to 2 hours
Chlorpheniramine maleate (P)	220 µg/kg prn	tid	30–40 minutes
Trimeprazine tartrate (POM)	500 µg–2 mg/kg prn	tid	30–40 minutes

*POM, prescription-only medicine

The action of beta-blockers may be more complex than was once thought. The decreased vigilance and reactivity associated with beta-blocker administration may be related to decreasing the proprioceptive afferent impulses to the reticular activating system, which is associated with maintaining a state of alertness.

In addition, beta-blockers that cross the blood–brain barrier can block serotonin receptors and thereby result in increased serotonin release; this can lead to some mood-stabilising effects.

Benzodiazepines

Benzodiazepines are GABA-agonists and hence increase the activity of this inhibitory part of the neurotransmitter system. The most frequently prescribed example is diazepam but other examples in UK veterinary behavioural medicine include alprazolam and clorazepate.

Diazepam has a short half-life of a few hours which limits its usefulness as a long-term drug in behavioural medicine but, in acute-phase management of sound phobias, it can be very effective.

The amnesic effects of benzodiazepines, which limit their use in long-term phobia management (owing to the animal's inability to benefit from behavioural therapy), make these drugs ideal as short-term therapy. Diazepam may be given at very low doses either before, during or after a phobic event because it causes retrograde amnesia. This can be very useful for blocking memories of individual events that occur during therapy and that might initiate a relapse.

It is important to consider the potential for human abuse and to be wary if prescriptions are being refilled too frequently, if the owner reports the use of increased doses to gain the same effect or if the owner repeatedly claims to have mislaid or lost medication.

There are reports that suggest diazepam is contraindicated in greyhounds and related breeds on the grounds of hyperaesthesia, ataxia and CNS excitation. Indeed, the potential for paradoxical excitement or hyperactivity in any dog in reaction to diazepam administration means that the first dose should always be administered as a test of response at a quiet time, with the owner present. Should agitation be seen, then diazepam must not be re-administered and alprazolam should be tried instead.

If used for long periods, benzodiazepines do carry a risk of withdrawal symptoms on cessation of the medication and so gradual decrease in dosage is recommended. Relapse is also a potential issue when using benzodiazepines; therefore, they should only ever be considered as a short-term approach to phobia cases.

Antihistamines

The most commonly used examples in treatment of sound phobia are chlorpheniramine maleate (chlorphenamine maleate) and trimeprazine tartrate (alimemazine tartrate).

Most phobic reactions are too severe for antihistamine use to be beneficial but in cases of mild reactions where some sedation is demanded, they can be useful.

There are relatively few contraindications, but antihistamines have been reported to be associated with a lowering of seizure thresholds (Table 8.6).

Long–term drug therapy as an adjunct to behavioural therapy

In cases where the phobia is seasonal, it is beneficial to start behavioural therapy at a time when the symptoms are less likely to be seen but this is not always convenient or feasible. Long-term drug therapy in phobia cases is used for several reasons:

- To improve response to behavioural therapy.
- To alleviate debilitating effects of phobia, such as contextual avoidance and generalised anxiety.
- To reduce further generalisation and acquisition of new phobias.
- To improve the welfare of the animal.

The delay in onset of action is considerably increased in these drugs in comparison to the short-term therapies and, in some cases, concomitant short-term therapy may be considered (Table 8.7).

Tricyclic antidepressants (TCAs)

The most commonly used of the TCAs in veterinary behaviour medicine is clomipramine which is available as a licensed product called Clomicalm®. The licence in this case relates to the specific condition of separation anxiety rather than sound phobia.

The use of the TCAs in the treatment of behavioural disorders is widespread but their use in phobia treatment is largely limited to the mild to moderate cases in which anxiety is a major factor. Individual TCAs vary widely in their specificity for blocking the re-uptake of norepinephrine versus serotonin and these differences can be taken into account when selecting medication.

Although chemically a member of the family of tricyclic antidepressants, clomipramine is technically classed as an SRI since it is moderately selective for the blocking of serotonin re-uptake. Its active metabolite, desmethyl-clomipramine, is responsible for the blocking of norepinephrine re-uptake and, overall, the drug has a blocking ratio that is 5:1 in favour of serotonin. All TCA drugs have a range of anticholinergic and antihistaminic effects that are largely responsible for adverse effects. More studies are needed on the potential role of TCAs in phobia management.

Selective serotonin re-uptake inhibitors (SSRIs)

These drugs are selective in their inhibition of serotonin re-uptake and they have been advocated for the treatment of

Table 8.6 Short-term drug therapy options in cases of canine sound phobia

	Contraindications – medical	Potential behavioural side-effects (not always seen)	Main expected behavioural effects	Indications – severity of phobia	Possible drug interactions
Acepromazine	Hypotension/respiratory, renal, hepatic or cardio-vascular compromise/ epilepsy/caution in brachycephalic breeds	Disinhibition of aggressive behaviour/ sensitisation to sound stimuli/ exacerbation of phobia/sound startle effect can lead to unpredictable behaviour	Sedation and removal of motor symptoms of fear	Not recommended for sound phobias	Potentiate the effects of some analgesics/ selegiline
Propranolol	Hypotension/cardio-vascular compromise/ renal or hepatic insufficiency/broncho-spastic disease/thyroid dysfunction		Removal of the somatic signs of fear/ attenuation of the fight/flight response	Moderate	Benzodiazepines/ antiarrhythmics/ sympathomimetic drugs/muscle relaxants
Diazepam	Hepatic compromise	Disinhibition of aggressive behaviour/ effect on short term memory/sedation limiting application of behavioural therapy	Sedation, blocking of short-term memory of the event and decreased conditioning of a negative association	Severe	Certain antibiotics/ anticholinergics/ neuroleptics/ antihistamines/ antidepressants
Chlorpheniramine maleate	Urinary retention/ glaucoma	Sedation limiting usefulness of behaviour modification	Sedation	Mild	CNS depressant drugs
Trimeprazine tartrate	As above	As above	As above	As above	As above

phobias with a panic component. They potentiate the effects of serotonin through increased serotonin output and through altering post-synaptic receptor sensitivity.

The most commonly used SSRIs in veterinary behavioural medicine are fluoxetine, fluvoxamine and sertraline, which have blocking ratios ranging from 15 to 150:1 in favour of serotonin. Those with increased selectivity (fluvoxamine and sertraline) have very little anticholinergic or antihistaminic effect and are therefore better tolerated. Specifically, the reduction in seizure threshold and effect on urinary retention is minimal in these drugs.

The drug sertraline has been used successfully in the treatment of sound phobias in dogs but it is not licensed for use in any non-human species.

The risks of behavioural disinhibition should be considered and TCAs, SRIs and SSRIs should not be used in cases where there is any history of canine aggression.

Monoamine oxidase inhibitors (MAOIs)

The licensed MAOI in veterinary practice is selegiline hydrochloride (Selgian®). This drug is licensed for use in behavioural disorders of an emotional origin, including fears.

Monoamine oxidase (MAO) is the enzyme mainly responsible for metabolising the monoamine neurotransmitters (norepinephrine, serotonin and dopamine). Two forms exist: MAOa and MAOb. MAOa is responsible for the breakdown of serotonin and norepinephrine; MAOb breaks down dopamine.

Selegiline, being a selective inhibitor of MAOb, increases the availability of dopamine for synaptic transmission. It is not totally selective and there is some inhibition of MAOa as well. For this reason, selegiline and TCA/SRI/SSRI drugs **must not be given concurrently**, or even within 2 weeks of each other. Apart from these neurochemical effects, selegiline also has antioxidant and neuroprotective effects that make it useful for the treatment of cognitive dementia.

Secondary adaptive mechanisms are believed to be important in the action of MAOIs and to result in a reduction in the number of beta-adrenoreceptors, alpha-1 and alpha-2 adrenoreceptors and 5-HT1 and 5-HT2 receptors.

Clinical experience suggests that selegiline is most effective in the treatment of sound phobias associated with behavioural inhibition and symptoms of social withdrawal.

In multi-dog households, selegiline has been associated with an increased assertiveness within the hierarchy and the literature suggests that selegiline should not be used in

Table 8.7 Drugs for long-term phobia therapy

Drug	Recommended dose	Delay in onset of action
Clomipramine (POM)	1–2 mg/kg b.i.d	4 weeks
Sertraline (POM)	1–2 mg/kg b.i.d	4 weeks
Selegiline (POM)	See data sheet	4–6 weeks

households where there has been pre-existing reporting of status-related behavioural issues between the dog and the owner.

SEPARATION RELATED PROBLEMS

A number of other problems are often confused with 'separation anxiety', some of which are covered in the chapter 'miscellaneous problems':

- Phobia problems (the dog has a fear of being trapped because it cannot access an escape route).
- Opportunistic destruction (bored, often young, dogs that experiment with stealing and damaging things as a pastime).
- Anxiety about the owner's return (dogs that have been conditioned to anticipate punishment by angry returning owners).
- Loneliness.
- Poor habituation to solitude.

All drug charts are intended only as a guide. Before deciding on medication, it is recommended that veterinary surgeons consult a comprehensive text on behavioural medicine for information on mode of action, limitations and contraindications. There are a range of doses cited in the literature and, where possible, the lowest effective dose should be used. Many of these drugs are unlicensed for veterinary use and will be used in an extra-label fashion. Owners must be made aware of this fact and informed-consent forms should be used. Veterinary surgeons should keep up-to-date with developments in respect of extra-label drug use and use medication and dose rates supported by current published literature.

Table 8.8 Long-term drug therapy options in cases of canine sound phobia

Drug	Contraindications – medical	Potential behavioural side-effects (not always seen)	Main expected behavioural effects	Indications – severity of phobia	Possible drug interactions
Clomipramine	Cardiovascular disease/ renal or hepatic compromise/glaucoma/ urinary retention/ pregnant and lactating animals	Disinhibition of aggressive behaviour/ mild level of sedation	Decrease in generalised anxiety	Moderate	MAOIs or antiepileptics/ antiarrhythmic drugs
Sertraline	Cardiovascular disease/ renal or hepatic compromise/ pregnant and lactating animals	Disinhibition of aggressive behaviour	Decrease in symptoms of panic	Severe – associated with panic	MAOIs or antiepileptics/ antiarrhythmic drugs/propranolol/ benzodiazepines
Selegiline	Cardiovascular disease/ renal or hepatic compromise/pregnant and lactating animals/ diabetes mellitus	Exacerbation of pre-existing status issues with owners/ increased assertiveness within canine hierarchy in household	Increased exploratory behaviour/ enhanced cognitive ability	Severe – associated with behavioural inhibition	TCAs/SSRIs/ antiepileptics/ phenothiazines/ alpha 2 antagonists

Noise phobia problems are quite common in the general canine population and dogs can easily develop a fear of being trapped if they experience a series of loud noises from which they cannot escape. Typically, this happens with dogs that are familiar with using a particular place at home and this 'escape route' either becomes inaccessible or the owners move to a home where there is no comparable hiding place. Dogs deprived of their natural hiding place within the home may try to get out of the house in order to 'get away from the noise'. The simple change of context from indoors to outdoors is sometimes enough for the fear to subside, but many of these dogs continue to panic. The dog will only calm down after the noises have gone away, whereupon they may revert to normal and be found happily wandering local parks looking for something to do. There are some cases where the dog comes to view the owner as its 'hiding place' so that, if the owner is away, the animal panics when it hears a loud noise. This is engendered by owners trying to soothe and comfort noise-phobic dogs when the phobia-inducing stimulus occurs.

Opportunistic destruction is very common and such dogs will raid bins and cupboards searching for food and things to destroy. These dogs often benefit simply from having some activities to do while the owner is away.

In some cases, opportunistic destruction is converted into anxiety about the owner's return. The dog is repeatedly punished by the returning owner for some misdemeanour but has no idea what the punishment is for. Dogs are not able to make associations between events that are separated by even a few minutes so they are unable to connect past misbehaviour with current events. It also has to be remembered that the owner's return is of great significance to the dog and it only takes a few occasions on which the owner has been verbally or physically threatening for the dog to come to dread the stress surrounding the owner's return. This creates anxiety and an anxious dog will often resort to self-appeasing oral displacement behaviour, such as chewing, because this makes them feel comfortable and more relaxed. The increasing destruction makes the problem worse because the dog experiences further punishment. These dogs will often attempt to appease the returning owner through acts of vivid submission such as rolling over or hunching and averting their gaze. Unfortunately, the owner usually misinterprets this as 'guilt' or an 'apology' but, being furious, then continues to corner and punish the dog.

Loneliness is a common problem amongst dogs that belong to working owners. Dogs are highly social animals and much of their individual confidence is determined by belonging to a stable social group. These dogs will often try to reunite themselves with their group by communicative patterns of barking and howling which are aimed at bringing the owner back. Many dogs simply do not habituate to being alone because they were not left by the bitch during rearing and the owners went out too infrequently for the young dog to adapt to solitude.

All of the above problems can be complicated by anxiety that is common in dogs that are not fully used to being left alone or who have had some kind of disruptive life event (like the death of an owner or re-homing), so dogs from rescue kennels are at increased risk of showing separation problems of one kind or another.

There is no reliable data on the exact proportion of animals that have each of these problems, as opposed to separation anxiety; true separation anxiety is probably relatively uncommon.

Separation anxiety is a very specific condition characterised by over-attachment, usually (but not always) to an individual person. The absence of that person causes the dog great distress even if the separation is brief. Anxiety can be defined as the 'apprehensive anticipation of threat or harm' and, since dogs with separation anxiety are concerned with the absence of the person to whom they are attached, we would expect signs of anxiety as that person prepares to depart.

DIAGNOSIS

Dogs with separation anxiety will tremble, pace, pant and show other signs of rising anxiety as the person gets closer to departing, which is easily seen if a number of video tapes are made of departures. Signs of anxiety persist throughout the time the owner is away. Barking and destructiveness may occur in bouts, with the dog stopping when it becomes fatigued but remaining anxious. Some anxiety will be seen even if the owner picks up a bunch of keys or puts on a coat when they are not going out. The dog will often anxiously shadow the individual they are over-attached to around the times when that person is likely to

---

Box 8.9   Typical signs of separation anxiety

- Anxiously following the person continuously (not anticipating food, attention, etc.), especially around the time they are about to leave.
- Tendency to maintain close physical contact with the person, even in otherwise non-stressful situations.
- Distress whenever the person is absent, even when other people are present.
- Over-enthusiastic greeting when the person returns, even after momentary absence.
- Destruction focused on escape (doors, windows, etc.)
- Hypersalivation, urination and defecation when left for longer periods.
- Distress vocalisation (screaming, incessant barking).
- Signs of rising anxiety with departure cues.
- Continuous distress while alone (dog does not settle).
- Repetitive unnecessary seeking of reassurance while the person is present.

go out. This often annoys owners, who respond punitively and therefore aggravate the situation.

Immediately after the owner has left, there is an initial 'panic' when the dog realises that the person has genuinely gone. There is often distress vocalisation, uncontrolled elimination and an attempt to escape from the house and follow the owner. If the dog does escape, it will remain distressed until it is reunited with the owner. Distress increases or remains the same throughout the period the owner is away.

Distress vocalisation must be differentiated from other forms of barking. Many dogs will bark or howl for short periods of a few seconds and then listen for a reply. They may try a variety of different barks and noises at a range of sound levels. These are deliberate and well-orchestrated attempts to communicate with the missing owner and bring them back and usually the dog will give up after a few minutes. Distress vocalisation is often much more extreme and disorganised, with the dog usually barking and screaming hysterically for long periods without a break.

Many dogs are anxious when left alone and this may increase their frequency of elimination. Where anxiety is mild, the dog will choose to use a specific latrine site, usually close to an exit point. In cases where anxiety is intense, the dog may urinate and defecate as it wanders around the house. The dog will spread this all over the floor as it continues to pace and there may be large amounts of drool mixed with the rest of the mess. This is more typical of genuine separation anxiety.

When the owner returns, the dog with separation anxiety is always overjoyed, even if the owner is angry and there is a history of the owner punishing the dog for its 'crimes' when they return. Dogs with other problems are usually either moderately friendly or submissive.

When the owner is present, dogs with separation anxiety will often maintain close physical contact, even in situations that are otherwise non-stressful. This behaviour is seen at the clinic and in the owner's home (Fig. 8.4)

Owners of destructive dogs may be tempted to confine them to an indoor crate, but this often merely contains the dog and localises destruction. Owners may not be aware that the dog is still extremely distressed and do not notice the damage the dog is doing in order to escape (Fig. 8.5).

When diagnosing the nature of a separation problem, it is best to think about the purpose of the dog's behaviour (self-appeasement, escape to get to someone or away from something, etc.) and the pattern it follows. This should usually be backed up by video evidence, especially where more than one dog shares the household. Owners frequently assume that the submissive or 'apologetic' dog is the one responsible for damage, but this is often not the case!

TREATMENT

Separation problems that do not involve anxiety or fear (boredom, opportunistic destructiveness, and loneliness) are dealt with elsewhere in the text.

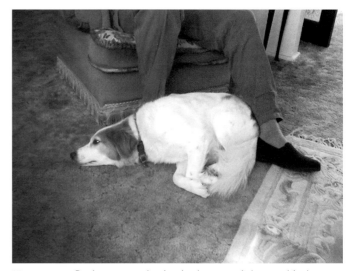

Figure 8.4   During a consultation in the owner's home, this dog continued to stay very close to the owner, even though this involved adopting a very uncomfortable position.

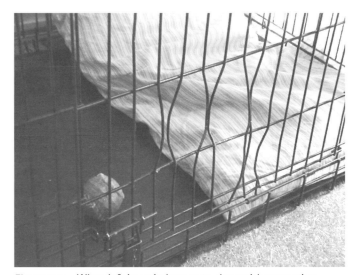

Figure 8.5   When left in an indoor crate, dogs with separation anxiety will make desperate attempts to escape, potentially damaging themselves.

Relieving anxiety about owner return

This problem is based upon a fundamental misunderstanding on the part of the owner who believes the dog understands that it has done something wrong, just because it is submissive when the person comes home. In fact, the dog is merely responding to the stimuli around it, including the person's posture, body language and tone of voice. Submission is a natural means of showing deference in order to limit the threat posed by another individual in a social group.

This misunderstanding of the effect of delayed punishment must be corrected or it will lead to other very serious problems. Likewise, owners must learn not to punish dogs when they are showing submissive behaviour because this may lead to much more serious displays of aggression

---

Box 8.10   Immediate action: anxiety about owner return

- Stop owner punishing the dog (physical and verbal) when they return home.
- Ignore dog for the first 10 minutes after coming home, regardless of whether it has done damage or not.
- Put the dog outside or in another room before cleaning up damage or mess.

Box 8.11   Treatment: dogs with anxiety about owner return

- Stop *all* forms of delayed punishment (punishment that occurs long after the event has passed).
- Stop *all* physical punishment (smacking, shaking, etc.)
- Install Dog Appeasing Pheromone (DAP®) diffuser close to dog's daytime resting-place.
- As the owner leaves the house, they should leave behind a number of things for the dog to destroy. These should be cleared up upon return.
- Perform multiple short departures every day (5 to 10 times as many as genuine departures). Duration should be randomly 0–10 minutes.
- The owner should ignore the dog for 10 minutes after coming home, regardless of what it has or has not done. The owner should try to act happy and relaxed but disinterested in the dog.

(Box 8.10). In these cases the dog has made an association between the absence and impending return of the owner and some kind of aversive experience related to punishment. For sensitive dogs this may be something as mild as sustained eye contact and scolding. The dog is apprehensive of the owner's response upon reunification and may be anxious whilst waiting for this event.

For these dogs there are several problems that need to be addressed:

- The dog's need for (destructive) self-appeasement behaviour.
- Conditioned emotional responses concerned with the owner's behaviour (raised voices, physical gestures of threat, standing or leaning over the dog).
- Conditioned emotional responses to the sound of the owner's return (footsteps, doors opening, etc.)
- Anxiety when the owner is out of the house.

All these elements must be addressed because these dogs are at significant risk of developing other fear and aggression-related problems, especially if they are not yet fully mature.

These dogs should be given a range of things to do that allow them to safely carry out destructive self-appeasement behaviour while the owner is out. This gives the dog an outlet for its emotional behaviour and reduces the

risk of the owner coming home to find personal property damaged.

The dog's needs are likely to be fairly specific and individual:

- Objects that retain the owner's body smell (shoes, clothes, objects they handled before going out).
- Things that maybe chewed or torn apart: texture and type of material is very important.

To be a successful diversion for the dog's destructive tendencies, the objects that the dog is given to destroy must satisfy the preferences that the dog has already shown.

For these dogs the main concern is not with being alone; it is with the owner's reaction when they return. So the primary method of treatment is to make repeated neutral presentations of departures and returns so that the emotional response to these events is extinguished. The emotional atmosphere around these events must become consistent and neutral from the dog's perspective (Box 8.11).

Processes of extinction take time and treatment may take several weeks to produce an effect. Most of these dogs are young and it should be anticipated that they may engage in opportunistic destruction until they have matured enough to lose interest in this habit. The fear and anxiety components of the problem may be reduced by the use of DAP®, which should be used alongside behavioural therapy until the situation is acceptable (1–2 months minimum).

Prognosis

These cases usually improve relatively quickly as long as the owner does not use punishment or draw the dog's attention to misdemeanours; and there is sufficient opportunity for the dog to carry out self-appeasement chewing without damaging the owner's property.

Relieving separation anxiety

Separation anxiety is a problem of hyper-attachment and this must be the main focus of treatment (Box 8.12). The reasons for excessive attachment must be dealt with, as must the range of conditioned associations that control the anxiety from which the dog suffers. Separation anxiety is a

---

Box 8.12   Immediate action: separation anxiety

- Stop owner punishing the dog (physical and verbal) when they return home.
- Ignore the dog for 10 minutes before departure and after return to the home.
- Make sure that the house is properly secure when the dog is left because it may escape and get injured.
- Consider using a dog-minder temporarily to help reduce stress.

---

condition in which the dog experiences enormous contrasts of emotion; when the person is present the dog has an ability to control its anxiety by maintaining proximity with the person, monitoring their activity and constant seeking of reassurance. The person is, in one sense, the medium through which the dog interacts with the environment. When the person is not present, the dog is very distressed and has no other strategy for coping so that, when the person returns, there is an immense sense of relief which only serves to clarify the distinction between their presence and absence. This level of dependence can also be flattering for the person, who may have their own reasons for wanting to feel 'needed' by the pet. For therapy to be effective all these issues must be addressed.

There are a number of elements to the problem of separation anxiety:

- Specific over-attachment to one person upon whom the dog places an excessive value and from whom the dog requires constant reassurance.
- Inability to derive equivalent reassurance from environmental stimuli that a 'normal' dog would find reassuring.
- An extensive collection of conditioned associations that the dog uses to predict the person's departure and which evoke feelings of anxiety.

The general principles of treatment are as follows (see Box 8.13 for a summary):

Make the subject of the hyper-attachment less valuable. Redistribute care giving (feeding, walks, grooming, play, etc.) to other members of the household so that the perceived value of the subject of hyper-attachment is reduced.

Reduce the contrast between times when that person is present and absent. Avoid all interaction around times of departure or return to the house. Reduce availability of attention and reassurance when the person is present; the owner must not respond to attention-seeking behaviour.

Teach signals that enable the animal to understand human interaction and terminate attention-seeking before anxiety or frustration set in. The dog must be taught a simple signal that a person may use to indicate that its attention-seeking is going to fail, so that frustration does not increase.

Prevent the dog from monitoring the person's activity. The person to whom the dog is hyper-attached should avoid allowing the dog to monitor their activity by maintaining physical contact (sitting on feet or in contact with the person's legs). Stop punishment of the dog when it shadows the owner. Delay the dog from following the person from room to room. Doors should be closed momentarily as the person goes from room to room.

Desensitise and countercondition responses to stimuli and events that are associated with the departure of the person or their absence. Many times each day

---

Box 8.13   Treatment: separation anxiety

- If other fear or anxiety problems are present, these may be a cause of excessive dependence on a person so they must be treated (fear of people, sonophobia, etc.).
- Identify the person who is the subject of the hyper-attachment.
- Redistribute care routine among other members of household.
- Increase the dog's activity, exercise and interaction with other dogs and people (where appropriate).
- Identify all departure cues to which the dog responds; desensitise and countercondition these.
- Reduce dog's ability to monitor the person's movements; encourage it to sleep away from the person and not in bodily contact with them.
- Ignore all attention-seeking.
- Measure the time period between departure and the dog's becoming distressed.
- Begin to practise multiple (10+ per day) unannounced departures that are shorter than this duration. The duration of each departure should be random and may be increased as the dog appears to cope.
- The daily routine should be consistent every day, even at weekends. Owners should not try to 'make it up' to their dogs by being around all weekend because they are less available during the week.
- Ignore the dog for at least 10 minutes after returning home, until it has fully calmed down.
- Leave food, chews and other distractions for the dog while the owner is not around so that, if it does calm down, it may find relaxation in these.
- Make the environment for the dog as appeasing as possible: use DAP®, leave items of the owner's unwashed clothes, isolate external noise, give the dog a comfortable den area, leave classical music or chat radio programmes playing at all times.
- Consider the use of anxiolytic medication.

---

pick up keys, put on a coat or shoes and then stay around the house. Once the dog is not reacting to these cues, they can be associated with other calming activities such as feeding.

Create an appeasing environment that satisfies some of the dog's needs to maintain emotional homeostasis. Provide the dog with a sense of continuity between the times the owner is present and away; for example, leave a quiet radio playing a talk or classical music programme (not loud pop music), leave a piece of the owner's clothing in the dog's bed, provide familiar objects as comforters, organise continuous replay of recordings of family conversation to give impression that people are at home.

It may be easiest to train the dog to be left in a location in which it is used to resting (e.g., the owner's bedroom).

Acclimatise the dog to brief, but randomly lengthening, periods of isolation. Measure the time period that elapses before the dog becomes severely distressed (maybe a few seconds). Practise going out many times each day for periods that are below this time limit. There should be no warning of each departure.

A calm and non-aroused posture may be clicker-trained so that it can be reproduced on cue. There should be practice sessions several times each day where the dog is cued to take up this posture and then continuously clicker-rewarded for staying calm while the subject of hyper-attachment walks around and in and out of the room, momentarily. The person doing the training must stay calm and relaxed, paying special attention to avoid giving additional cues that encourage anticipation of reward. Gradually the person spends more and more time out of the room.

Pheromonotherapy

DAP® is a useful and safe adjunct to therapy. It provides relief from anxiety and should be installed at resting 'dog height' in an accessible location next to where the dog is to be left. It must not be placed high up or behind a cupboard because the dog may climb or destroy furniture to get to it (Box 8.14).

Drug therapy

SRI and SSRI drugs produce a suppression of isolation distress vocalisations in a number of animal models of anxiety. There have also been successful trials of the SRI clomipramine for the treatment of separation anxiety in the dog. Psychoactive drug therapy may be combined with pheromonotherapy for increased efficacy.

Clomipramine is the only licensed drug in this class, but fluoxetine and other SSRI drugs can provide similar benefits. Any individual SRI or SSRI drug will have a response rate of around 70%, so it is not uncommon to have to switch from one drug to another if there is no response after 8–12 weeks.

Clomipramine is only moderately selective for serotonin re-uptake inhibition, and produces numerous anticholinergic side-effects that may make it unsuitable for certain cases and a thorough medical work-up should be carried out before prescribing it.

These drugs should never be used without a behavioural modification plan because their efficacy is limited. During treatment, owners should notice significant changes in general anxiety and signs of hyper-attachment. Drug therapy may be withdrawn when signs of hyper-attachment are reduced but it must be withdrawn slowly to avoid relapse and dysphoric side-effects.

> **Box 8.14　Common errors when using Dog Appeasing Pheromone (DAP®) for separation cases**
>
> - Diffuser is switched off overnight or when dog is not at home: DAP® takes time to build up in the atmosphere and this will limit the pheromone's effectiveness. Diffuser must remain on at all times.
> - Diffuser is plugged in too high up (kitchen wall sockets are at waist height): The dog must be able to lie down comfortably or sleep close to the diffuser or it may not have an effect.
> - Diffuser is hidden behind furniture or is situated in a room to which dog cannot gain access at all times; this may increase the dog's sense of isolation and the dog may destructively attempt to get to the diffuser.
> - Diffuser is sited too close to open patio doors or windows so DAP® levels in the home never build up to effective levels.
> - Number of diffusers is below the manufacturer's recommendations for the area treated: owners may need to install several diffusers in different parts of the home to provide good coverage.

Prognosis

The prognosis for dogs with separation anxiety is variable. Treatment depends upon an enormous amount of work from the owner and a lot of support is needed to get them through. Some owners may be overwhelmed by the amount of work needed. It is very hard to use purely behavioural therapy for dogs that are very distressed and spend a lot of time alone. Many dogs, therefore, have to be given drug therapy which creates compliance issues for some owners.

In successful cases the treatment period is typically 4–6 months.

ADVICE SHEETS THAT MAY BE RELEVANT TO THIS CHAPTER

In Appendix 2:

1. Using a houseline
3. Reward and punishment
6. Muzzle training
9. The 'come away' command
11. Attention-seeking and the 'no' signal
12. Click-touch training
13. Preparations for phobic events
16. Environmental enrichment for dogs
17. Using food rewards for training
18. Food for work
19. Introducing the clicker

Chapter **9**

Canine compulsive disorders

INTRODUCTION

'Stereotypical' is an adjective used to describe repetitive, ritualised, out-of-context locomotor behaviour. In a scientific and welfare context, *stereotypy* was the term applied to the continuous rhythmic pacing, circling, running and shuffling behaviour seen in some zoos, production and laboratory animals. Use of the word 'compulsive' was introduced when a range of other behaviours were recognised to be broadly related to the stereotypies but could not be captured within that definition because they were non-locomotor. These included repetitive vocalisation, licking, self-mutilation and static, continuous behaviours such as staring into space or holding an object or part of the body in the mouth. Now the term compulsive is often used as a general term for all behaviours of this class.

Not all animals that carry out apparently stereotypical or compulsive behaviour are suffering from a compulsive disorder. There are many behavioural, neurological and medical conditions that can cause these types of behaviour and these must be completely ruled out before a case is categorised as a compulsive disorder.

Compulsive disorder is typical of what has become accepted in human psychiatry and veterinary behavioural medicine as a 'syndromic diagnosis'. Syndromes are clusters or groupings of medical or behavioural signs that are seen to consistently occur together. In human medicine and psychiatry, syndromes are the product of the analysis of the common factors of thousands of cases but they still have no defined aetiology. Investigation into the aetiology underlying syndromes will inevitably lead conditions such as compulsive disorder to be broken down into one or more aetiological diagnoses.

Something is known of the aetiology of obsessive–compulsive disorder (OCD) in man, but the evidence is mostly circumstantial. For example, the current working hypothesis is that there is some underlying 'dysregulation' of the serotonergic system. This is supported by the positive response of human patients to treatment with serotonin re-uptake inhibitors (SSRIs), the presence of indicators of abnormal serotonin turnover in cerebrospinal fluid samples of sufferers and the comorbidity of OCD with other anxiety and depressive disorders. Specific serotonin receptor agonists can exacerbate symptoms of compulsion, and serotonin re-uptake inhibitors relieve them. However, as is the case with models of anxiety and depression, the situation is far more complex than this. We know that interference with other neurotransmitter systems (dopaminergic and opioid) can also have an effect on compulsion and stereotypy.

Veterinary behavioural medicine has been strongly influenced by attempts to compare compulsive disorders in animals with OCD in man. To understand this, it is worth briefly considering the human experience of OCD (Table 9.1).

In OCD, obsessions are unwanted and intrusive thoughts occur in the form of ideas, images or impulses. The patients are not delusional and have full insight into the fact that these thoughts are purposeless and inappropriate. Obsessions are often highly unpleasant in nature, being concerned with themes of injury or harm, danger, doubt, loss, contamination and even uncontrollable impulses to act aggressively. There are common classes of obsession within the human population but the precise nature of obsessions is highly specific to the individual.

Compulsive behaviour arises from the need to control, satisfy and alleviate the concerns arising from the obsessional thoughts. The patient experiences urges to do things in order to lessen their feelings of anxiety or dysphoria. Those with obsessions relating to disorder might compulsively collect and tidy things; those with recurring doubt may continually recheck things. These behaviours become patterned into 'rituals' and there is often a superstitious fixation with the number of repetitions of this ritual that will guarantee protection from the consequences of the obsession. For example, soon after waking, a patient may get a feeling that this is an '8' day. To combat an individual intrusive thought, the patient will be compelled to repeat each ritual exactly eight times when they experience an obsessive thought. The performance of the ritual must be absolutely perfect or it 'does not count' and the patient may become very distressed if unable to perform the desired

number of perfect repetitions. They may also panic if the means to satisfy the obsession is not available.

It is clear that, although compulsive disorder in animals is also concerned with ritualisation and repetition of behaviour, human OCD also involves all sorts of thoughts, preoccupations and attempts at rationalisation that cannot exist in animals and do not fit with the type of behaviour they perform. Hence the term *obsession* cannot be easily applied in animals.

There may be some common neurophysiological or biochemical defect that produces disorders in man and animals, but human attempts to rationalise, adapt to and compensate for their own motivations and behaviour makes human OCD a more complex condition.

There are a number of theories about why compulsive disorders develop in animals. They mainly revolve around ideas about how individuals cope with arousal and anticipation. These are psychological states that are vital to normal behaviour and are linked to anxiety and normal expectations of reward. If we anticipate threat or danger, then the emotional flavour of the anticipation is negative and we experience anxiety, which is unpleasant. The intensity of the anxiety depends upon the level of arousal we experience and the aversiveness of the outcome we anticipate. Anticipation of a positive outcome can also become unpleasant if arousal is intense and prolonged and the actual outcome is in some way less positive than was expected. When the outcome is less rewarding, or never happens, then frustration is the result. Frustration and fear are essentially the same emotional state in animals. People label them differently only because they can interpret an emotional state in the light of events that led up to it. Both anticipation of threat or danger and anticipation of frustrated non-reward are therefore negative emotional experiences involving anxiety.

Most dogs have a normal ability to cope with arousal, anticipation and frustration and do not develop problems, even after prolonged confinement, isolation or behavioural conflict. However, the rate of repetitive behaviour in kennelled dogs is known to increase after even short periods of 2–3 weeks. This is temporary, and the majority of dogs revert to normal when they return to their home environment.

Compulsive disorder appears to develop when the dog discovers that multiple repetition of a ritualised behaviour produces a reduction in arousal and frustration. The behaviour that becomes ritualised is often related to behaviour that the dog is already highly motivated to perform. This can be species- or breed-specific behaviour, or behaviour that has been learned through previous reinforcement. Typically, the behaviour corresponds with modified displacement or self-appeasement behaviour or frustrated escape behaviour. Once repeatedly performing the ritual, the reduction of arousal the dog experiences is a powerfully motivating reward. Many situations in life involve anxiety, behavioural conflict or frustration and the individ-

Table 9.1 Similarities between human OCD and veterinary compulsive disorder

OCD	Compulsive disorder
35% of first-degree relatives are also afflicted.	Incidence higher in certain breeds and lines.
Consistent improvement with SRI/SSRI treatment.	
Evidence for reduced serotonergic transmission in basal ganglia.	
Imbalance of serotonin vs. dopamine transmission in basal ganglia.	
Often comorbid with other anxiety disorders and depression.	

ual may learn that carrying out repetitive rituals provides a faster, more reliable and perhaps more effective escape from these negative emotions. The trouble is that, in compulsive animals, the threshold to trigger the behaviour becomes progressively lower so that the animal appears to lose the choice over whether or not to perform it.

So, to begin with, the dog may only tail-chase in one context, with a very small number of intense triggering events but, over time, the compulsive behaviour becomes more widespread. For the dog with separation anxiety, the compulsion might begin with some tail-chasing as the owner leaves or is not present but then expand to times when the owner's attention is otherwise directed, such as when the phone is answered. Eventually, tail-chasing becomes such a reliable means of reducing arousal and the threshold is so low that tail-chasing interferes with the dog's ability to carry out normal behaviour. It substitutes for play, contact from the owner and a whole host of other normal interactions in a variety of contexts. Many types of behaviour may become compulsively repeated (Figs 9.1–9.3).

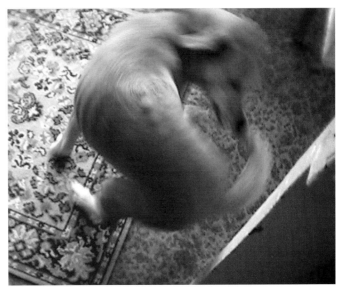

Figure 9.2   Compulsive tail-chasing is well coordinated and often rapid. This dog would tail-chase for up to 60 minutes until physically exhausted.

DIAGNOSIS

Medical issues

The diagnosis of compulsive disorders in veterinary patients is hampered by the fact that we have to base our conclusions on what we observe. The patient cannot report physical sensations such as pain. This makes it very easy to mistakenly label behaviour as abnormal and compulsive when it is a normal and predictable response to disease.

Compulsive disorder is a syndromic diagnosis and it is essential that other aetiological diagnoses must be investi-

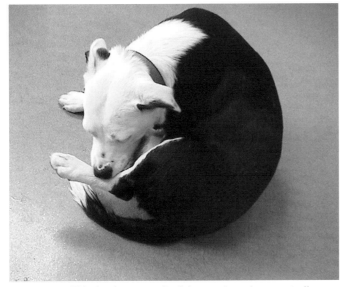

Figure 9.1   This dog has caused a lick granuloma by repeatedly licking its hock area.

gated first. This is because compulsive disorder is so easily confused with other neurological or medical disorders that produce similar signs and there are so many medical contributory factors to the genuine condition (Table 9.2). Also, because there is the likelihood that the animal will be treated with psychoactive drugs, medical investigation must be thorough and include:

- physical examination
- neurological examination
- haematology and biochemistry
- imaging and other investigations that may be needed to rule out medical disorder.

Medical problems can be divided into two categories:

1. Disorders that can produce repetitive or apparently compulsive behaviour that might resemble those seen in stereotypical and compulsive disorders; for example:

   - cognitive dementia
   - epilepsy
   - encephalitis
   - hydrocephalus
   - portosystemic shunt
   - injury, localised and referred pain (e.g., spinal disc lesion)
   - neurological abnormality (neurogenic pain, loss of sensation)
   - sensory abnormalities (keratoconjunctivitis sicca, haemorrhage in aqueous humour).

2. Disorders that contribute to the development of genuine compulsive disorder, such as:
   - cognitive dementia

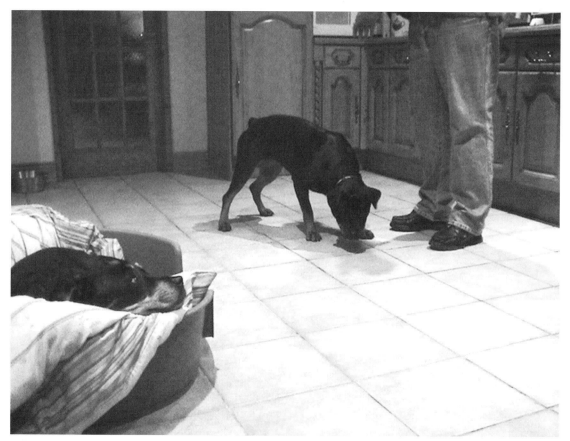

Figure 9.3 Compulsive animals are capable of responding to external stimulation. In this case, the dog is compelled to chase shadows and light spots. This behaviour often attracts the attention of other dogs and may be alarming to them.

- metabolic disease known to contribute to anxiety (hypothyroidism, etc.)
- neurological abnormality (neurogenic pain, loss of sensation)
- sensory deficit (contributing to anxiety).

Any medical maintaining factors should be ruled out or treated before any other kind of therapy commences; otherwise anticompulsive medication may be merely covering up signs of treatable organic disease (Box 9.1).

The role of learning

Early experience is important in preventing all kinds of anxiety disorder. The puppy that has been properly acclimatised to living in an intensely sociable and complex domestic environment is attracted to, rather than afraid of, novelty and is accustomed to periods of solitude. This greatly reduces the risk of developing behavioural problems, including compulsive disorder, and results in dogs who have learned to cope with the normal range of stimulation, arousal, frustration and behavioural conflict.

Normal learning can produce behaviour that is remarkably similar to compulsive disorder. For example, dogs are able to simulate a wide range of medical signs in order to get attention. If being lame has gained a great deal of sym-

pathy from the owner, then the dog is quite capable of mimicking lameness in order to get more. The same may be true of the dog that learns to tail-chase, groom excessively

Box 9.1 Medical factors contributing to development of compulsive disorder
Conditions that interfere with the ability to respond to a situation:
Impaired perception
Impaired mobility
Conditions that increase the need for self-appeasement behaviour (grooming, licking, etc.):
Painful conditions
Anxiety
Sensory loss
Conditions that increase general anxiety:
Metabolic disease (hypothyroidism, etc.)
Cognitive impairment

Table 9.2 Differential signs of pacing and circling

Compulsive disorder	CNS lesion	Pain (local/referred)	Cognitive dementia	Epilepsy
Direction of circling is consistent	Always circles towards the side of the lesion	Direction of pacing/circling may vary	Direction of pacing/circling may vary	Behaviour may vary
No neurological signs	Neurological signs contralateral to direction of circling: • Reduced menace response • Dilated pupil • Localised loss of sensation (face) • Altered locomotor reflexes (unilateral)	Localised ipsilateral neurological signs may be present (e.g., if pain due to spinal lesion)	Symmetrical neurological signs may be present in several areas including symmetrical sensory loss (central blindness/deafness)	No neurological signs
Normal gait and coordination	Ataxic gait (unilateral proprioceptive losses) even outside bouts of pacing or circling	Gait may be affected by unilateral lameness	Symmetrical gait abnormality (shuffling, hypermetria)	Gait may be uncoordinated during a seizure
Normal awareness	Reduced general awareness	Normal awareness	Markedly reduced general awareness	Marked changes in awareness before, during and after an episode of circling
Behaviour may be provoked by external events (loss of attention, sound, presence of unfamiliar people, etc.)	Behaviour appears 'unprovoked' by external stimuli	Behaviour may be provoked by external events (those causing painful activity), or the animal may suddenly start to pace/circle without an apparent external trigger	Behaviour may be provoked (e.g., by sudden, unexpected noise) or unprovoked (generalised nighttime pacing and circling)	Behaviour most common on transition from non-aroused to aroused state (e.g., waking). May occur during physical or emotional stress
Behaviour is often fast and very highly coordinated. Within a bout, each repetition is very similar to the last	Behaviour is slow and clumsy	Behaviour is purposeful and well coordinated	Behaviour is vegetative and purposeless	Behaviour is well coordinated but sluggish and a dog may stumble over objects

or bark rhythmically in order to get a response from the owner. Remember that all the dog may require is that it becomes the focus of the owner's interest for a fraction of a second; momentary eye contact may be enough reinforcement to increase future expression of the behaviour. If the owner shouts at the dog, then it has still gained some sort of attention although the overall effect may be to increase the dog's anxiety and hence its need for further reassurance. The severity of the behaviour depends on the reliability and intensity of reinforcement from the owner, as well as the value the animal places on getting attention.

This kind of attention-seeking behaviour only occurs when the person is present but not directly attending to the dog. Such dogs will often learn not to seek attention when

the person is genuinely busy cooking or gardening, for example. This is fundamentally different from compulsion arising out of hyperattachment (separation anxiety) because, in these cases, the behaviour may be seen at any time when the owner is unable to attend to the dog, including times when they are away.

Assessment

A list of typical compulsive behaviours is included in Table 9.3.

Dogs with compulsive disorder show normal levels of awareness throughout their behaviour, which differentiates them from dogs with epilepsy or cognitive impairment.

Table 9.3 Common stereotypical and compulsive disorders

Type of behaviour	Example	Breed predisposition
Oral	Flank sucking Self mutilation: • Lick granuloma • Tail biting • Foot chewing Repetitive self-grooming Repetitive licking: • Self • Objects • Other animals (including owner) Pica	Doberman pinscher Labrador retriever
Locomotor (no external stimulus)	Circling Tail-chasing Spinning Freezing Repetitive pouncing Fly snapping	Bull terrier (English, Staffordshire) King Charles spaniel
Locomotor (responding to external stimulus) Other	Fascination with reflections and shadows: Shadow and light spot chasing/pouncing Repetitive play with water surfaces Vocalisation: • Repeated ritualised barking or whining Staring into space	Border collie and related dogs (including crossbreeds) No specific breed

They may, however, be very difficult to interrupt and, if manually restrained, they may become aggressive. If the compulsive behaviour is forcefully interrupted, then the dog may show an even more furious bout of the behaviour as soon as the restraint is released. Once distracted, these dogs may show a preoccupation with returning to the compulsion; glancing back at the tail, for example. Between bouts of compulsive behaviour, the dog will appear completely normal and the transition to and from compulsive behaviour is usually quite sudden and abrupt, without prodromal or postictal signs that are present in epilepsy.

As the compulsive disorder becomes worse, the range of situations in which compulsion is seen grows wider. Whilst initially often linked to one context, the behaviour generalises to other contexts. In severe cases, compulsive behaviour will substitute for normal behaviour and will interfere with eating, social interaction and exploratory behaviour.

The current severity and initial response to treatment give some indication of prognosis and it is essential to gather baseline information about the level of expression of compulsive behaviour so that the owner is able to observe and track subtle changes (Box 9.2).

Box 9.2 Assessment of severity of compulsive disorder

Interrupting the behaviour

How easily may the dog be interrupted when behaving compulsively?
Once interrupted, is continuous distraction required to prevent the dog from returning to compulsive behaviour? Is compulsive behaviour more intense after a period of distraction?
Does the dog show aggression or irritability when interrupted?

Number of different contexts in which the stereotypy occurs

Number of different events or stimuli that trigger a bout of compulsive behaviour

How much time is spent in compulsive behaviour?

How often does the dog behave compulsively in a given day (or on average during a week)?
How long do bouts last and approximately what proportion of the dog's waking time is spent in compulsive behaviour?

To what degree does compulsive behaviour compete with or substitute for other normal behaviour?

Does compulsion interfere with normal behaviour? (e.g., eating, resting, play, interaction with people and other animals)
Does the dog behave compulsively in preference to performing normal behaviour?

Progression

Over what time period has the compulsion developed? How has it progressed?

Dogs that show compulsive behaviour in multiple contexts, with the behaviour substituting for a number of normal behaviours and being hard to interrupt, are seriously affected.

TREATMENT

Compulsive disorder is both debilitating and progressive and it should be treated aggressively from the outset (Box 9.3).

Treatment should involve:

• alteration of environment to reduce or remove maintaining factors

- a comprehensive behavioural plan
- complete review of medical management (pain relief, management of concurrent conditions whether thought contributory or not)
- use of an appropriate psychoactive medication (where necessary).

Box 9.3   Immediate intervention: compulsive disorder

- Identify and, where possible, ask the owner to avoid triggering stimuli and events.
- Stop the owner from punishing or intervening to stop the behaviour, as the dog may become aggressive.
- Clear the environment of items in which the dog may become entangled if it is circling or tail chasing (dogs may strangle themselves).
- Alter environment to include greater stimulation and distraction.

Environmental and management modification

Environment and management conditions are responsible for maintaining the dog's general level of arousal and anxiety. If this level is close to the threshold above which the dog begins to show compulsion, then even minor events may be enough to trigger a bout of compulsive behaviour. If the environment is sufficiently stressful, and the dog's threshold is low enough, then compulsion may be almost continuous. This is the situation that is seen in many production and zoo environments.

It is important to provide an environment that minimises stress (Box 9.4).

Predictability and controllability are vital; the dog must be able to tell when events are going to happen and have some control over them. It is useful to fix a strict routine for daily activities that creates a profound sense of order. This ritual of daily life reduces unpredictability and anxiety. All events should occur in a predetermined order relative to one another. The daily routine should include:

- several periods of physical exercise (increasing exercise may help some dogs)
- opportunities to interact with other dogs (as long as this is not stressful)
- several regular feeding times and the use of a multitude of activity feeders
- regular play sessions, interspersed with training
- controlled, timed interactions with the owner.

This routine should be maintained every day, even at weekends, until the level of compulsiveness is reduced by behavioural therapy. Then the owner can begin to introduce subtle changes in routine so that the dog learns to become increasingly adaptable.

Any obvious stressors should be minimised:

- External noise that is a cause of anxiety or fear (loud noises, traffic, people's voices on the street, etc.)
- Triggers off territoriality (delivery via letterbox, delivery people approaching the house).
- Conflict with other dogs in the same household (dispute over food, toys or attention, hierarchical conflict with other dogs in the home)
- Emotional behaviour by the owner (anger, shouting, etc.)

Environmental enrichment

The dog's environment must be made more engaging so that its time and energy budget are used up constructively. Activity feeding is a good way to do this but using a single feeder is not enough. The dog needs a multitude of food-finding activities, starting with ones that do not increase frustration. The complexity and difficulty of the activity feeders can be increased as the dog adapts to this form of feeding. A handout with suggestions for activity feeding is included in Appendix 2.

Box 9.4   Summary of environmental changes

- Provide the dog with a quiet and calm refuge or resting place where it may go to at any time and will not be disturbed.
- Reduce any known sources of conflict with other animals in the home (e.g., hierarchical disputes, competition over food, toys or attention).
- Stop punishment and threat (scolding, smacking, etc.)
- Reduce human emotional displays that create stress (displays of anger such as shouting).
- Reduce incidence of noises that may increase anxiety (loud music, video games, noisy children playing, etc.)
- Broaden the range of non-stressful activities in which the animal may engage but which do not provoke the compulsive behaviour (new games, visits to new places, greater social contact).
- Introduce activity feeding: Buster Cube®, activity ball, scatter food in garden, hide food around house/garden.

Behavioural therapy

Any event that produces a rapid increase in arousal or intense anticipation and frustration may result in a bout of compulsion. Common triggers include:

- telephone ringing or being used
- front doorbell ringing
- visitor coming into the house
- beginning or end of play

- beginning or end of interaction with owner
- reaction to noises and events outside the house
- owner departure.

Owners should make a detailed list of triggering events so that any common factor, such as loss of attention, can be identified. Wherever possible, exposure to these triggering events should be minimised so that new responses to them can be trained in a controlled way.

The aim is either to associate the event or cue with the rewarded performance of another behaviour (response substitution) or to countercondition the emotional response to it.

- *Response substitution:* a calm behaviour (sitting or laying down) is clicker-trained: the training method of 'shaping' is used to train the dog to adopt an unaroused, non-anticipatory state, lying down with low muscle tension, low vigilance and low heart rate. The dog is continuously reinforced while it adopts this behaviour on cue (e.g., a verbal signal). The dog is then rewarded for doing the same when the cue is given in the presence of a mild version of one of the triggering events. The intensity of the triggering event is gradually increased during these training sessions. The dog is then rewarded for adopting the same state spontaneously, without a verbal cue, when experiencing increasingly intense presentations of the triggering event.

- *Counterconditioning:* starting with mild presentations of the stimulus, it is associated with another event that is both satiating and results in low arousal (e.g., feeding).

All training must be carried out in a range of contexts to avoid it becoming context specific. For some triggering events, the animal may need to be desensitised before beginning response substitution or counterconditioning.

Clicker-training is superior to other forms of training in this context because it may be used to reduce anticipation. The click is used to pinpoint the rewarded behaviour, which may be shaped to include a decrease in muscle tension, heart rate or non-attendance to the trainer or other events. The trainer makes no intentional movements that indicate that a food treat is to be given until after the click has been given. They must not reach for or touch food until after observing the correct response from the dog and then making a click. The dog is forced to duplicate and refine its behaviour in order to get further clicks. Using clicker-training, it is relatively easy to train the dog to adopt a non-vigilant and non-anticipatory waiting state on cue.

The clicker-trained waiting state may be associated with contexts as well as individual events so that the dog learns to become less aroused and anxious in a range of familiar situations. The dog might be regularly taken for short periods to an environment where it has previously behaved compulsively and trained to adopt calm behaviour for repeated reinforcement. This will reduce the general level of arousal the animal experiences in that context.

Some events that trigger intense and uninterruptible compulsiveness may need to be broken down into a chain of stimuli that can be individually associated with other behaviour. For example, the sound of footsteps on the street, the sound of a gate opening, further footsteps leading to the house and then the sounds of a doorbell. This sequence of cues predicts the arrival of a visitor and contribute to a gradually rising level of arousal that precedes this event.

Certain events and human interactions often provoke a bout of compulsiveness because they always cause arousal or end in frustration. A good example is when a dog greets someone. It begins to get the anticipated reward of attention but, just as its level of arousal increases and its greeting behaviour becomes more intense, the person terminates the greeting. This is apparently a no-win situation. If we intensify the response to the greeting, then the dog's arousal increases and frustration is greater when the interaction comes to an end. If we do not respond at all, then the dog is left in a state of frustration anyway because the attention-reward it anticipated while waiting for the person to enter the home is denied. Other interactions, such as play, involve unavoidable increases in arousal as they start, and then a degree of frustration as they come to an end. The answer is to use rewards other than attention that can be given at high intensity without causing excessive arousal and anticipation.

The beginning and end of these arousing activities may need to be ameliorated with a calming training episode. It is therefore useful to precede play or greeting with an intense period of clicker reinforcement of a trained 'waiting state' that curbs arousal and anticipation and to finish play in the same way. For example, the owner uses a clicker-training routine to reduce arousal before the door is opened and the guest is admitted to the house. In the case of play behaviour, the game is repeatedly interrupted with short periods of training every few seconds so that arousal does not become excessive. It should be terminated with the delivery of a chew, activity feeder or some other distracting non-interactive activity. In this way frustration is minimised. A general method for controlling arousal during play is included in a handout in Appendix 2.

General anticipation can be reduced by giving a clear signal before all interactions begin. For example, the dog might be asked to sit or lie down before receiving attention and the owner announces what they are going to do before stroking the dog. In this way the dog's level of anticipation is reduced because each interaction is named and highly-structured. The dog knows exactly what is going to happen. The end of an interaction is also signalled in a way that the dog understands, rather than the owner simply withdrawing contact and wandering away. Clicker-training can also aid this. A 'no' signal may be conditioned so that the dog understands that interaction is over. Use of this method helps to reduce frustration. The dog may also be taught to stay calm whilst being stroked or handled. Similar methods can be used to condition a response to other forms of interaction. Handouts for both these clicker-training techniques are included in Appendix 2.

Behavioural therapy can be gradually withdrawn once the level of compulsive behaviour has settled down to an acceptable level (Box 9.5).

Psychoactive medication

Drugs should definitely be considered for cases where:

* the condition is severe:

    compulsive behaviour is seen in multiple contexts
    compulsive behaviour substitutes for a wide range of normal behaviours

* the condition is longstanding
* the compulsive behaviour is difficult to interrupt or maintain distraction from.

They may also be considered when progression has been rapid and the situation is continuing to worsen.

The decision to use medication for less severe cases may be based on the efficacy of a trial of behaviour modification. If environmental enrichment and behavioural modification produce good and persistent benefits, then continued behavioural therapy may be sufficient. However, if there is only a moderate response to therapy after 12 weeks, then the use of drugs should be reconsidered. As with all dogs with this condition, there is a strong possibility that these dogs will become worse over time which may force the need to use medication in the future.

Many different classes of drugs with completely different neurotransmitter effects have been shown to have an effect in treating compulsive disorders. The only consistent fact is that none of them has achieved a very high response rate, which further indicates the complexity of the neurochemistry of the condition. The only group of drugs that produces useful and reliable effects that are consistent with current hypotheses about aetiology of compulsive disorder are the SRI and SSRI drugs. The others will be mentioned for interest and completeness and because some may be used as adjunct therapy.

Opioid antagonists

Examples of opioid antagonist drugs include naloxone, naltrexone and nalmefene. These drugs were originally found to be successful for the treatment of stereotypies in tethered sows. They have been moderately successful in small-scale trials with self-mutilatory compulsive disorder in companion animals but they are of no practical use because the drugs have such short half-lives. There is insufficient evidence to support their use.

Typical and atypical antipsychotics

This group includes the neuroleptics haloperidol and pimozide, as well as the atypical antipsychotic risperidone. In human medicine, these drugs are sometimes used as augmentation therapy for refractory OCD after multiple failure of response to SRI/SSRI drugs or after relapse. In this role they are used in conjunction with an SSRI, primarily for cases of comorbid Tourette syndrome or where there are signs of tics and psychotic episodes. Pimozide is used to augment an SSRI where there is poor response to the SSRI alone.

These drugs are generally not suitable for veterinary use because they have poor safety profiles and there are no accepted dose rates. Also, most the comorbid indications for using these drugs have not been identified in veterinary patients.

Azapirones

Buspirone is a partial agonist of the serotonin-1a receptor. Normally, serotonin binding to the presynaptically located form of this receptor causes a reduction in the further release of the neurotransmitter into the synaptic cleft: a form of negative feedback. Buspirone blocks this and thus raises synaptic serotonin concentration.

On its own, buspirone has no role in the treatment of compulsive disorder but there have been trials testing it as an augmentation treatment with a variety of SRI and SSRI drugs. Results have been extremely variable in man with some trials showing no benefit over placebo.

Box 9.5   General summary of behavioural therapy for compulsive disorder

* Create a regular daily routine and stick to it.
* Increase the dog's level of mental and physical activity.
* Train and then consistently use specific cues that indicate the beginning and end of specific kinds of interaction (play, stroke, etc.)
* Train a 'calm' response on cue, and associate this with each of the stimuli and contexts that currently cause compulsive behaviour.
* Use training to control arousal at the beginning and end of exciting activities, like play. Interrupt these activities with short bouts of training to stop arousal becoming excessive.
* Train dog to remain calm during interaction so that these become less arousing and therefore less frustrating when they finish.
* Desensitize and countercondition dog to cues that provoke the behaviour (departure cues, ringing phone, unfamiliar person present, etc.)

Other drugs

Phenobarbitone is sometimes mistakenly prescribed for compulsive disorder, either alone or in combination with propranolol. There is no evidence that phenobarbitone will have any effect for genuine compulsive disorder and it is the author's experience that it can make the problem worse. Of course, phenobarbitone and other antiepileptic drugs are used for cases of repetitive behaviour that result from seizures.

Dietary modification or supplementation

L-tryptophan may be used to augment SRI or SSRI therapy if given in conjunction with a low protein diet. Giving a low protein, high carbohydrate diet is known to increase active transport of dietary serotonin precursors across the blood–brain barrier and this too might be expected to help with dogs that have a poor or marginal response to several SRI or SSRI-type drugs.

Serotonin re-uptake inhibitor (SRI) and selective serotonin re-uptake inhibitor (SSRI) drugs

The mainstay of drug treatment for compulsive disorder is with SRI and SSRI drugs. A particular feature of these drugs is that there is a significant delay between the start of therapy and signs of efficacy. Indeed, some owners may report that there has been an immediate response to therapy but this usually indicates that the patient is suffering from side-effects. SRI and SSRI drugs increase synaptic serotonin levels, which in turn leads to adaptation of the neurotransmitter system through the up and down regulation of different receptor and secondary messenger systems. This involves protein synthesis which takes at least 3 weeks to accomplish. So these drugs cannot produce significant beneficial changes within a month and may take 6–8 weeks to show true efficacy. Adverse effects of these drugs are due to their immediate impact on histamine and acetylcholine transmission which gradually wanes after the first 7–10 days.

The first drug to be used extensively in man was clomipramine, an SRI. This produced good effects and was, for a time, the drug of choice. However, more modern alternatives have become available that produce at least equivalent anticompulsive benefits, but with fewer adverse effects.

Recently developed SSRI drugs are more selective for serotonin over norepinephrine and have little or no anticholinergic or antihistaminic effect. They have less effect on seizure threshold and urinary retention and are generally less sedative. The general advice in man is to start therapy with an SSRI drug (fluoxetine, fluvoxamine, paroxetine or sertraline). If there is a failure to respond, then this is switched to another SSRI or to the SRI clomipramine.

Dose rates are generally a little higher for treating compulsive disorder than for other conditions but it is better to switch to another drug if there is a poor response. Increasing the dose of an individual drug beyond the normal dose range merely risks producing more side-effects. These drugs can also have a general inhibiting effect even on normal behaviour, which is obviously undesirable.

Various augmentation strategies are used for refractory cases in man, including using antipsychotic drugs or buspirone with an SSRI. The results have been very variable and given that most of these drugs are not safe for use in veterinary patients, these combinations are not an option within general practice.

On a much more positive note, the most successful augmentation strategy used in human psychiatry is to use behavioural modification which is automatically part of the approach we use in veterinary behavioural medicine.

Response to treatment

Compulsive disorder does not respond to therapy with SRI/SSRI type drugs in a straightforward manner:

- The response to SRI/SSRI drugs is inconsistent. In man it varies from around 40–60% for a single agent which means that, even if the diagnosis is correct and therapy is entirely appropriate, a significant number of patients will not respond at all.
- For those patients that do respond, there is usually only a partial reduction in compulsive behaviour (30–50% in man, typically higher in dogs).
- Response to treatment can only be evaluated after at least 12 weeks of continuous therapy.
- Improvements in expression of compulsion are independent of changes in mood (anxiety, etc.)
- Relapses are common and drug therapy may need to be changed regularly.
- Even short breaks in therapy with these drugs can significantly impair future response to treatment with that agent.

Remember that the relatively poor recorded responses to therapy reflect the use of these drugs in isolation, without behavioural therapy. Improvement is considerably greater when drug and behavioural therapy are combined.

With such apparently inconsistent responses to treatment, it is essential to collect baseline data on the level of compulsive activity.

This should include:

- videotape of the compulsive behaviour
- tests of interruptability of the behaviour
- comparative photographs of any lesions.
- structured observation by owner (interruptability, frequency and duration of bouts of compulsion, number of contexts within which it occurs).

Similar information must be collected for comparison at regular intervals so that treatment can be reviewed. These are not cases that can be treated and forgotten.

Medication with psychoactive drugs should be seen as a way to reduce the inflexibility and rate of expression of compulsive behaviours so that environmental change and behavioural modification can be more effective. It must never be used on its own.

Duration of treatment will vary. There is a general tendency for compulsive behaviour to become worse during the dog's life unless living conditions are substantially changed before the threshold for compulsive behaviour becomes excessively lowered. If there is a response to therapy at 8–12 weeks, then progress should be reviewed regularly (monthly). A minority of individuals show a complete cessation of compulsive behaviour after a few months and can be weaned off drugs if there is a period of more than 8 weeks without any evidence of compulsive behaviour. Alternatively, owners may be happy to accept that a degree of compulsiveness will always remain but wish to stop drug therapy because signs have improved to an acceptable level. In these cases, the drug must be withdrawn slowly so that recidivism is avoided and so that drug therapy can be more rapidly reinstated if a relapse occurs during withdrawal. Dogs that relapse in this way should be reintroduced at the full drug dose and may have to stay on it for a long period. Some individuals become resistant to treatment if it is reintroduced after a relapse and they will benefit from a switch to another drug.

Drug withdrawal

For short courses a gradual withdrawal, giving a 25% dose reduction each week for 3 weeks, and then stopping.

For longer courses, 1 week of withdrawal is allowed for every month of treatment. The withdrawal period is divided into three sections and dose is reduced by 25% for each section. Alternatively, dosing frequency is reduced.

Pheromonotherapy

There have as yet been no specific trials on the efficacy of Dog Appeasing Pheromone (DAP®) for the treatment of compulsive disorder but the chemical is thought to increase acceptance of environmental stimuli and events. It may help where social problems exist between conspecifics and it would be predicted that DAP® might have a beneficial effect on cases of self-mutilation. The author has found some success in combining DAP® with behavioural and psychopharmacological approaches in some cases.

PROGNOSIS

Intermittent relapses are common with this condition so owners must be aware that they may have to use drugs and an intensive course of behavioural therapy again in the future. The prognosis is poor for dogs that continue to live in stressful or impoverished environments, as it is for long-standing cases where compulsive behaviour substitutes for a wide range of normal activities.

Dogs with a long history of severe compulsion may benefit from lifelong treatment with psychoactive drugs and will require regular reviews and changes in therapy to maintain improvement.

LICK GRANULOMA AND SELF-MUTILATION

Diagnosis

Compulsive self-mutilation must first be differentiated from conditions that cause localised pain or loss of sensation. This is particularly important for dogs that have been docked or have had a history of tail trauma and now tail biting. Post-amputation neuromas might be an initiating factor in this kind of tail-chasing and self-mutilation.

Dogs will also repeatedly lick and groom areas as a form of self-appeasement when they are in chronic pain but the site that is licked may be quite distant from the part of the body that is causing pain.

Lick granulomas are common in large-breed dogs; the condition exhibiting sexual dimorphism in favour of the male. There have been theories that self-mutilation is related to a different neurotransmitter defect from locomotor stereotypies. The theory was that the dopaminergic system was involved and that once the animal began to cause actual tissue damage, then endogenous opioids (endorphins and enkephalins) produced both analgesia and euphoria. Despite this, clinical experience is that self-mutilatory compulsive disorder responds just as effectively to SSRI drugs as does locomotor stereotypy. It may well be that endogenous opioids are produced and that they do cause analgesia, which is why the damage can be very severe in some cases, but there is no evidence to date that there is a special neurochemical dysfunction.

Treatment

The treatment of self-mutilation involves healing the lesion as well as preventing the motivation to maintain it or create a new one. These lesions are often deeply infected and chronically inflamed. The lesion should be managed in the same way as any other area of chronic inflammation and infection (Box 9.6).

Self-mutilation is episodic for many dogs, recurring occasionally throughout life. Between episodes the dog continues to groom more regularly than normal but without causing any damage. Episodes of actual trauma often start very suddenly and, within a short time, the dog has created a new wound or granuloma. In some individuals, the condition progresses in the same way as other compulsive disorders; substituting for normal behaviour, occurring in more contexts and becoming less interruptible.

Box 9.6   Treatment of lick granuloma

- Swab lesion for culture and sensitivity tests
- Treat with appropriate antibiotic (topically and systemically)
- Use topical anti-inflammatory drugs
- Local excision of tissue to reduce excess granulation tissue that is interfering with re-epithelialisation
- Use of appropriate dressing to suppress granuloma formation and encourage epithelialisation
- Consider laser treatment to speed up epithelial growth at edge of lesion
- Protect lesion from continued trauma (Elizabethan collar, neck brace, flavour deterrents)
- Use SSRI/SRI at least until one month after lesion has fully healed
- Same behavioural interventions and environmental changes are appropriate for compulsive self-mutilation as for other compulsive behaviour

Prognosis

As with other compulsive disorders, self-mutilation commonly recurs. Treatment may need to be reviewed regularly to prevent repeated bouts.

Prevention of relapse or recidivism depends on the same environmental modification as for other kinds of compulsive disorder.

ADVICE SHEETS THAT MAY BE RELEVANT TO THIS CHAPTER

In Appendix 2:

1. Using a houseline
6. Muzzle-training
9. The 'come away' command
11. Attention seeking and the 'no' signal
12. Click-touch training
13. Preparing for phobic events
16. Environmental enrichment for dogs

Chapter 10

Canine elimination problems

INTRODUCTION

The normal development of elimination behaviour is as follows:

- 0 to 3–4 weeks: Elimination is stimulated by perineal grooming by the bitch. The bitch cleans the puppy and removes its waste.
- 3 to 5 weeks: The puppy starts to move away from the nest to eliminate.
- 5+ weeks: The puppy chooses a fixed latrine location which becomes more specific with time.

Full house-training involves several processes:

1. Learning to ignore the sensation of a full bladder or bowel.
2. Learning what kinds of substrates and locations provide suitable toilets.
3. Learning to eliminate on command.

Like children, many young animals are highly sensitive to bowel and bladder-filling signals so they will feel that they need to go to the toilet more often than an adult might. If access to a preferred latrine is restricted, dogs will gradually learn to disregard such sensations because they have to withhold urine if a latrine is not available. If there is continuous free access to a toilet location, perhaps with a back door open into a garden during the day, then the puppy may remain oversensitive to these signals because it can eliminate whenever it wants to and may not learn to disregard the more painful sensation of having a properly filled bladder. These puppies may wake their owners regularly during the night wanting to go to the toilet or may find an indoor latrine which they use whenever outdoor access is restricted. The same problem is encountered when owners give puppies a temporary indoor toilet to use.

Latrine selection is guided by maternal behaviour but also depends upon the kinds of substrate and location that are available during development. Puppies can learn quite fixed location and substrate preferences by the time they are 12 weeks old so it is important to start to train the right choices at an early age. If this is not done, then they may learn troublesome preferences, such as a desire to eliminate on paper, carpet or hard floors, before they are homed. This is another reason for early homing (at 7–8 weeks), so that the owner can train the preferences that are most compatible with domestic living.

The first location choice the puppy makes for itself is to find a latrine away from the communal resting area (nest). If puppies cannot do this because they are confined to a kennel or single room, then they will learn to overcome natural resistance to soil in a communal rest area. This presents problems later on because confinement to an indoor kennel will not cause the older dog to withhold urine and faeces.

The process of house-training dogs is actually very straightforward in nearly every case but still the old idea of rubbing a puppy's nose in its mess persists and causes problems. Excessive or delayed punishment of behaviour risks the puppy developing fear or mistrust of the person and will have no beneficial effect on house-soiling. Dogs are not capable of learning the consequences of their behaviour unless they are caught in the act of doing something. Punishment that is delayed by even a few seconds will be incomprehensible to the dog who will just assume that the person is unpredictable and aggressive. This can cause problems of submissive urination, fear, anxiety and aggression. House-training should always be accomplished through positive reinforcement (Box 10.1).

GENERAL ASSESSMENT

Some basic clinical data should be gathered in all cases:

- medical history
- physical examination: including abdominal palpation, internal examination of rectum, and external examination of urinary tract
- measurement of daily water intake
- comprehensive urinalysis
- inspection of a faecal sample
- neurological examination of detrusor and other reflexes
- other investigations where indicated by historical and physical findings (e.g., radiography, cystography, ultrasound, haematology, biochemistry).

Specific points of note are:

- incontinence (nocturia, urine dribbling while recumbent, etc.)
- polyuria or polydipsia, which will increase urine throughput, frequency and urgency of elimination (this must be investigated fully)
- faecal consistency. Hard faeces may cause pain on elimination and are a potential indication of endocrine disease or dehydration. Soft faeces increase urgency and frequency of defecation
- diseases that may affect mobility and limit animal's ability to reach a suitable latrine

- cognitive impairment
- sensory loss.

Clinical signs should be investigated as with any other medical disorder. There is no point in assessing behavioural aspects of a house-soiling case until medical underlying factors have been fully investigated. Do not assume that the owner of a house-soiling puppy will spontaneously bring your attention to the fact that it has never passed a normal solid stool, even though that is an obvious barrier to house-training.

Elimination problems must be differentiated from scent-marking problems which have a quite different motivation. Both male and female dogs will scent-mark, with the rate of marking depending upon reproductive status. Males and females will over-mark spots that have been previously scent-marked by another dog. They will also frequently scent-mark after meeting or seeing another dog.

The behavioural history should pay special attention to:

- the dog's rearing environment and early house-training
- age of onset of the condition
- pattern of elimination (where, how often and when)
- volumes of urine passed (as an indication of infection or obstructive disease of the urinary tract)
- the events that immediately precede elimination (presence of another dog or person, owner's return home, touching by the owner, etc.)
- the animal's behaviour before and after it has eliminated (excited, happy, anxious, fearful, withdrawn, etc.)
- the owner's response when the puppy has soiled in the house
- the puppy's feeding pattern (how many meals? Fed ad libitum?)

Once medical causes have been ruled out or treated, then a range of behavioural diagnoses may be made:

- *Incomplete house-training:*
  Inappropriate substrate or location preference.
  Inadequate or inappropriate house-training.
  Poor management or change in management.
- *Emotionally related urination:*
  Due to anxiety.
  Excitement urination.
- Submissive urination.
- Scent marking.

Box 10.1   Immediate action: house-soiling

- Stop excessive punishment such as smacking, shouting or 'rubbing the dog's nose in the mess' as these will make the situations worse.
- Stop delayed punishment.
- Use a good cleaning routine.
- Keep the dog supervised and take it to the toilet regularly.

Box 10.2   Cleaning routine

- Mop up waste.
- Clean the area with warm soapy water or preferably a weak solution of a biological detergent (applied to a test area of flooring or fabric first).
- Rinse with water.
- Lightly apply an odourless spray-on disinfectant solution.
- Apply a spray-on odourless biological deodoriser if necessary.
- AVOID using bleach or strongly-scented disinfectants or cleaning solutions as they may identify the area even more strongly as a latrine.

INCOMPLETE HOUSE-TRAINING

Many dogs are, in fact, not house-trained despite the fact that they do not soil the house very often. It is usually clear from the history that the owners had difficulty with house-training for one reason or another, or that husbandry of the dog has in some way sidestepped the issue of house-training.

Typical problem scenarios include:

- The dog that is reared or kennelled for a period in a large concrete kennel with full-time access to a concrete run. The dog loses indoor/outdoor discrimination and develops a preference for a hard stony or concrete substrate regardless of where it is. These dogs often soil on hard floors and tiled surfaces.

- The dog that is 'sent' into the garden to go to the toilet (perhaps after asking to go out). The dog then becomes distracted, perhaps territorialising, investigating or playing in the garden. The owner has not supervised the dog and is unaware that it has not eliminated. Within a few minutes of returning to the house, the dog feels a sudden urgency to eliminate and urinates on the floor.

- The owner puts the dog outside for an hour or two several times each day, typically at times when it might normally be expected to eliminate. The dog has to eliminate outside because that is where it happens to be when it needs to pass urine or faeces. This dog may start to soil the house regularly, and even develop a preference for doing this if the owner cannot maintain this routine of putting the dog out.

- The owner has provided an 'emergency' indoor toilet for the dog, such as a pile of newspapers. The dog has never learned to ignore normal bladder or bowel-filling signals and goes to the toilet whenever it experiences even mild discomfort. It may even have a substrate preference for this 'emergency toilet'.

Punishment is an important factor. Physical punishment should never be used with dogs because it can condition aversive associations between an approaching or touching hand and an experience of fear or pain. These dogs may misinterpret hand contact as a threat, which risks a bite.

In house-soiling cases, all forms of punishment that produce a strong avoidance or submissive reaction should cease (even a raised voice) because:

- anxiety may increase the need to eliminate, making the problem worse.
- the dog may associate punishment with the act of eliminating whilst in the owner's presence. It is much more difficult to house-train a dog that sneaks off to soil in a private corner every time the owner is not looking, or cannot be rewarded for appropriate behaviour because it is terrified to eliminate whenever the owner is in sight.
- methods that do not involve positive punishment work just as effectively but with less risk of adverse effects.

Treatment

An owner handout for basic house-training is contained in Appendix 2. The aim is to train a location and substrate preference using reward-based training. In the case of a dog with a house-soiling problem, the aim is to train a new set of preferences that conflict with those that create the conditions for house-soiling.

The animal must associate going to the toilet in a specific place, preferably on command, with getting the rewards of praise, freedom to explore, play and food. A clicker-training method is best because it offers the easiest way to indicate that complete bowel or bladder emptying is the rewarded behaviour.

Clicker-training is also particularly useful in cases where a problem has developed through over-punishment. The click is an impersonal signal which can be delivered from a distance and is a noise which has only ever been associated with a rewarding outcome. So the owner can reward the dog for good eliminative behaviour without having to linger in close proximity or display a potentially unsettling level of interest in what the dog is doing. The house-training method on the owner handout can be adapted to suit such special cases (see Appendix 2, Sheet 19).

To be effective, the location chosen as the dog's preferred latrine should be recognisably different from other locations. Wringing out urine from house-soiling accidents on to the chosen spot will create the right odour mark and it helps to pick a spot that is identified by a landmark such as a nearby bush or tree. It is also important to pick a substrate that is dissimilar from any that the dog might soil on in the house. Concrete is very similar to a tiled floor and decking feels rather like floorboards. Dogs that have been reared in a concrete kennel with a concrete run are already at a disadvantage because they have begun to learn a potentially inappropriate substrate preference.

Grass is often a good substrate but owners who do not have a garden or who live in a flat without easy ground-floor outdoor access may need to provide an artificial grassed area as a training latrine; for example, a large but low-level, grass-filled planter in a corner of the patio or on a balcony with drainage.

House-training depends upon limiting the dog's opportunity to mess in the house through a combination of constant supervision and confinement to a place where it will not soil. Most dogs will not soil close to their bed so confinement to a small bed area, such as an indoor kennel, may be effective. The dog must be trained to accept confinement before doing this (see Appendix 2). In some cases a dog will show an absolute preference for one location and substrate, such as the kitchen floor, so confinement to a carpeted lounge or bedroom will prevent elimination when the dog is alone. However, you need to be confident of success before you suggest this.

This method may be effective for dogs that have lost their inhibitions about soiling in their own bed or rest area and will soil in an indoor kennel.

Some owners may have to accept that there is no practical way to stop occasional accidents in the house and they will have to depend upon positive reinforcement to house-train the dog. If training is done well and latrine sites in the house are easily cleaned, then these dogs will still become properly house-trained within a few weeks (Box 10.2).

Furniture and flooring can become damaged by urine and also contaminated by urine odours that can be hard to remove. Some surfaces absorb urine and faeces odours, making cleaning pointless. Property should be properly protected and absorbent surfaces should be properly water-proofed and sealed (Box 10.3).

In some cases, it is useful to use mild punishment to interrupt the dog as it prepares to or starts to eliminate in an inappropriate location. The punishment must be of the remote kind; that is, not associated with the presence of a person. It should be only just powerful enough to interrupt elimination without causing an escape response or other obvious signs of fear or anxiety. Shouting at the dog or yelling its name may condition negative associations leading to fear and more secretive house-soiling. A clap of the hands is usually sufficient to stop the dog without alarming it. The dog is then calmly taken to its latrine location to be rewarded for finishing off what it was doing, but in the right place.

Sound-based remote punishment devices, such as a tin full of pebbles or specially designed loud aerosol are frequently cited as mild forms of punishment, but they should be used with caution. From the human perspective they may appear to be mild but, in comparison to animals, our hearing is insensitive and confined to a much narrower sound spectrum. To some dogs these sound devices may be very alarming so such punishments should be introduced with care. Other forms of remote punishment, such as a water pistol, may work but

---

> ### Box 10.3 Protecting the home
>
> The following are some suggestions for temporarily protecting property that is at known risk of contamination with urine or faeces:
>
> - Fill all cracks in woodwork, surfaces and edges or corners with a waterproof sealant; for example, at junctions between different kinds of flooring, skirting boards and between wooden flooring tiles.
> - Remove or scrape away urine-damaged wood and material.
> - Over-paint surfaces with several coats of organic solvent-based varnish or paint to block the odour of urine that may have already become absorbed into wooden objects.
> - Clean and use waterproof grout or mortar between floor tiles.
> - Use an appropriate sealant or chemical treatment to protect cork, terracotta, and other porous floorings.
> - Protect upholstered furniture with a covering of heavy grade polythene.
> - Remove loose covers, wrap furniture and cushion covers with heavy grade polythene and then replace covers.
> - Put a waterproof plastic cover over mattresses and bed bases.

it is actually very difficult for owners to use them without being seen and therefore becoming connected with the event.

Prognosis

The prognosis for incomplete house-training problems is good unless the dog has been reared without an opportunity to learn normal preferences. The prognosis is more guarded for dogs that have been reared or kept in a confined area so that they have had to overcome the usual aversion to soiling close to a resting place, or for dogs that have developed a substrate preference for indoor flooring.

ANXIETY URINATION

Anxious dogs can experience loss of control due to intense emotionality. Dogs with separation anxiety have a primary over-attachment to their owner and will soil whenever isolated from them. These dogs will sometimes urinate and defecate as they run around in a state of 'panic' and distress immediately after the owner has left. Owners come home to find the floor covered in urine and faeces that the dog has trodden around.

There are other causes of this pattern of soiling; for example, dogs that become intensely anxious when they are confined in a place where they anticipate a phobic event. In more moderate cases, the anxiety merely increases the frequency and urgency of elimination.

Anxiety disorders are a common problem in the geriatric age group. These may be new problems resulting from cognitive impairment or debilitation, or may be re-emergence of old problems with which the animal is now less mentally equipped to cope. Periods of illness or stress may make the dog more emotionally reliant on the owner who may, in turn, become more attentive and supportive. Problems of anxiety are complicated and incorrect diagnoses are common, so these cases must be carefully investigated.

EXCITEMENT URINATION

In man, it is known that certain emotional states can cause a temporary loss of bladder control. A good example is enuresis risoria ('giggle incontinence'). This condition affects both children and adults and, whereas other forms of childhood incontinence such as nocturia are limited to childhood, enuresis risoria continues to affect a significant number of sufferers throughout adulthood. There appears to be no functional or anatomical urinary tract defect associated with the condition so it is assumed that the loss of control relates to some central emotional effect, perhaps originating in the limbic system.

Excitement urination also affects both young and mature dogs that have no obvious physical cause of incontinence, so the conditions may be similar. Excitement urination is very frustrating for owners and there is a temptation to punish or threaten the dog as it begins to eliminate. In any case, it is likely that the human observer will be unable to disguise their irritation. Unfortunately, this often triggers another problem: *submissive* urination.

Diagnosis

Excitement and submissive urination can initially be discriminated because, in excitement urination, there is no attempt to show a submissive body posture. However, once the dog regularly tries to appease the owner's anger, then the two conditions start to overlap. There may still be an obvious shift in behaviour from excitement to submission in response to the owner's behaviour.

Treatment

It is essential to clarify the conditions that lead up to the excitement urination:

- Identify the level of arousal that precedes urination (by observation of the dog's behaviour).
- Try to identify two or more obvious behaviours that the owner can easily recognise as indicators that the dog is becoming over-excited.
- Detail all interactions that result in over-excitement (touch, eye contact, verbal signals of attention).

The general approach is to desensitise and countercondition the animal to all the situations and interactions that currently provoke over-excitement. To do this, the owner must display an awareness of what it is they are doing to provoke the dog. The level of greetings and interactions with the dog must be downgraded so that the dog never reaches the threshold of excitement for urination. Over a number of training sessions, the owner should find that the intensity of contact needed to provoke excitement increases.

At the same time, the dog should be conditioned to perform more relaxed and restrained greeting behaviour in these situations so that it can meet people without becoming over-excited. Tricyclic antidepressant and selective serotonin re-uptake inhibitor drugs can prove beneficial in these cases if they are refractory to behavioural modification alone. The mechanism may be through the side-effect of increasing urinary sphincter tone or through a central effect on mood (Box 10.4).

Prognosis

The prognosis for these cases is good, although treatment may take time. A poor prognosis arises from a lack of owner patience and compliance or if a physical problem is present, such as incontinence.

SUBMISSIVE URINATION

This is commonest in younger animals and happens in response to situations in which the dog anticipates a need

---

Box 10.4 Treatment: excitement urination

- **All punishment of the excitement urination must cease.** Owners must take care not to show expressions of anger or disgust which may evoke submissive urination.
- Clearly identify to the owner those behaviours that indicate that the dog is becoming so excited that it may urinate.
- The owner must reduce the intensity of all interactions (such as greetings) so that the observed level of excitement remains well below this level.
- Contact should be immediately and abruptly withdrawn if the dog approaches the state of over-excitement that will lead to urination (or if urination begins). The person should turn their head away from the dog and withdraw all contact.
- The dog must be desensitised to the intensity of greeting and other behaviours that trigger excitement.
- The dog should be taught to associate staying calm when touched with the delivery of a food reward (see Advice sheet 12 on 'click-touch' training in Appendix 2). Touch may then be used to calm the dog in other situations.

to demonstrate appeasement. Most commonly, this is upon reunification with a higher status member of the group, be that a person or another animal. It can also occur in response to social signals that indicate threat or those where the other individual's intention is to reaffirm a status relationship by provoking a gesture of submission. The latter is most common between conspecifics. There may, as in other forms of emotional urination, be an actual loss of bladder control due to the intensity of emotional state, but the act of urination may also be an intrinsic part of the submissive gesture.

Diagnosis

Diagnosis is based upon an analysis of the following.

1. The situations in which the urination occurs:
    - during greetings
    - when the person is standing over the dog
    - touching of the head or neck
    - when punished (verbal or physical)
    - during eye contact.

2. The dog's other body and facial posture around the time of urination.

3. The behaviour to which the dog is responding (that of other animals and people).

    Dogs with a problem of submissive urination will adopt a typical posture during the interaction:

    - tail curled under, often with the tip wagging
    - low, hunched body posture
    - head turned down or away
    - rolling over onto the side or back.

    This is rarely a static posture, as the dog will often writhe or crawl around so as to stay within the field of vision of the person or animal to whom they are submitting. The aim is to draw attention to the sustained and absolute nature of the submission. Dogs that have developed submissive urination after punishment of excitement urination will often start by being very excited and then show submission when the owner attends to or goes to greet them. This is an attempt to appease an anticipated threat. They may also alternate between excitement and submission in response to owner behaviour. Uncertainty about the owner's reaction in certain situations will also raise levels of anxiety.

Treatment

Owners must avoid using body language and types of contact that promote submission of any kind. If they are already interacting with the dog when it starts to become submissive, then they must withdraw attention, turn away and ignore the dog without showing any anger or irritation.

A clicker method can be very useful for training new greeting behaviour with the lure of food and dogs can be conditioned to remain in a non-submissive posture when touched or spoken to. For example, the dog is given a click

each time it remains sitting and does not submit when touched gently on the head or neck (Box 10.5).

Prognosis

Dogs that have been severely punished have a more guarded prognosis, as do dogs that have other anxiety and fear problems. Otherwise the prognosis is good. Treatment may take several weeks or months according to severity.

Box 10.5   Treatment: submissive urination

- **Never** punish submissive urination.
- Stop all interactions that evoke submission. This may mean stopping all greeting behaviour to begin with.
- If dog begins to show submission then break off interaction.
- When greeting, get closer down to the dog's level and touch the chest or chin rather than top of the body.
- Only show greeting when the dog is not in a submissive posture.
- Condition a new greeting behaviour (using the lure of play or food).
- Condition new responses to touch (see Advice sheet 12 in Appendix 2).

MARKING BEHAVIOUR

Marking involves leaving a signal that acts as a complex 'calling card'. The chemical composition of the urine, which includes both metabolic waste products and pheromonal chemical signals, carries information about identity, gender, reproductive state and health. Both male and female dogs scent-mark in order to announce information about themselves that may help them to maintain territory or secure a mate.

Urine marking is different from other forms of (normal) urination in that:

- frequency is higher
- volume is smaller
- placement is different (the individual chooses places that are likely to be noticed, urinating high up against vertical surfaces in the case of the male dog).

Diagnosis

There are typical situations in which marking occurs:

- Communicative signalling:
  after meeting, seeing or hearing a conspecific (or some times a person)
  territorial boundary marking.
- Emotional:
  response to anxiety or acute frustration.

Intact males tend to mark more often and neutering them will substantially reduce the level of normal territorially and socially motivated scent marking. As with non-sexually motivated mounting behaviour, neutering will not necessarily have any positive effect on marking that is due to anxiety or frustration. In fact, the problem may be worse because some males show more signs of anxiety after neutering. Care should also be taken when deciding to neuter a male that has concurrent intraspecific aggression problems with another male in the same household. Inappropriate neutering may cause greater aggression between the dogs. Any male dog may scent-mark more frequently in the presence of an intact bitch in oestrus.

As would be expected from the function of marking behaviour, intact bitches urine-mark more frequently when they are in oestrus. This urine is loaded with chemicals that announce the bitch's impending availability to mate and it should be cleaned away with a spray containing biological washing powder or liquid mixed with water. This prevents the lingering odour from attracting a garden full of fighting and posturing male dogs. The same method of cleaning is recommended whenever a bitch approaching or in heat urinates in a public place, because the remaining presence of bitch urine odours can give dogs a reason to fight. Neutering a bitch will suppress this pattern of urination. It may also reduce anxiety in cases where anxiety is observed to increase during the onset of oestrus or during pseudopregnancy. Care must be taken to ensure that prolactin levels are low after neutering, either by careful timing of surgery or the judicious use of antiprolactin drugs such as cabergoline.

Dogs that mark for non-communicative purposes, as a response to frustration or anxiety, will not respond to neutering.

Treatment

As mentioned previously, neutering is appropriate for communicative scent marking. Where indoor scent marking is a response to external events such as the presence of other dogs, then the first step is to reduce the number of triggering events:

- Block views of the areas where the trigger stimulus appears.
- Keep windows and exterior doors shut and use music to block out sound.

If the precise stimuli that trigger a scent-marking event can be identified, such as the noise of people talking outside the house or the noise of dogs barking, then it may be possible to desensitise and countercondition the animal to these stimuli. A recording of the noises might be used.

If anxiety is an underlying element, then all factors that contribute to it should be identified:

- Reproductive hormonal status (high follicle stimulating hormone or prolactin levels)
- Metabolic disease (e.g., thyroid dysfunction)
- Pain and debilitation

- Cognitive impairment
- Sound sensitivities and phobias
- Fear or phobia of other dogs, people or other animals
- Conflict between dogs sharing the home or visiting it.

These problems should be dealt with separately. Dog appeasing pheromone (DAP®) is a safe way to help to reduce anxiety and may help to reduce indoor scent-marking behaviour.

Scent marking is a socially suppressible behaviour, so a high-ranking dog within the group may challenge another lower-ranking dog for doing it. Scent-marking dogs are therefore very sensitive to verbal and physical punishment from their owner and will simply shift the timing and pattern of marking to avoid provoking a reaction from the owner. Whatever punishment is used, it must not be connected with the presence of the owner.

Remote forms of punishment may be used but the same problems exist as ever. Punishment should only be just sufficient to interrupt the behaviour without causing fear or distress. If there is an emotional basis to the problem, then fear or anxiety caused by inappropriate punishment will make the situation worse.

If punishment is to be used at all, then it should be combined with rewarding for scent marking that occurs in other more acceptable contexts. Owners may walk their dogs and clicker reinforce them for scent marking in the same places on every walk, or they may set up a series of markers in the garden that indicate places where the dog may spray. To make this easier, it is best to choose and duplicate the kinds of garden objects that the dog has formerly sprayed against. The dog may be walked around the garden several times each day and impassively clicker-reinforced whenever he sprays on the marked objects. The trainer should interact as little as possible during the training, food should not be used as a lure and the trainer must not give any signals that enable the dog to predict and anticipate the click. In this way, the behaviour is likely to become controlled by contextual cues and not related to the presence of the owner.

A good cleaning routine is essential to remove any urine that may attract re-marking by the dog or, more seriously, over-marking by other dogs in the home. A weak solution of biological detergent in water can be applied from a sprayer bottle after any residual urine has been wiped away. Bleach and scented disinfectants should be avoided. As with other elimination problems, heavy wax polish, varnish, waterproof paint and crack sealant should be used to prevent urine soaking into walls, cracks and flooring.

In cases where anxiety is an underlying factor in scent marking, psychoactive drugs may be appropriate, or DAP® may be used (Box 10.6).

Prognosis

Reliable improvements depend upon proper treatment of the factors underlying the problem. Dogs that have used scent marking have a significant risk of recidivism.

Box 10.6   Treatment: urine marking

- Avoid direct punishment.
- Investigate and deal with social and other problems that are the motivation for the behaviour.
- Follow appropriate cleaning routines (not pine disinfectants or bleach).
- Use mild remote punishment to interrupt marking.
- Reward marking in an appropriate outdoor place.

Box 10.7   Treatment: urinary incontinence

- Complete review of health and current treatment (including pain management).
- Neurological investigation of bladder and sphincter function.
- Investigate and treat or correct functional bladder abnormalities.
- Review level of cognition (treat as necessary).
- Change lifestyle to reduce weight if dog is obese.
- Train to eliminate on command so that minimal urine is left in the bladder at rest times.
- If possible, train dog to request to go outside to eliminate.
- Increase number of opportunities to eliminate so that bladder does not become over-full.
- Train dog to use a specific bed that is easily cleaned and washed.
- Consider changing the type of bed so that sleeping posture does not favour leakage.
- Regular urinalysis to detect early signs of reflux cystitis (owner may be provided with stick tests).

INCONTINENCE

Dogs with incontinence are often referred for behavioural therapy. It is quite easy to write off cases of dogs that dribble urine in their sleep or while resting as insignificant. However, incontinence is a life-threatening condition. Many owners will tolerate almost any level of debilitation in their pets but will draw the line at the perceived loss of dignity associated with incontinence.

A very good indication of the way the owner feels about this situation is the time it takes from first noticing incontinence to the date of presentation at the clinic. The owners who wait longest probably have the lowest expectation of successful treatment and are closest to considering euthanasia, which is why they delay seeking treatment. These dogs have very few chances left and may be suffering from a number of other concurrent and contributory medical problems for which the owner has been too scared to seek treatment.

So an elderly dog with cognitive impairment, PU/PD and arthritis should not simply be put onto drugs to improve urinary sphincter competence. This will, at best, offer a temporary solution. This dog is likely to attain full continence for only a few months before a relapse and would be better served by a complete physical and behavioural 'overhaul'. All medical and behavioural issues should be tackled (Box 10.7).

These are perfect examples of the kind of case in which the intervention of a trained veterinary behaviourist can offer the best hope for a good long-term prognosis.

ADVICE SHEETS THAT MAY BE RELEVANT TO THIS CHAPTER

In Appendix 2

3. Reward and punishment
15. House-training
17. Using food rewards for training
18. Food for work
19. Introducing the clicker

Chapter **11**

Canine aggression problems

INTRODUCTION

The main focus of legislation for the control of dogs in the UK has been the protection of the public from dog bites. Unfortunately, dog bite statistics indicate that the majority of attacks are not by unfamiliar dogs but by family pets or dogs that are well-known to the victim. Children are most at risk, with male children having the highest risk of all. The implication is that the behaviour of the victim is an important factor in dog bite attacks and that many bites could be avoided if dog owners were better educated about the behaviour of their own pets.

Most dogs give out a large number of warning signals long before a bite occurs, even if the owner is not aware of them. Owners may not be aware of these signals either because they are ignorant of normal dog behaviour or because the dog's communicative system has been impaired by selective breeding or deliberate surgical alteration (e.g., docking).

The lack of a tail, mobile facial features and a physique that cannot express variations in threatening or submissive behaviour places a dog at a serious disadvantage in its interaction with people and other dogs. Such animals often appear to react suddenly or more violently because they are unable to deliver vivid signals that would normally accompany or precede growling, barking or snapping. Clearly, an inability to display intention, including the delivery of effective appeasement signals, would lead to an increased incidence of conflict, a conclusion that appears to be borne out in evidence of intraspecific aggression in dogs.

'Aggression' is merely a term used to describe a group of behaviours; it does not explain the cause of or motivation for the aggression. It is too easy to talk about an 'aggressive dog', as if aggressiveness is the major feature of an individual dog's personality. In fact, most aggressive dogs are only aggressive for a small part of the time in discrete situations. The rest of the time they may be completely amenable. Aggression is therefore not a diagnosis; it is simply a description of a particular behavioural response to a complex emotional condition.

IMMEDIATE INTERVENTION

Aggressive behaviour can lead to litigation against the owner of the animal, the behaviourist or referring veterinary surgeon. The veterinary practice that is first contacted by the owner of an aggressive dog is under an obligation to provide sensible safety advice to help prevent injury to persons or damage to public property. Owners *must* therefore be given suitable advice at the time of first contact with the practice (e.g., muzzling).

Treatment offers hope of future improvement of behaviour but it may take many months to produce a result. It may be impossible to get an immediate appointment with a suitably qualified behaviourist and so there may be a delay of several weeks between first presentation of the case and the beginning of therapy.

This is a very high-risk period because often the dog has only been brought to the practice because of some serious incident and the risk of further bites or attacks is high.

At the time of first contact, the primary responsibility of the behaviourist or veterinary surgeon is to give advice to prevent risk of injury. Failure to give the right advice at this time is likely to lead to litigation and it must be remembered that claims for dog bite injuries may run into tens or hundreds of thousands of pounds.

One significant factor is that the simple act of asking for help often releases a lot of tension for the owner, which may reduce their vigilance and sense of risk. This increases the probability of further aggressive incidents, at least in the short term. It is therefore vital to counsel owners that they must take appropriate preventative measures.

The significance of barking, growling, lunging, snapping, nipping and biting as part of a continuum of aggressive behaviour must be explained so that the owner fully understands the risk. The targets of all these types of aggressive behaviour (people, children, other animals) and the contexts in which aggression occurs must be identified.

Owners must be advised to use all appropriate measures to prevent risk of injury; for example:

- stop using punishment
- wherever possible, avoid allowing the dog to come into contact with the potential targets of aggression

- where contact with a target is unavoidable, the animal must be supervised by a responsible adult, controlled and muzzled at all times
- situations in which aggression has been seen should be avoided
- where it is impossible to avoid such situations, the dog must be supervised by a responsible adult, under control and muzzled
- check and secure fences to prevent escape from the property
- use locked gates and doors to prevent people or other animals from entering areas where the dog is loose or unsupervised
- remove obvious sources of conflict, such as food bowls, toys and chews that the dog may attempt to guard
- avoid triggering or intensifying aggressive behaviour (punishment, eye contact, sudden or threatening movements).

Muzzling is a very worthwhile safety precaution but dogs must be trained to accept a muzzle or they may become aggressive when one is fitted, or they may persistently try to remove it. Basket muzzles are preferred over close fitting fabric types because they offer the best protection from bites whilst allowing the dog to breath, pant and communicate freely. No muzzle is absolutely secure and, in some cases, double muzzling is required; a fabric muzzle worn under a basket type muzzle. Muzzles should not be used as a substitute for other forms of control and an aggressive dog should not be considered safe to be off leash simply because it is muzzled.

Owners must be made aware of their legal position. In the UK, the Dangerous Dogs Act enables a court to issue a control or destruction order against a dog, as well as fines or other punishment against the owner. This act applies to all types of dog, not just those, like the pit bull terrier, that have been specifically proscribed as 'dangerous'. The court is not obliged to consider any mitigating circumstances (such as illness or provocation), expert opinion or testimony to the dog's character. They are only concerned with the physical and witness evidence that an injury has taken place. In this way, the dog is treated much more like a criminal person but with reduced opportunity for mitigation. Where it is considered a matter of public safety, action under this act may be instigated by the police without a supporting complaint by a member of the public. Again, all that is required is factual evidence of a bite incident which may be provided by a hospital department. Indeed, hospital emergency departments now routinely inform the police of any dog bite injury. There does not need to be a past history or pattern of aggressive behaviour; one incident is enough. An injured party may seek compensation through the civil courts, regardless of whether a criminal prosecution has been successful. An owner may be liable for injury or damage to property consequent to the behaviour of the dog. The personal cost of the consequences of a dog bite may therefore be very serious, in addition to the distress of seeing the harm that a dog has done to someone.

RISK ASSESSMENT AND PROGNOSTICATION

Before treating aggressive dogs, it is essential to make an accurate assessment of previous aggressive behaviour and produce some predictions about future risk and prognosis. Unfortunately, there is inadequate scientific data to provide a reliable means of predicting the likelihood of future bite incidents.

Important questions to consider are:

- Will this dog bite (again)?
- What harm may it do if it does?
- Can the cause for the aggression be treated?
- What ongoing risk will the dog present after treatment?
- Whilst treatment proceeds, can people and animals be kept safe from the dog?
- Are the owners willing and capable of accepting and managing the immediate and long-term risks?

Since so much depends upon the owner's ability to handle and manage the dog, it may not be possible to give an accurate judgment of risk until therapy has begun. This is why follow-up is absolutely essential for these cases (Box 11.1). If the owner is unable to comprehend the risk the dog presents, or is unable to follow simple safety advice, then the risk may be too high for the case to be safely treated (Box 11.2).

TREATMENT VERSUS REFERRAL

There should be no pride attached to the decision of whether or not to treat aggression cases because this is a specialised area of behavioural medicine that carries risk for all involved.

In general practice, the veterinary surgeon's primary responsibility is to make sure that aggression cases are identified as early as possible, that owners are provided with suitable safety advice and that the various options of treatment and referral are made clear. Poor or dangerous advice may be costly to the practice or damage its reputation. Success with aggression cases is unlikely to do anything for a practice other than bring forth more aggression cases.

The same rules apply to behavioural cases as with any other. If diagnosis or treatment are beyond the knowledge and ability of the practitioner, then the case should be referred. Beyond this, there are other indicators that referral may be the best option:

- The owner is unreliable or shows little grasp of the actual risk that their dog presents.
- The dog has inflicted, or is likely to inflict, serious injury to a person.

Box 11.1   Follow-up for risk assessment

- Treatment of aggression cases is absolutely conditional on owners following the advice they are given in the treatment plan.
- At the first consultation the owner must be given a simple set of safety measures to lower risk of further incidents (muzzling, supervision, isolation of the dog from contact with at-risk individuals, etc.)
- The owner should also be set some training tasks to complete.
- With high-risk cases, follow-up should be soon after the initial consultation (within 2–3 weeks).
- Reassessment must concentrate on compliance with the safety measures and the owner's ability to complete the tasks. If the owner has been unable or unwilling to carry out safety measures, this indicates that future risk for this case will be high. This is particularly true if the owner is allowing at-risk individuals, such as children, to be in unsupervised contact with the aggressive dog against safety instructions.
- Treatment should only proceed if the owner can be persuaded to follow advice

---

Box 11.2   Predictability of aggression

Aggression is often labelled as 'unpredictable' when this is rarely the case. Usually there is a discernible pattern to the dog's behaviour:

- Warnings the dog has given (growl, stare, etc.)
- Avoidant behaviour the dog has carried out
- Timing (certain times of day)
- Related to events or activities (territorial trigger, arrival of a visitor, play, grooming, feeding, owner departure from the house, etc.)
- Presence of certain stimuli (a noise, another dog, unfamiliar people, etc.)
- In response to the actions of a person (raised hand, getting dog off sofa, taking food from dog etc.)

To safely treat aggressive dogs, the motivation for every aggressive incident must be thoroughly understood and a pattern of behaviour identified if possible. The owner should be asked to describe what happened at each event and not to interpret what happened. The first priority is to use this information to prevent injury. If attacks were unpredictable, then this would constitute a serious and unavoidable risk that would not be acceptable.

- Vulnerable individuals are involved (children, disabled, elderly).
- Multiple or complex problems are present.
- The risk the animal presents is not easily reduced by obvious changes in management.
- The owner is already awaiting prosecution relating to the aggressive behaviour of their dog.

With a potentially dangerous animal, it is vital that the person who assesses and treats the case is of sufficient calibre and experience. The practice will remain liable if a referral is made to an inexperienced or untrained 'behaviourist' who does not have appropriate insurance and who subsequently gives advice that leads to an injury.

THE SEQUENCE OF AGGRESSIVE BEHAVIOUR

Owners often report that a dog has only just started to become aggressive because it has recently bitten someone, when in fact it has been showing aggressive behaviour such as growling, barking or snapping over a long period. Alternatively, the dog may have been showing avoidant or inhibitory behaviour, the meaning of which has not been understood. In both cases, the final aggressive outburst was predicted by a pattern of preceding behavioural signs.

Once a dog has become aggressively aroused, there is a normal progression from body stiffening, through growling, snarling and snapping to an actual bite (Fig. 11.1). Dogs who bite or snap will have previously shown a large number of less obviously threatening behaviours, such as growling. People either disregard these behaviours or do not understand their significance. In some cases they may actually taunt the dog deliberately or react punitively. The person's reaction will determine whether, next time, the dog shows more intense aggression or gives less warning signals before biting. Of great importance is the fact that any situation where a dog growls is one in which it may go on to bite if the problem is not properly resolved. The

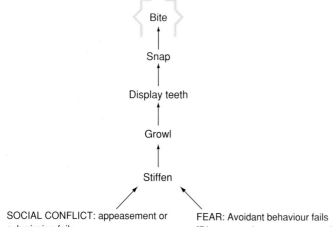

SOCIAL CONFLICT: appeasement or submission fails
[avert gaze, active submission, etc.]

FEAR: Avoidant behaviour fails
[Distance maintenance, escape]

Figure 11.1 Sequence of aggressive behaviour.

owner must therefore not only detail all bite incidents but also all the situations in which the dog growls, snarls or snaps. These will give a much more complete picture of what motivates the aggression, especially if there has been only one incident of an actual bite.

Before becoming aggressive, the dog's initial response to threat may be submissive or avoidant. The dog may show a typical submissive expression or body posture or it may try to escape from the situation. If the dog's attempts to avoid conflict are ignored, the dog will become aggressive. Good examples of this are when a person corners a dog to use physical punishment after the dog has tried to submit or escape, or dogs that roll onto their backs and then snap or bite when a person reaches down to stroke them. This latter example is a typical common misunderstanding of submissive behaviour.

Learning plays an important role in the development of aggressive behaviour. If on previous occasions a dog has shown avoidant or appeasing behaviour in a conflict situation and this was not successful, then this strategy may be abandoned in favour of a more assertive and offensive pattern of aggression. Good history-taking should reveal that the dog's behaviour has changed from predominantly avoidant or submissive to threatening. Dogs may also learn aggression to manipulate the outcome of a situation in their favour. If growling or snarling always causes a person to withdraw, then the dog may use these communications in a wider range of situations in order to control interaction with the person.

CLASSIFICATION OF AGGRESSION

The main motivations for aggression are:

- competition to gain an immediate share of resources or to gain the status that will guarantee permanent control over them
- self-defence or defence of the group
- defence of resources that are already held by the individual or group (including territory).

These motivations exist in every dog but whether they surface as aggression depends on the availability of resources, the dog's traits of personality, its ability to communicate, its experience and the behaviour of social partners (including people).

The classification of aggression is therefore fraught with difficulty, as each individual possesses a mix of self-defencive, resource-guarding or competitive motivations which may have changed or developed over time. Several forms of problem aggression may be seen in the same animal. Rather than label an individual as suffering from territorial aggression, it is therefore more important to understand the motivation for the behaviour and how it developed. For example, the territorial dog may be primarily motivated by a fear of the people it attempts to repel from the border of its territory. This dog may have a history of a fear of people that stretches back to its puppyhood.

Of necessity, this chapter falls into the convention of considering aggression within certain classes but the practitioner must always be aware that only in the simplest cases will the dog fit into one class without aggression in any other circumstance. There are no short cuts and it is essential always to gather a complete history to make sure that other problems are not overlooked.

Predatory behaviour and play-biting do not constitute genuine forms of aggression. If genuine aggression does arise during play then it is probably due to fear, competition or possessiveness and hence dealt with under one of those headings. Predatory behaviour does not involve any communication with the victim, any self-defence or competition with it and is purely a part of hunting behaviour. Play-biting and predatory behaviour are discussed in the chapter on miscellaneous problems.

METHODS OF TREATMENT

General preparation for treatment should include training the dog to perform basic commands such as to sit, lie down and recall, preferably using a clicker method. Generally, unruly dogs may benefit from training of 'no signals', 'play signals', and games that demonstrate owner control over play, such as the games for reducing possessiveness. Information about these methods is included in Appendix 2.

Specific behavioural methods of treatment are desensitisation, counterconditioning and instrumental procedures and are used in the treatment of most aggression cases. The 'come away' command can be trained and then used to control fearful dogs as they encounter situations that might otherwise evoke aggression. Conditioned punishment, such as the use of a rattle can or training discs, may also be used to disrupt aggressive behaviour as it commences so that more desirable behaviour can be commanded and then reinforced. Unconditioned punishment, such as hitting or shouting at dogs, or punishment that produces fear and stress have no place in the treatment of any behavioural problem although it may be difficult to persuade clients not to punish their dogs in these ways in the heat of the moment. There may also be considerable peer-pressure from friends or human victims of aggression that the dog should be physically punished for its misdemeanours. Clients must be convinced to resist such pressure because the aim is to treat the dog and not to make its problems worse.

FEAR-RELATED AGGRESSION

For a description of behavioural signs of fear see the section in Chapter 3 on canine communication. Fear is at the root of many aggression problems and expressions of fear are often seen in possessive or so-called 'dominance' aggression cases. Unfortunately, fear is often overlooked as an underlying motivational or maintaining factor in aggression cases which means that they are inappropriately treated and people may be injured (Box 11.3). It is therefore

Box 11.3　Immediate action: fear-related aggression
Owners must take the following actions:

- Identify all fear-eliciting events and stimuli.
- Take measures to avoid these events and stimuli.
- Keep the dog under complete control and supervision whenever encountering the fear-eliciting event or stimulus.
- Stop using a choke chain.
- Introduce a face harness (Halti®, Gentle Leader®) in conjunction with a half-check collar. The leash must be attached to BOTH for security.
- Train the dog to wear a muzzle, which may then be used to further increase safety in unavoidable situations where aggression may arise.
- If the dog is fearful of people, do not allow them to try to befriend the dog using food treats or try to interact with it in any other way.
- Do not threaten or punish the dog when it is frightened or aggressive (this may cause redirected aggression or increase fearfulness).

important not to take a superficial view of aggression cases based upon the most obvious features of the dog's behaviour or the owner's interpretation of events.

When recording information about aggression cases, it is important to get witnesses of the events to describe the precise posture and signalling used by the dog. Very often there is a gradual change in behaviour over the course of a number of incidents such that fearful behaviour is very much more obvious in the earliest ones. In the later incidents, the dog's actions may be much less hesitant or avoidant because it has learned that there is nothing to be gained from delaying a full-on aggressive assault.

As mentioned previously, aggression is most commonly expressed towards fear-evoking stimuli when avoidant or appeasing behaviour has failed. Typically, the dog has shown this type of non-confrontational behaviour on more than one occasion, but each time the threat has persisted or increased. The dog may actually have been harmed as a result of attempting to avoid conflict. Alternatively, the dog has been attacked without warning and therefore it has been unable to mitigate the threat through its own behaviour. Lastly, many dogs change from avoidant to more offensive behaviour as they reach maturity. Whilst young they may be reluctant to socialise with people or other dogs, trying to avoid interaction by running away or hiding behind the owner or a conspecific. As the dog matures, these puppy-like behaviours are replaced with adult attempts at self-defence. As an adult, the dog cannot rely on others in its group to defend it, so the burden is on the individual to defend itself. Instead of retreating the dog may then resort to attack.

There is a considerable variation of breed-specific response to threat or fear, which leads to a misunderstanding of the behaviour of certain breeds of dog. Terriers are very often labelled as dominant because they appear to be very confrontational and bold. In fact, terriers simply have a different response to fear. Many terrier types have been selectively bred to have traits such as 'gameness' and tenacity and they are expected to deal with aggressive prey at close quarters. In situations of fear, such as when handled in the veterinary practice, these dogs may react aggressively. Experimentally, this breed difference in behaviour has been demonstrated. When presented with a novel and fear-eliciting stimulus, certain breeds favoured inhibited behaviour and might even become catatonic if sufficiently frightened (e.g. a beagle); but a range of terrier-type dogs showed the opposite reaction, becoming highly aroused and agitated. We see this often in terrier-type dogs with sound sensitivity problems. Rather than hide, as most dogs do, they run around and bark.

Other breed-specific behaviour is also important. Collies and other herding-type dogs will often fall back onto herding behaviour when frightened. They will herd and dart at the thing that frightens them, perhaps nipping and lunging at it. A good example is the collie who jumps at and tries to chase traffic, joggers and cyclists.

Dogs with fear-related aggression often have a history of a lack of socialisation and habituation to environmental stimuli during the sensitive period or they have experienced lengthy periods of isolation when they did not come into contact with people, noise, complex environments or other animals. They often have a number of fear-related problems, such as sound sensitivity, which have a direct impact on the fear aggression problem. The noise-sensitive dog may, for example, be more aggressive or fearful in certain environments where there is a background of noise. Exposure to sensitising contexts such as a noisy or busy training class may encourage the development of complex fear problems (Box 11.4).

Box 11.4   Prevention of fear–related aggression

- Puppies must not be reared in a non-domestic environment.
- Dogs should experience a wide range of social contact with different people and other animals from the earliest age to maturity.
- They must be exposed to a full range of domestic and environmental stimuli (noises, objects, locations).
- The presence of people should be always be associated with reward.
- Owners should avoid exposing immature dogs to situations where they may be attacked by people or other animals.
- Dogs should not be forced to confront situations that they find frightening.
- Verbal punishment should be just forceful enough to stop behaviour, never enough to elicit fear.
- Physical punishment must never be used.

Diagnosis

Fear can be seen in the characteristic pattern of avoidance behaviour, body language and facial expression. The body may be hunched or crouched so as to appear smaller and less threatening. A fearful dog may snarl or growl but, typically, the gaze is averted and side teeth displayed. Ears will be flattened and head held low. The dog will try to move away from the threat if this is possible. If it is confined, then it may try to repel the threat by lunging forward and retreating whilst barking or snapping.

Dogs with fear-related aggression will show observable signs of fear at the time of presentation or during the early stages of developing a problem. Behaviour becomes more complex and less easy to identify as fearful as it is affected both by learning and experience.

Treatment

The method of treatment of all fear problems is essentially the same, depending as it does on desensitisation and counterconditioning. Using fear-related aggression towards people as an example, the process is as follows:

- Identify the general class of target (in this example 'unfamiliar people').
- Grade the response to target according to appearance or behaviour. Some dogs are more aggressive towards men or children and may react differently according to their clothing, what the person is carrying or how they are moving. List all those features which affect the dog's response so that they can be introduced during training.
- The dog is then trained to adopt a calm state on cue in a range of different contexts when the fear-eliciting stimulus is *not* present; this includes those where the stimulus would typically be encountered. This training may be combined with a 'come away' signal so that the dog learns to look away from the thing of which it is fearful and come to the owner where it will be rewarded for remaining calm.
- Find a group of willing volunteers who will be able to act as stooges for training.
- Training is begun with the least fear- and aggression-evoking examples of the class, at a distance which does not trigger aggression. For more information on this see Chapter 8.
- Each time the stooge appears at a distance, the dog is given a game or a handful of food. This begins with the person at a distance that normally does not evoke any aggression. After a number of repetitions, the dog should show positive anticipation of play or food when the person appears at this distance.
- The training is repeated with a number of stooges at a gradually decreasing distance.
- An instrumental procedure may now be introduced in which the dog is rewarded for performing the 'come

away' command that has already been trained. The dog is repeatedly rewarded whilst it stays sitting and calm throughout the period that the person is present.

- Over a number of sessions, that person is brought closer, making sure that, at no point, fear or aggressive arousal is elicited. They may also walk or run around faster, make noises, move about or carry items in a way that would previously have evoked more fear and aggression. These changes are introduced gradually, systematically and with sufficient distance to avoid aggression or fear.
- Training only continues with other progressively more fear-eliciting persons as the dog ceases to respond to the less evocative ones.

Training may be used in real-world situations only once the dog is fully counterconditioned not to respond to any of the previous triggers for aggression as simulated by the volunteers must, and in any case, proceed with immense caution.

Advice sheet 9, with instructions for training a 'come away' command, is included in Appendix 2.

By identifying the elements of a person's appearance that the dog responds to, it is possible to do a lot of training with a limited number of volunteers who can be dressed or disguised. Above all, in this example, it is important to note that 'unfamiliarity' is an element of the fear so the volunteers must not try to befriend the dog at any stage during training. Familiar individuals may be used during training only if they can be disguised or kept at a distance so that the dog cannot recognise them.

The person training the dog must not give praise or reassurance when the dog becomes aggressive; instead they must try to control the dog using the commands that have been taught. The tone of voice must remain the same throughout, never becoming threatening. Clicker-training is a very useful method of training to use because the click is identical on each occasion and does not carry any emotional complication. It is also easy to give repeated clicks and food rewards whilst the dog remains calm, each click pinpointing a rewarded behaviour which will be recorded in the dog's memory.

This process of training can be lengthy, especially with severe cases. Owners must be prepared for months of hard work which also requires considerable follow-up. The clinician must be confident that the owner will not take risks and that their coordination, timing and control of the dog is perfect. Some practitioners work with rehabilitation trainers who specialise in supervising these kinds of training sessions and can offer more cost-effective support in conjunction with the supervising behaviourist.

DAP® may be used to assist therapy for fearful dogs but its effects are limited by the diffusion of the pheromone chemical. Drugs such a selegiline may be used to reduce apprehension or to increase confidence in dogs that have become inhibited. Drugs should always be used with care in aggression due to the risk of disinhibition and of increasing the dog's confidence to carry out an aggressive attack (Box 11.5).

Box 11.5   Treatment of fear-related aggression

- Explain to the owner the signs of fearful arousal and other behaviours that will enable them to understand and predict the dog's behaviour more effectively.
- Avoid fear-eliciting situations.
- Identify and grade the stimuli and events that evoke fear.
- Desensitise and countercondition the dog to fear-inducing stimuli and events, starting with stimuli that evoke the least response.
- Train a 'come away' command and teach the owner to use this to control the dog during training, once initial desensitisation and counterconditioning are complete.
- Identify contexts and other stimuli that contribute to raised fearful arousal.
- Desensitise and countercondition the dog to these contexts and stimuli.

Prognosis

This depends to a large extent on the owner's expectation. It should be possible to reduce expressions of fearful aggression to the point at which the dog appears to react normally and non-aggressively in most circumstances. Whether it will be possible for the dog to interact directly and at close range with the things it fears, without any risk of aggression, is more difficult to assess at the outset and is easier to judge as treatment progresses.

As with other aggression problems, a poorer prognosis is associated with dogs that become aggressive more rapidly and with less warning, and with longer standing cases. Dogs that begin to show overtly aggressive behaviour before reaching maturity also have a poor prognosis.

STATUS-RELATED AGGRESSION

The term *dominance* has generally been applied to this class of aggression, which is something of a misnomer because dominance and aggression do not automatically go hand-in-hand. In wild and feral canine groups there is a need for order. The whole group contributes to maintaining territory, finding food and catching it but without some kind of hierarchy, there would also be constant competition for mating rights or the spoils of a hunting expedition. The solution dogs have adopted is a kind of hierarchy with separate male and female lines within the group. This avoids direct competition between the two genders which would threaten the long-term survival of the species. At the head of this social structure are an alpha male and alpha female. These individuals are described as dominant because others submit or defer to them in situations of conflict. The popular misconception is that canid society, especially that of wolves, is filled with conflict and fighting when they are, in fact, altogether more complex and cooperative.

This idea that 'dominance' is achieved by aggression and force perhaps reflects our own attitudes towards hierarchical relationships more than it does the situation in canine social groups. In fact, successful leadership within the canine group is only guaranteed to those individuals who have the greatest social ability.

The successful male dog is therefore the one that has proven its physical strength during play, mock fights and minor battles with other dogs. At the same time, this dog will have made alliances with many members of the group who have accepted its pre-eminence in exchange for gaining a share of the resources they need. An unnecessarily brutal and competitive individual who tries to monopolise resources is very unlikely to achieve significant rank because it will have few supporters when a genuine conflict emerges. Instead, it may be mobbed, injured or driven out.

There are costs and benefits from holding the highest rank. The main cost comes from the effect of stress on health; dominant dogs suffer more disease and die younger. The main advantage to being an alpha dog is to have reproductive rights within the group. So there is a trade to be made; a short life but offering the greatest opportunity for transmission of genetic information to the next generation. For the lower-ranking individuals there are advantages too. They benefit from the stability and lack of day-to-day competition within the group. They may live longer, they may achieve higher rank later, when they may mate and produce offspring and, because they are closely related to the highest-ranking dogs, a proportion of their genes will be carried forward to future generations by the successful matings of the dominant dog. In order to benefit from this situation, high-ranking dogs need to make sure that they are in the best position to capitalise on their mating rights so they take conflict with other dogs very seriously. One misjudged fight could easily destroy the mating potential of a high-ranking dog that has spent its whole life trying to achieve status. So a well-fed high-ranking dog will not pick a fight over food with a lower-ranking but hungry one, just to assert itself.

Of course, fighting is seen in dog groups. Beta-rank members often act as enforcers, controlling access to the alpha members and defending their own position in the group. Below them there will be constant vying for rank. However, these dogs have known each other all their lives and they have gained a very good understanding of each other's strengths and weaknesses through play, mock fights and observation of fights between other dogs. There is no need to fight constantly.

There *are* situations in which high-ranking dogs do get involved in genuine physical conflict. However, these are not merely fights or brawls; they are highly structured and both participants have a multitude of communicative opportunities to diffuse the situation or break off the battle with little cost to themselves. Both animals are well aware of the cost of raising the intensity of the conflict and much of the 'fight' is actually a display that is designed to intimidate rather than injure.

So hierarchical relationships in dog groups are a way to create a cooperative social order, which holds a group together and enables the needs of individuals to be met. It is also a way of supporting the diversity of hunting skills, sociability and other behaviours that are needed through changing environmental stresses. If we look at our relationships with dogs from this standpoint, it is perhaps easier to understand how things have gone wrong and what needs to be done to resolve situations in which competitive and status-related problems have developed. Rather than talk in terms of dominance, it is better to consider status and competition. The boundary between competition and status-related problems is a subtle one. For competition to exist, there merely have to be resources which two individuals value highly enough to compete for them. The issue of status emerges when the overall pattern of the dog's behaviour indicates that it perceives its rank entitles it to control over certain situations and resources. People may be entirely unaware that they are providing the dog with inappropriate information about its rank, or indeed that a rank relationship is developing, until it is too late. Once the dog perceives its relative status to be high, then it may not accept certain classes of interaction because these have a symbolic meaning within a status relationship. People may unwittingly fall foul of this, which leads to dangerous conflict (Box 11.6).

Diagnosis

Cases should be assessed to rule out more basic motivations for the behaviour before suspecting an issue of status; above all looking for signs of fear within the current behav-

---

Box 11.6 Immediate action: status–related aggression

- Identify situations in which conflict occurs.
- Identify and protect at-risk individuals. Isolate them from conflict with the dog.
- Stop confrontation.
- Stop punishment.
- Stop provocation.
- If there is a family member to whom no status-related aggression is shown, then that person must be responsible for controlling and looking after the dog. This person must always be present if the dog is with other people.
- This person may train the dog to accept a muzzle so that it may be muzzled in any risky situation where exclusion of the dog is impossible.

iour or during its development. Status need not be involved if the dog only shows aggression whilst competing for or defending a single type of resource. If the devotion to controlling that resource seems excessive, then this may be indicative that other medical or behavioural problems exist. For example, a medical condition that might increase hunger, or an over-attachment to one human individual whose attention is monopolised and guarded from others in the house (Box 11.7).

Status-related aggression should only be diagnosed if the dog shows a consistent pattern of controlling behaviour which is not linked to previous punitive confrontations with the owner. There should also be a consistently expressed pattern of dominant body postures and communications from the dog, which have *not* evolved from earlier fearful ones.

Status-related aggression may be indicated by a consistent pattern of:

- unidirectional social contact: the dog initiates and demands attention or other forms of social contact but objects when 'lower-ranking' individuals attempt to initiate an interaction
- confident aggressive display: head held high, body rigid and erect, direct staring eye contact with erect and forward-facing ears, incisors and canines bared
- attempts to adopt dominant postures over people: e.g., standing over someone whilst growling
- aggressive responses to human interactions that might symbolise a challenge to the dog's status (eye contact, leaning over the dog, hugging the dog, stroking or placing hands on the head, neck and back of the dog)

> **Box 11.7   Preventing status-related problems**
>
> - Control the resources the dog needs without excessively restricting access to them or competing for them.
> - Initiate activities (play, feeding, attention giving) very regularly and on your own terms without forcing the dog to demand them.
> - Do not respond to demands.
> - Do not use force to take food or toys away from the dog.
> - Do not play excessively physical games that give the dog information about your strengths and weaknesses. Play should always involve a toy.
> - Play should be cooperative, allowing the dog to win some of the time, but ultimately ending with the person terminating play in possession of the toy.
> - Give clear signals at the beginning and end of play so that frustration is avoided.
> - Do not use physical punishment because this creates fear and mistrust. It also teaches the dog to engage in a form of conflict. Ultimately all dogs have better weaponry than we do and they are confident to use it.

- control of access to space: e.g., aggressive response when moved, stepped over or asked to leave a particular place
- aggressive responses to interference in its activities: aggressive when pulled away from or interrupted whist carrying out activities
- aggressive control of a wide range of resources.

It is therefore absolutely essential to gather objective information about the problem. Many owners can only interpret what has happened in terms of dominance because this is the only term that they have heard. Detailed notes must be made of all of the aggressive incidents in which injury has occurred. All other situations in which agonistic signalling has occurred (aggressive growling, barking, snarling, etc.) should be listed and the dog's behaviour and body language throughout the incidents should be detailed (facial and body postures, eye contact, reaction after the incident is over).

Status-related aggression should only be considered where there is an existing relationship between the dog and the persons involved. Opposition to control in stressful situations, such as at the veterinary clinic, is not a sign of dominance and is merely an expression of self-defence.

Treatment

In a status problem, the dog enforces a set of rules and has a scale of responses to their infringement. The first step is therefore to define the circumstances in which aggression is seen and all of the various triggering events. This provides a basis for avoiding confrontation with the dog and increases safety. Punishment and confrontation must be stopped.

The dog's perception of its status is dependent on symbolic behaviours that indicate control, which may be manipulated by us to alter the balance of power in the relationship.

Rules of interaction must be:

- The dog is taught basic obedience commands such as 'sit' and 'lie down'.
- The person must not respond to any of the dog's demands (for play, attention, food, etc.), no matter how solicitous the dog becomes. Instead, the person gives a signal that tells the dog that it is being ignored.
- Every day the dog must be given many opportunities to obey one of the basic obedience commands in order to get food, attention or some other interaction. If it does not respond, then the person ignores the dog and withholds the reward. All members of a household must behave in the same way.
- It is very important to start by training the dog to respond to the signals that are going to be used because this reduces the potential for frustration and irritability. A typical way of doing this is to use the

clicker-training method indicated in Advice sheet 11, Appendix 2, about attention-seeking and the 'no' signal. This trains the dog to leave a person alone, using a clear signal that has been conditioned as part of a game that the dog can easily understand and enjoy.

- At no point should food or attention be offered to the dog as a lure in order to encourage it to comply with a command. The dog is likely to see an outstretched hand holding a treat as an invitation to compete for a resource that the person is deliberately withholding and aggression may be the result. Instead, the person should call the dog and ask it to do something before making any move to provide the reward. Clicker-training offers an ideal method of training these dogs without offering lures or using physical contact.

If the dog is aggressive when handled or moved, a houseline may be employed to enable persons to control the dog's movements without presenting a challenge (see Advice sheet 1 in Appendix 2). The use of a houseline should be supported with reward-based training to reinforce responses to commands that enable the person to control the dog without confrontation. This might include training the dog to get up, move on and off chairs or in and out of the house on command. In all cases, the commands must be delivered in the same relaxed tone of voice without any threat or anger which might signal conflict. Once again, clicker-training is an effective method of teaching these commands as it does not involve using food as a lure or any kind of physical contact which might place the person at risk of being harmed.

If the dog is amenable to play and does not interpret any part of play behaviour as a threat, then this may be another important activity to control. Owners may employ the methods included in Advice sheet 8, Appendix 2, so that the dog learns to respond to the person's emotional signals. Owners should be encouraged to learn and use playful meta-communications, such as the play bow, to initiate and maintain play.

If there are specific stimuli or events that trigger an aggressive response, then these should be carefully desensitised and counterconditioned (Box 11.8).

Prognosis

Indicators of high risk or poor prognosis include:

- dogs that have inflicted serious injury or may do so in the future
- dogs that give little warning or which progress to an attack very rapidly
- the presence of at-risk individuals (children, elderly, disabled), especially where they are the main target for the aggression
- dogs that appear to behave in a provocative manner, deliberately setting up situations over which they may aggressively take control
- dogs that control the person's movement about the home and may therefore place them at risk during an emergency
- owners who behave inconsistently or who cannot resist using punishment or confrontation.

Most dogs with status problems are actually quite willing to accept a change of status, as long as access to resources remains adequate and predictable. In fact, many of these dogs are less anxious and stressed when their rank has been properly confirmed.

Box 11.8 Treatment of status–related aggression

- Avoid confrontation (staring, pushing the dog around or using stern commands).
- Do not use punishment.
- Stop responding to demands for interaction (feeding, play, attention). This may involve teaching a non-confrontational 'no' signal, as described in Advice sheet 11, Appendix 2.
- People must start and end all interactions. They must ask the dog for an act of obedience before interacting with the dog, allowing it access to a resource or giving something it wants.
- All interactions must be ended with a non-confrontational signal that tells the dog that the interaction is over.
- Use houselines and other methods to retain control over the dog in key situations.
- Restrict access to privilege (depends on individual case): do not allow the dog onto furniture, into bedrooms, etc.
- Train the dog to obey a wide range of commands so that it can be told to go in and out of the house, or get on and off furniture without perceiving this to be a confrontation.
- Exercise control over all of the dog's behaviour by using commands.
- Introduce and use a face harness (Halti®, Gentle Leader®) in combination with a half-check collar. The leash should be attached to BOTH for security. This kind of harness provides greater control.
- Desensitise and countercondition responses to triggers for aggression (with extreme caution).
- If the dog stares at, or otherwise begins to threaten a person, it should immediately be called away.
- Due to the risk of disinhibition, drug therapy should not be considered for this condition, other than under the direct supervision of a veterinary behaviourist.

Cases must be followed up very regularly (monthly, followed by 2-monthly) to reassess risk and make sure that owners are applying the plan correctly. Owners must report to the person supervising the case if there is any concern that the training methods are increasing the risk of aggression.

Owners must be aware that they can never revert to the way they behaved before because the dog must always have its rank confirmed by their behaviour.

A minority of dogs with status problems are not willing to accept a lower rank. These dogs may constantly seek to test or circumvent the new rules and will actively seek to create new opportunities to assert themselves. This may be because people have been inconsistent in the past and the dog has not built up enough experience of the new rules for it to accept them as permanent. It may be because the owner is not actively offering opportunities to interact or gain access to resources in exchange for deference, so the dog's needs are not being met. If the owner's implementation of the behavioural modification plan is not at fault and the dog is genuinely unwilling to accept a change of status and is becoming more aggressive, then euthanasia may be indicated.

REDIRECTED AGGRESSION

When aggressively aroused, the dog is in a self-protective state and ready to repel a threat from whatever origin. In some cases, the dog will direct its aggression to a target other than the original stimulus that caused the aggressive arousal. This we call 'redirected aggression'.

There may be several factors underlying apparently 'redirected' aggression:

Overwhelming motivation for self-defence: the dog mistakenly treats the target of its redirected aggression as if it were part of the assumed threat.

Frustration: the target of the redirected aggression in some way limits or interferes with the dog's ability to carry out self-defensive behaviour. For example, the owner restricts the dog's movement using a collar and leash or directly intervenes in a fight.

Fearful association: the target of the redirected aggression has previously threatened the dog in similar situations and is therefore perceived to be part of the threat. For example, owners who have hit or shouted at a dog whilst it has been defending itself in a similar situation, or who generally apply strongly punitive methods of control and discipline.

It is therefore important to analyse all the situations in which the dog has carried out redirected aggression.

Redirected aggression is a common complicating factor in other forms of aggression and the risk it presents should be assessed before treatment of other aggression problems begins. It is not safe for owners to carry out training for an inter-dog aggression problem if their dog may, at some time, threaten to cause them serious injury (Box 11.9).

Diagnosis

In redirected aggression, the dog becomes aggressively aroused by a stimulus or target other than the person that it attacks. Initially, the aggression is directed towards the stimuli that caused the aggressive arousal, but rapidly this switches to the person exerting control or attempting to punish the dog. Redirected aggression involves a significant amount of learning and the dog may begin to show aggression towards the handler in anticipation of threat from them, based on previous experiences (Box 11.10).

Treatment

The precise kind of provocation for the redirected attack is important. If the owner can avoid performing the triggering behaviour, then the situation may be safe to do training to desensitise and countercondition the dog to the stimuli that provoke aggressive arousal. However, if merely by restricting the dog on a leash the owner becomes the target of its fury, then training will be hampered unless the dog can be made safe (such as by being muzzled).

To prevent redirected aggression, owners must avoid interfering in fights and the use of physical punishment. Either will lead the dog to consider the person to be a potential part of the threat.

The main form of aggression must be identified and treated without placing anyone at risk. Situations in which

---

Box 11.9   Immediate action: redirected aggression

- Identify all situations in which redirected aggression occurs.
- Avoid these situations until the dog can be safely controlled or has been muzzled.
- Stop using a choke chain.
- Introduce a face harness (Halti®, Gentle Leader®) in conjunction with a half-check collar. The leash must be attached to BOTH for security.
- Train the dog to accept a muzzle and put this on well before any triggering situation is encountered.
- Do not try to apply a muzzle when the dog is aggressively aroused or is about to become so.
- Stop punishment.

Box 11.10   Prevention of redirected aggression

- Treat fear and other aggression problems as soon as they appear.
- Do not use threats, punishment or coercion to stop aggressive behaviour.
- Do not use painful methods of control such as choke chains.
- Do not use painful methods of training such as shock collars.
- Do not encourage territorial behaviour of any kind.

redirected aggression occurs should be avoided. Once the stimuli that elicit aggression have been identified, these should be carefully desensitised and counterconditioned.

Prognosis

The prognosis is good as long as the underlying aggression problems can be treated and the owner ceases all punishment. Dogs that have begun to redirect their aggression towards nearby persons who have made no attempt to control or punish them, have a poor prognosis. They may require very little provocation to redirect aggression. Dogs that present a significant risk of inflicting serious injury also have a poor prognosis.

POSSESSIVE AGGRESSION

Dogs may try to retain possession of objects or food for a number of different reasons. These may be divided into two groups, according to where the value of the object lies:

1. **Item has intrinsic value**: The object has some value which is independent of any social interaction. These are generally survival resources such as edible food items or locations where they may be found.
2. **Item has extrinsic value**: The object has no intrinsic value but possession of it may be a means of eliciting play or attention, or of demonstrating social status and control

The strength of motivation to possess the object depends upon the level of the intrinsic or extrinsic value it holds, which is in turn affected by other factors. For example, a dog that is suffering from a medical disorder which increases hunger will be more likely to guard food. Sudden

---

Box 11.11 Immediate action: possessive aggression

- Avoid sources of conflict: hide toys, tidy away things the dog may steal, do not give high-value chews or food items that the dog may guard.
- Do not allow at-risk individuals (children, disabled, elderly people) to approach the dog when it has something that it may guard.
- Supervise the dog at all times when it is with people who may be at risk.
- If there is aggression around food, give several smaller low-value meals each day and do not handle or approach the dog while it is eating.
- Do not punish or challenge the dog while it is eating or guarding an object.
- Do not try to take objects away unless the dog is at risk of seriously harming itself and you are willing to accept that you may be bitten.

---

changes of this type should be regarded as a potential sign of illness. Conversely, owners should be warned that polyphagic dogs with a history of food-guarding may become more determined not to give up stolen or scavenged food items.

The extrinsic value an item holds is generally learned through interactions with other individuals. In dogs of less than 5–6 months of age, the extrinsic value of items is primarily concerned with attracting play or attention. These young dogs often learn that people will show an interest in them when they pick up a particular item. The dog is incapable of discriminating between its own toys and other items around the home; it merely discriminates between them on the basis of the person's response. Mature dogs may place value on an object according to the attention that possessing it commands, but also because retaining possession of it may symbolise status or control over other individuals that are equally determined to take it away.

The dog may thoroughly enjoy being chased around the home as the owner tries to get the TV remote control back, which is rewarding. Even the fact that the previously disinterested owner has started to pay attention to the dog will be enough to reward the behaviour. This situation may develop into the basis for a severe behavioural problem. If, when the item is finally taken away from the dog, it is physically punished then this will instil fear. The dog will not understand why a previously playful situation has ended with threats, especially if it has used appeasement and playful meta-communication throughout. Alternatively, the dog may come to regard possession of the object as the only reliable means of prolonging interaction with the owner, so it becomes highly determined not to give it up.

Actual loss of the object is therefore associated with two punishing experiences: the end of interaction with the owner (a form of negative punishment) and some kind of chastisement (positive punishment). In some cases, the motivation to hold onto the object is purely fearful because the dog anticipates punishment as soon as it gives the object up. The motivation to hold onto the object and thereby avoid this situation will be very intense.

As the dog matures, other factors come into play. At around 6 months of age, dogs may start to compete with conspecifics and people over food objects. At this age dogs are becoming independent and would, in a feral situation, begin to take over the task of feeding themselves. They would naturally come into competition with conspecifics and there is therefore an expectation that anyone approaching them while they are eating may, in fact, have the intention of taking the food away. Many owners will deliberately take away food bowls and chews if a dog growls at them but, unfortunately, this merely reinforces the dog's motivation to guard.

Food is a survival resource and some dogs can become extremely aggressive in food-guarding situations. Thus, extrinsic value has been added to a resource that was already valuable enough and the dog has learned to regard people as potential competitors for resources. This problem can be entirely avoided if owners regularly go to their puppies to give them titbits while they are already consuming food, but this routine must be maintained from a few weeks of age right through to maturity.

As dogs approach maturity, their response to threat also changes. There is a transition from appeasement and withdrawal to aggression. If owners have punished a submissive puppy when taking an object away from it, this dog may start to show overtly aggressive behaviour in the same situations when it reaches maturity.

When assessing these problems, it is also vital to see or get a good description of the dog's behaviour when it is guarding the object or food and details of a number of similar incidents throughout the dog's life. This will help to indicate whether the dog is behaving competitively or through fear. In most cases, there will be avoidance or fear-related behaviours which are an indication that the dog perceives the situation as threatening. If the dog also shows appeasement or avoidance to certain gestures, such as a raised hand, this indicates that punishment has been used. Sadly, dogs can learn this kind of response even after only one punitive incident. Dealing with the fear, anxiety and loss of trust involved in these cases is important (Box 11.11).

Diagnosis

Food-related possessiveness

It should be obvious that food is being guarded but, in fact, often the owner is not aware of the connection between the presence of food and aggression. This is especially true if the dog has been guarding food that has been dropped, stolen or hidden. Food-related possessiveness should be suspected if aggression often occurs at times when people have food that might be dropped. Children often drop or lose possession of food, which the dog then immediately begins to guard (Box 11.12).

Object possession

Similar comments apply as in food-related possessiveness (Box 11.13).

Box 11.13 Prevention of object guarding

- Create structured play activities for the dog.
- Limit access to interactive toys (toys that people use to play games with their dog). These must be brought out and offered by the owner, as a solicitation to play. After play they must be put away.
- Play must involve the dog repeatedly giving up the toy to get a food reward and continuation of play.
- If the dog will not drop, then play must end and the person should walk away and ignore the dog.
- This works even better if several people are involved. If the dog will not give up the toy then play is continued between the people with another toy and the dog is ignored. To rejoin the game the dog must give up possession of the toy it has. In this way possession of a toy immediately devalues it.
- Games should end with the dog having a small chew or some food treats.

Box 11.12 Prevention of food-related aggression

- Give weaning puppies multiple food bowls distributed around the nest area so that the perceived value of food resources is low and competition does not occur.
- Right from the moment a puppy joins the family, owners should regularly approach it whilst it is eating to give additional titbits. This routine should continue from puppyhood until maturity.
- People must never take food bowls or chews away if the dog growls at them and must not scold the dog for doing so.
- If the dog steals and tries to eat something potentially damaging to it then minimal force must be used to get the item away. The dog should be given another (better) food item as a replacement immediately after giving it up.
- Offer advice on potential food-related problems at puppy classes and 6-month health check.

Treatment

All situations that lead to possessive aggression must be identified and, where possible, avoided. Steps should be taken to assess and to reduce risk.

Items that have high intrinsic value must be devalued or removed. This might mean feeding a bland and less desirable diet in several smaller, and hence less valuable, meals or not giving highly-prized chews such as rawhide or bones. Objects that are likely to be stolen or guarded must not be left around for the dog to pick up.

Aggression around the food bowl

Any medical motivating factors should be investigated. In young dogs, persistent gastrointestinal parasitism or disease are potential issues as they may affect hunger or absorption of nutrients from the gut. As an immediate safety measure, the dog may be fed away from contact with people or other animals. Indeed, where there is competition between animals over food it is best to feed them separately anyway.

Owners must stop confrontation over food and give the dog several smaller meals of a diet that it finds less attractive. Dried food of low palatability is often the best choice.

In mild cases where there have been no bites, no punishment and the dog shows growling only as it eats, ignoring the dog and not reacting to it may cause the problem to subside. Where growling is intense or the dog turns away from its food to growl or bark at a person, but there have been no bites or any signs that there might be an attack, then the method described in Advice sheet 4, Appendix 2, may be followed.

Where the dog is targeting vulnerable individuals, has already bitten or has started to guard space around its feeding area, this should be regarded as serious and expert help should be sought.

Aggression over food outside the bowl (chews, stolen food items, etc.)

The nutritional and health status of the animal should be checked. If scavenging and stealing has begun suddenly or started in a mature dog, disease should be suspected, especially if signs of endocrine disease, PU/PD or polyphagia are present.

If the dog aggressively guards chews that have been given by the owner, then these should either be withdrawn or reduced to such a size that they may be consumed in less than 2 minutes. The dog can then be given chews when it is on its own in the garden.

The value of chews may be reduced by giving ones the dog is less enthusiastic about or by cutting down their size and increasing the number of smaller chews given over the course of the day. If the dog regularly hides food items and then guards the location where they are stashed, then they must not be given again.

The dog should be taught a 'leave command' (see Advice sheet 20, Appendix 2) and a drop command using a range of objects. The leave command is used to prevent the dog from picking things up. Once the dog will drop toys and other objects in order to get a food reward, this may be extended to low-value food items. The dog is asked to drop the item, given a food reward when it complies and then given the item back. The food reward that is given must be of higher intrinsic value to the dog than the food item it has to give up. In this way, the dog learns that giving up the item does not mean permanently losing out and is, in fact, the key to gaining access to even better food treats.

This can then be extended to more and more contentious items. The clicker method is particularly useful for this kind of training as it is possible to click to pinpoint the exact moment when the item is dropped so that the act of dropping is rewarded.

Some dogs will have become sensitised to eye contact as a gesture of threat, or may associate certain verbal signals or tone of voice with impending threat. For these dogs, it is important to start training using a new command and using no sustained eye contact. It may help if the dog is given a large amount of conventional reward-based training of basic obedience commands in which eye contact is made only at the time when a reward is being given.

Object (non-food) possession

First, the original motivation to possess the object must be identified; this will involve a description of a large number of incidents tracing back to the beginning of the problem.

If the motivation was originally to get attention or play, then the object may be devalued by giving the dog alternative methods for getting these rewards and by controlling play (see Advice sheet 8 in Appendix 2).

A large amount of time should be spent training the dog to retrieve items on command and to drop them at the person's feet so that this becomes a routine part of the dog's repertoire. Once the dog understands the 'drop' signal and the things it has formerly guarded have been devalued, it should be possible to extend the 'drop' training to items that the dog has stolen or wishes to guard.

Any guarded items should be listed and then put into order of how much the dog values them. Training begins with the lowest value items and proceeds to the more valued ones as the dog shows absolute compliance with training. This training must be carried out in a number of dissimilar contexts to avoid context specificity.

If the motivation for guarding is an attempt to demonstrate or maintain control of situations, then underlying problems in the relationship with the owner must be addressed. It is most likely that other behavioural problems will be present so the whole situation must be investigated.

Early intervention in these problems is very important because the information the dog learns about its relationship with people and other animals will have a long-term effect on the way that it behaves.

Prognosis

Prognosis is determined by:

- age of onset of problem; early onset has a poorer prognosis
- owner response; punishment impairs prognosis, as does deliberately provocative or competitive behaviour
- duration of problem; prognosis becomes worse for long-term cases where there have been many incidences of guarding behaviour
- number of situations in which guarding is seen
- targets of aggression; children and the elderly are more vulnerable to injury
- severity of aggression; number and type of bites at each incident
- level of provocation required to trigger aggression; prognosis is poor if the dog requires no direct

provocation to trigger an attack; for example, if someone walks past the dog without attending to it.

- amount of warning signals issued before a physical attack; dogs that give little warning have a poor prognosis.

TERRITORIAL AND PROTECTIVE AGGRESSION

The dog's survival is dependent upon defending and being defended by the group and protecting access to the area of territory which contains the resources the group needs for survival. In terms of the companion dog, the group includes other residents in the house and familiar individuals. The territory might include the owner's property, the street area close to the home, the car and any number of other places. The territory is not restricted to the land covered by the deeds of the owner's house.

In wild or feral situations, there will be ongoing negotiation of territory dimensions between nearby groups of dogs. The severity of aggression between groups will depend upon the level of territorial infringement and the motivations of the opposing groups. It would be unwise to engage in a bloodthirsty fight over a patch of peripheral territory that contains little of any value, but the same encounter would be very different if it occurred close to the central or most valuable area of territory.

In the domestic context, the dog may see many people and other dogs passing by its property, either on the street or on footpaths near to the garden, which heightens the sense of territorial threat. When the dog mounts a ferocious territorial defence, the opponent always appears to retreat, which only serves to reward the dog with success. Delivery people who come to the door are amongst the worst problems for the territorial dogs because they come right up to the boundary of the territory and then go away again. This heightens the need for the dog to guard against these people and the dog may get the impression that, if it were not around to guard the door, these people would certainly break in. Many territorial dogs do not enjoy the duty of guarding the home; they do it because they have to. In fact, it may be immensely stressful for them.

There can be serious consequences for the dog's behaviour in other situations. For example, some dogs will carry out ferocious attacks on other dogs who they see passing their house on a daily basis. These are individuals who have shown an ongoing intention to enter the territory and the dog may recognise them as a serious threat in whatever context they are encountered. This reaction may generalise to other animals who look similar (Box 11.14).

In protective aggression, the dog will guard a person or persons that it regards as valuable or the source of valuable resources. The pattern of aggression is very similar to territorial aggression, but with the person as the focus of the dog's guarding behaviour (Box 11.15).

Diagnosis

Territorial aggression

Territorial aggression is usually seen only in specific familiar locations that the dog has adopted as its territory. This usually means the owner's home and garden. It may also include land adjoining the owner's property, including the street outside. Some dogs will territorialise familiar parks and other homes or places that they regularly visit. Territorial aggression is not generally seen in novel or unfamiliar locations, although this may be complicated if the dog also has fear-related aggression (Box 11.16).

Box 11.14   Immediate action: territorial aggression

- Secure the perimeter of dog's territory (lock gates, check fencing).
- Do not allow visitors to meet the dog at any boundary of the territory (fence, gate, front door).
- The dog must NEVER meet people on its territory unless under the supervision and absolute control of the owner.
- Train the dog to accept a muzzle.

Box 11.15   Immediate action: protective aggression

- Identify and avoid all situations in which the dog shows protective aggression.
- Train the dog to wear a muzzle and use this to reduce risk if the dog must be exposed to situations in which it may become aggressive.
- Follow advice on preventing territorial aggression.

Box 11.16   Prevention of territorial aggression

- Minimise territorial triggers.
- Do not reward the dog for territorial aggression.
- Put the dog out of the way when visitors enter and leave the property.
- Do not allow the dog to spend time patrolling and guarding the boundary.
- Provide outlets for normal behaviour to reduce boredom.
- Encourage all visitors to the home to give the dog food rewards and engage it in play.
- Block views of roads and alleys that the dog shows an interest in guarding.

Protective aggression

Dogs with protective aggression will only show aggressive behaviour when the person they are guarding is present. However, this is also complicated by the common comorbidity of fear-related aggression (Box 11.17).

Box 11.17   Prevention of protective aggression

- Do not allow one person to take over the entire caregiving routine for the dog. If the dog lives with a single person then friends and family who visit should feed, groom and attend to the dog while they are present (as long as the dog does not have fear-related or other aggression problems).
- Train the dog to carry out behaviours such as 'sit', 'wait' and 'heel', and use these to control its behaviour when on a walk.
- From an early age, encourage unfamiliar people to throw the dog extra-tasty food treats.
- Do not encourage territorial behaviour at home.

Treatment

Territorial aggression

It is essential to reduce the number of triggers for territorial behaviour so that the dog is placed under less stress and there is less opportunity for rehearsal of territoriality. A list of suggestions is included in Box 11.18, and in Advice sheet 7, which can be found in Appendix 2.

There are usually a series of territorial triggers that cause the dog to become increasingly and aggressively aroused as people approach the territory of the house.

There will be a number of specific stimuli which elicit territorial behaviour, such as the sounds of footsteps outside or the doorbell. The dog may be desensitised and counterconditioned to these stimuli, or the stimulus may be changed for another that evokes a different response. For example, the sound of a new doorbell might be associated with feeding time so that when this bell is finally installed to replace the old one, it does not evoke the territorial response. A gravel pathway might be paved to reduce the sound of footsteps that aggravates territoriality.

Territoriality in the home is frequently supported unintentionally by owner behaviour. When the dog goes to bark at the door, the behaviour has several functions. It is an alert signal for other members of the group, it is a call for reinforcements and it is a warning to the intruder that they should leave.

When the owner goes to the door after the dog has barked, they are reinforcing two of these motivations. When the person goes away this reinforces the other.

Box 11.18   Reducing responses to territorial triggers

- All deliveries should be made to a delivery box as far away from the house as possible, preferably out of sight of the dog.
- The views from vantage points must be blocked so that the dog cannot see what is going on outside the house.
- Apply translucent plastic to windows that directly overlook areas that the dog territorialises so that it cannot see whether people are coming or going away.
- Keep windows shut to prevent the sounds of passersby entering the house.
- Leave a radio or other sound source playing to block out external noises.
- The dog must not be present when people are entering or leaving the house and should be shut away at these times. The owner should call the dog away from the place it is guarding rather than pull it away.
- Use dog-appeasing pheromone in accordance with the manufacturer's instructions.
- In some cases, it may help if delivery people always put a large treat through the letterbox for the dog, so that it associates their presence with the arrival of a food treat.
- Do not shout at the dog when it goes to bark.

To successfully reduce territoriality in the home, the dog must learn that its territorial behaviour does not recruit support from others in the home. Where several dogs behave as a group, supporting each other's territorial behaviour, then it is often best to start training with the dogs individually before training them as a group.

Owners can follow a training exercise several times each day that teaches the dog that its territorial behaviour is fruitless. A volunteer comes to the door and rings the bell. When the dog rushes to the door nobody reacts and, after a few seconds, the owner doing the training calls the dog away from the door. When the dog comes away it is repeatedly rewarded with food, play and attention. If it goes back to the door it is called away. All this time, the volunteer remains on the doorstep until the dog has fully calmed down. Then they may go away, but if at any point the dog begins to bark again they must come back.

Most dogs find this confusing at first because barking is having the opposite effect from what they are used to; the person stays or even comes back when the dog barks and the owner does nothing to deal with the situation but instead rewards the dog for coming away and not barking. On the first occasion that this routine is practised, it may take a long time (up to 40 minutes) for the dog to calm down. After that, the dog will calm down progressively faster as long as the number of training sessions outnumbers the actual territorial events by a factor of at least 3 to 4 times. In other words, the new strategy proves to be more consistently appropriate than the old one.

If there is trouble calling the dog away from the door then the owner may need to practise doing recall training for food rewards in a number of less challenging situations until the dog's response is generally improved.

In some cases, the owner may need to train and use a conditioned punishment, such as a rattle can or training discs. Using the training method described in Advice sheet 14, Appendix 2, the dog is taught to associate an otherwise innocuous sound (the rattle of the can or discs) with failure to get an anticipated reward. This sound is then used to show the dog that its behaviour of barking at the stooge at the door is failing. This enables the dog to make a more rapid judgment to stop barking and return to the owner for a food treat.

The effect of this, in combination with the other advice on territorial triggers, is to reduce the necessity for intense territorial behaviour (Box 11.19).

Box 11.19 Treatment: territorial aggression

- Reduce territorial triggers and opportunities to territorialise.
- Do not allow the dog to meet visitors at the territorial boundary (garden gate, front door, etc).
- Desensitise and countercondition the dog to stimuli that evoke territorial behaviour.
- Train the dog to come away from the boundary when it is alerted to become territorial by a volunteer outside the house. (See text.)

Protective aggression

Dogs with protective aggression usually show territorial behaviour too. This must be addressed. The care-giving routine for the dog should be divided amongst a group of people that the dog already trusts and against whom it shows no territorial aggression. This includes feeding, grooming and play.

The owner should train a set of basic obedience commands and then use these to control the dog's general behaviour when it is on a walk. The owner must also avoid showing fear or anxiety and instead try to remain calm and happy in all situations, so that the dog does not get the impression that they are worried and need protection. If the dog has shown aggression towards people when on walks, then it is sensible to train it to wear a muzzle in these situations.

The dog may be desensitised and counterconditioned to the presence of people that it considers to be a threat to its owner by using similar methods to those listed under fear-related aggression. It may be trained to obey a 'come away' command, which places the owner back in control of the dog's behaviour. In some circumstances, a conditioned

punishment may be used to suppress vigilant behaviour, such as watching passersby or other dogs, as this is a prelude to protecting the owner. The rattle noise is delivered each time the dog stares at the target. Use of punishment in this way should be carried out with great care (Box 11.20).

Box 11.20 Treatment: protective aggression

- Treat any territorial aggression problems first.
- Reduce the 'value' of the person the dog guards by distributing the care-giving routine amongst a group of other people (friends, family). See text.
- Use sensible safety precautions to protect people (muzzle in public places, etc.)
- Desensitise and countercondition the dog to stimuli that evoke protective aggression.
- Train the dog to perform a 'come away' command so that the owner can take control of its behaviour.
- The owner must conceal their anxiety or fear and try to act happy and confident at all times.

Prognosis

The prognosis for territorial and protective aggression depends greatly on the management of the dog. No dog that has shown territorial behaviour should ever be allowed to meet people on its territory without the supervision of the owner. They can never be trusted to make a correct decision in these circumstances.

It is the owner's responsibility to secure their property so that the dog does not present a threat to anyone. Gates must be locked and fences made escape-proof. Protective dogs may need to be constantly muzzled in public.

Electric fences that employ a shock collar to deter a dog from approaching or leaving the boundary of the property do not constitute a secure means of protecting persons from dogs that show territorial behaviour.

MATERNAL AGGRESSION

The hormone prolactin drives maternal aggression, causing the bitch to be protective of her puppies and the resources she needs to rear them. This aggression may be quite intense and out of character for the bitch who may ferociously guard food, bedding and other objects. The level of aggression may fluctuate during the day, making the bitch's behaviour highly unpredictable.

Maternal aggression is also influenced by the bitch's previous experience, so care should be taken not to expose her to events or stimuli that she has previously found stressful or threatening because these also may trigger aggression. Not only could she become dangerous, but also this gives the puppies an opportunity to witness and perhaps model behaviour that we would rather they did not acquire.

The risk of maternal aggression is not confined to the bitch rearing puppies.

After every season, a bitch will have a rise in prolactin which can cause:

- increases in general depression, restlessness, irritability, competitiveness and anxiety
- maternal behaviour: nest-building, collecting and mothering of objects
- lactation.

Many bitches do not show the well-known and most obvious signs of false pregnancy and instead just show the general personality changes listed above. They may therefore become generally more aggressive (Box 11.21).

Box 11.21   Immediate action: maternal aggression

- Identify any stimuli or events that may increase the bitch's anticipation of a threat to her puppies (noises she reacts to, people, etc.)
- Isolate the bitch and puppies in an area of the home where she is calmest and to which only individuals that she trusts have access.
- Do not try to separate the bitch from her puppies, or get between her and them.

Diagnosis

Maternal aggression is seen only in bitches with pre-weaning puppies or experiencing false pregnancy. Maternal aggression may be confused with other resource guarding and possessive behaviour if it is caused by false pregnancy. A physical examination, the timing of sudden onset of the behaviour relative to the most recent oestrus and a history of behavioural changes accompanying false pregnancy should confirm the diagnosis. Prolactin levels and associated aggressive behaviour may persist indefinitely in the neutered bitch which was thought to be hormonally neutral. Previous medical and behavioural history should cause suspicion that the current problem is, in fact, partially caused by elevated prolactin (Box 11.22).

Treatment

Maternal aggression is likely to be repeated at every season and every false pregnancy, so bitches with this problem should be neutered. Since prolactin levels persist indefinitely if there is no functioning ovarian unit to terminate production, bitches should be treated with an antiprolactin drug (cabergoline) to prevent this (Box 11.23).

Box 11.22   Prevention of maternal aggression

- Bitches that are not to be used for reproduction should be neutered.
- Those allowed to reproduce should have the best parental temperamental history and be thoroughly socialised and socially referenced.
- The bitch should be provided with a quiet and calm nesting place that is used exclusively for puppy rearing.
- Unfamiliar people must not be allowed into the nest area while the mother is with her pups.
- Once the pups have become mobile and it is clear that the bitch shows no defenciveness, then controls may be relaxed.

Box 11.23   Treatment of maternal aggression

- Practise sensible safety measures.
- Do not breed from the bitch again or allow her to have further false pregnancies.
- Neuter and treat with an antiprolactin agent (cabergoline).

Prognosis

The prognosis for bitches with maternal aggression is excellent, as long as further incidents are prevented and any underlying hormonal factors are dealt with.

PAIN-RELATED AGGRESSION

Pain may be an underlying factor in many more aggression cases than we realise. Chronic low-grade pain increases irritability and self-defensiveness and reduces the threshold for aggressive behaviour. As social animals that live in a status-related hierarchy, dogs are under pressure to conceal any discomfort they experience so that others in the

---

Box 11.24   Immediate action: pain-related aggression

- Identify the source of pain and treat appropriately.
- Teach the dog to accept muzzling so that painful procedures may be carried out without risk.
- Do not use force or heavy restraint when carrying out procedures as this may sensitise the dog to other forms of handling.
- Carry out a trial of a memory-blocking agent (diazepam/alprazolam) to be used to prevent recollection of painful incidents after they have happened (see Chapter 6).
- Do not use punishment.

group do not take advantage of the situation to compete with them for rank or resources. A dog that is in pain may not be able to manage a sustained challenge from another member of its group, so it is likely to become more offensive when threatened in order to give the opponent less opportunity to discover its weakness.

The circumstances of an acutely painful incident will be remembered by the dog so that it may become alarmed and aggressive when certain stimuli are presented in the future. For example, many dogs become alarmed when they see a syringe or hear a syringe case being opened.

Certain conditions may lead to sudden jolts of pain which the dog may associate with the event that immediately preceded it; spinal pain, abdominal pain, and inflammatory joint disease are examples. A dog that is playing and experiences a sudden spasm of abdominal pain may falsely associate that pain with the actions of its playmate, leading to aggression then and in the future. Young dogs with a history of chronic diarrhoea or vomiting should be treated so that they do not make these kinds of associations.

Where pain may result from a surgical procedure it is absolutely imperative that appropriate analgesia is given (Box 11.25).

Box 11.25   Prevention of pain-related aggression

- Condition the dog to associate handling and minor procedures with reward from an early age.
- Condition positive associations with the locations in which procedures are carried out (veterinary clinic, grooming parlour, kennels, etc.)
- Use care and minimal handling during procedures.
- Do not use coercion or punishment if the animal is less than compliant.
- Use proper perioperative analgesia.
- Treat painful conditions at an early stage (e.g., gastrointestinal disease in young dogs).
- Use anaesthesia for potentially painful procedures.

Diagnosis

There may be a history of concurrent painful disease. Where the dog has a co-existing painful condition this should at least be considered to be a maintaining factor in aggression. However, many painful conditions are difficult or obscure to diagnose.

Treatment

No behavioural modification should be started until the source of pain has been investigated and treated, especially where chronic disease is suspected. The protocol for treatment depends upon the amount of warning and the level of aggression the dog shows.

All procedures that evoke aggression should be listed. These should then be divided into their individual steps so that counterconditioning can be carried out for each step. For example, stroking down the leg towards the foot, then touching the foot, then holding the foot and finally picking the foot up. Each step is repeatedly associated with the delivery of a reward if the dog shows no sign of aggression, moving on to the next step as each is completed.

This process will be made easier if the dog is first taught a non-confrontational 'no' signal (see Advice sheet 11, Appendix 2) so that this may be used to indicate to the dog that any objection will not be rewarded. If the dog objects the person turns away and quietly says 'no'. They then wait for a few seconds before repeating the step again.

It will also help to follow the advice on the click-touch training handout (Advice sheet 12, Appendix 2) as a precursor to actual training as this method can be modified to train tolerance of procedures.

Many dogs are able to distinguish between training and real examination or handling during procedures. The dog may learn to tell the difference from changes in the owner's body tension, tone of voice or the part of the dog's body that they are looking at. For example, the dog may tolerate handling of its foot while the owner is looking at its neck or face, but then becomes aggressive as soon as the owner looks directly at the foot that is being held.

In these cases, the owner also needs to build up confidence so that they do not give out signals that alarm the dog. The click-touch approach should be used for several weeks before actual training starts to build up a strong association between non-threatening touch and reward. The dog is trained to wear a basket muzzle with a small hole cut in the front so that food treats can still be given. This allows training to proceed with less risk of the owner becoming tense or of the dog biting.

Training must be carried out in a number of contexts to avoid context specificity and to make sure that the dog is tolerant of handling in the kinds of situations where it is most likely to occur, that is, at the veterinary practice or grooming parlour. Although no clinical trials have been carried out, it is the author's experience that DAP® helps to speed up the process of training dogs to tolerate handling and can be used in the veterinary clinic to help training transfer to that context. A DAP® diffuser is used in the room at home where the dog undergoes training (or a DAP® collar is used if this is available). When the dog goes for training at the clinic or groomer, a DAP® diffuser is installed there and left running for at least an hour before the dog arrives. When it arrives, the dog is allowed to sit near to the diffuser at the practice for a period of at least 5–10 minutes before training begins.

Some dogs show acute apprehension merely of the context of the clinic, and it is worth bringing the dog to the clinic repeatedly just to have food rewards and a game while the DAP® diffuser is running. Actual training can begin once the dog is relaxed in the clinic and shows no sign of apprehension.

Until the dog is fully conditioned to tolerate handling again, painful procedures should be avoided. If restraint or a procedure is essential, then fast-acting memory-blocking drugs may be given after the event to prevent recollection so that the dog does not build up additional negative associations. Low-dose benzodiazepines work well in this situation but must only be given *after* the procedure is complete, otherwise disinhibition of aggression might occur. Once dosed with a benzodiazepine, the dog should be kept under minimal stress until the drug has worn off (≥4 hours).

Once treatment is complete, the dog will always be susceptible to relapses and owners should continue to do regular training to maintain tolerance to handling (Box 11.26).

Box 11.26   Treatment: pain–related aggression

- Treat the cause of pain.
- Avoid painful procedures and restraint.
- Countercondition response to handling and procedures.
- Use an adapted muzzle for safety if necessary.
- Use DAP® to improve response to training.
- Use memory-blocking drugs to prevent recollection of any essential procedures that must be carried out before behavioural treatment is complete.

Prognosis

Owners with dogs that have shown pain-related aggression must be careful to maintain strong associations between various forms of handling and reward. These dogs are inclined to relapse if they experience pain in the future. The prognosis, as always with aggression cases, depends upon the degree of warning the dog gives and the speed with which it shifts to offensive aggression.

AGGRESSION BETWEEN FAMILIAR DOGS (SHARING A HOME)

The main motivations for this form of aggression include:

- competition over resources (including owner attention)
- status-related conflict.

Complicating factors are:

- punishment of puppies or juvenile dogs by adult dogs
- self defensiveness (e.g. due to illness).

Older dogs will often bite puppies or younger dogs around the muzzle area in order to punish them. Usually, the puppy has persisted in an interaction that the older dog

---

Box 11.27   Immediate action: aggression between familiar dogs (sharing a home)

- Dogs may need to be kept apart to avoid further fights.
- Remove common access to resources the dogs compete for (toys, food, etc.)
- Dogs must meet only when supervised and under control (on leash or muzzled).
- Owners must be warned of the potential for redirected aggression. Fights must be broken up by calling or distracting the dogs into another activity, or by the use of loud noises or water to disrupt the fight. Use of leashes as lassos may enable the dogs to be pulled apart, but owners should avoid handling the dogs while they are fighting because they may be severely injured.

---

does not want, despite numerous warnings. In these situations, aggression can be reduced by giving the adult dog time away from the puppy so that it is not being used as a 'baby minder' for the young dog. The owner should divert the puppy from doing things that annoy the older dog by calling it away to play or do something else. Mild chastisement may also be used to interrupt the puppy, but not to frighten it. Once the adult dog has some support from the owners and can spend periods relaxing away from the young dog, the situation usually subsides.

Self-defensive behaviour is common in diseased or debilitated dogs, or those who have been constantly threatened by another dog in the household. If space is restricted and the victim cannot move far enough away from the aggressor to avoid threat, then it may become self-defensive. The same situation occurs if the aggressor is unwilling to accept the victim's repeated submission or appeasement behaviour. Where self-defensiveness is caused by illness, the dog should be treated but, in some cases, permanent management may be necessary, such as in the case of blind, deaf or otherwise permanently disabled dogs.

Diagnosis

Competition for status or resources is the commonest cause of disagreements between dogs that share a home.

Resources may include:

- people (attention, etc.)
- food
- toys
- space
- resting areas
- specific locations (bedroom, kitchen, a place close to the owner).

Conflict may be confined to times when a particular resource is available, with dogs showing no animosity towards each other at any other time. However, it is important to make notes of all situations where dogs challenge each other through eye contact or posture and to detail the general pattern of dominant and submissive behaviours between them. Competition for resources is influenced by the availability of a resource, the value that each individual places on it and any existing status relationship between them. This is important because a dog that experiences hunger due to metabolic disease may compete excessively for food or chews; or a dog with an attachment problem may attempt to monopolise contact with a particular person, even if this risks a status conflict. If the availability of a resource changes, such as when a member of the family leaves home, the dogs may also be brought into conflict. Pressure on one resource is likely to spill over into fights at other times if a high-ranking dog perceives that its status is being undermined in a way that will affect access to other resources.

If competition develops into a wider conflict over status then other behaviours are seen, such as one dog controlling the other's general activities around the house and its access to certain areas. One dog may shadow the other, preventing it from doing certain things and repeatedly using dominant displays to demand submission. The same dog may also keep account of the other's activities so that violence explodes out of apparently minor disagreements after an accumulation of other infringements has been logged. This situation may be highly stressful for both dogs.

Status-related problems are often made worse by interference from the owner who wishes to keep the relationship between the dogs 'fair', or who wishes to punish the dog that is seen as the aggressor. This makes it impossible for the dogs to reach a settlement over who has the higher status (Box 11.28).

Treatment

Mild punishment aggression used by adult dogs to discipline juveniles should be differentiated from fear-related and more serious status-related conflict. The general relationship between the dogs and their behaviour at around

the time of each incident should make this distinction straightforward.

Where illness exists, or one individual has been injured or frightened during fights, an element of self-defensiveness will be present. This involves fear and anxiety.

All avoidable sources of competition should be removed. If serious injuries have resulted in fights, the dogs may need to be isolated from each other for a period to prevent further fights and to allow them to settle down.

The dog with the highest rank should be identified from the total pattern of submissive, dominant and avoidant behaviours seen between the dogs, together with the current priority of access to resources. Owners need to be educated so that they can identify, record and respond to the more subtle signs of conflict between the dogs. Any medical problems should be treated as they will have a negative effect on the status of affected animals.

The dog with highest status should have its rank supported by all family members, giving it priority of access to resources and chastising the subordinate dog for any infringement of the status relationship before a conflict ensues. This means that the subordinate dog will have to accept a lower quality of life while the social order is being stabilised. Some loss of privilege will be permanent. Owners may not be able to accept this, but many will understand that both dogs are actually more content now that there are fewer altercations, and they can both get some share of what they need (Box 11.29).

Box 11.29   Maintaining stable-status relationships

- The dog with highest status should be given preferential access to resources: going ahead of the other dog through doorways, getting food first, having priority of access to owner attention and certain locations.
- The lower-ranking dog is trained to sit and wait while the higher-ranking one gets food and other privileges first.
- At the very first sign of conflict, the owner must intervene to chastise (mildly) and isolate the lower-ranking dog. This will impress upon it that the status of the dog of higher rank is supported by an alliance with the owner.

DAP® has proved beneficial in reducing intraspecific aggression within the household. The reason is not clear but it may be that DAP® makes the dog behave in a more juvenile manner. Certainly, dogs with this problem that are treated with DAP® appear to become more playful and willing to offer submission to each other. DAP® is also thought to reduce anxiety.

Anxiety may also be reduced if the lives of the dogs are more structured and involve a greater amount of training. Essentially, the dogs are expected to perform obedience tasks in order to gain attention, food and access to

---

Box 11.28   Prevention of aggression between familiar dogs sharing a home

- Avoid keeping two or more dogs of the same gender in the same household.
- Avoid same gender pairings from the same litter or breed.
- Choose dogs of very different sizes.
- Neuter early, especially where females are kept together.
- Use antiprolactin drugs to treat false pregnancy at the earliest opportunity and to reduce prolactin at neutering.
- Determine the status relationship between dogs and reinforce rather than interfere with it.

resources from the owner. This may also raise the owner's status so that the dogs mutually adopt a lower rank.

Status conflicts often start because two dogs are of similar motivation, size and physical ability so that it is hard for them to accept differential status. The risk of this is increased when the owner picks two males or females from the same litter. Neutering one male in a pair (the subordinate one) will help to increase the physical difference between them. The feminising effect of neutering may also help to reduce conflict.

Aggression between females is potentially far more damaging and problematic because it often involves absolute resource control that is not settled by a stable status relationship. Bitches vary in their level of competitiveness and aggressiveness according to reproductive state. From the time of the rise in follitropin (follicle stimulating hormone, FSH) to the end of oestrus, bitches may be antagonistic towards each other. They may also be aggressive during any period of raised prolactin. Bitches often synchronise their oestrus, which adds to the possibility of aggression at this time.

During oestrus, pregnancy and false pregnancy the bitch's perceived resource demands increase. Demands may exceed the available space and resources, so that the competitor bitch would normally be driven away. This cannot happen in a domestic environment so the fights may be intended to eliminate the threat posed by the other bitch, either by crippling or killing her. If, as is likely, aggression is worse around the time of each oestrus or during the periods of false pregnancy, then the first step to treating aggression between bitches is to neuter them. An antiprolactin drug such as cabergoline should be used as a precaution. This creates a stable platform upon which the other behavioural modification can be based. Owners who are unwilling to neuter bitches that have shown a clear worsening of aggressive behaviour due to hormonal effects, should be warned that even intensive behavioural therapy may produce only a temporary resolution and that vicious fights may re-occur at the next oestrus or false pregnancy.

One problem with treating intraspecific aggression is that some degree of fighting may be inevitable during treatment. Often the shock value of each fight is greater to the owner when the time period between fights becomes longer. This can be disheartening and alarming to owners who cannot face seeing any further aggression and cannot understand why fights are still happening occasionally after 2–3 months of treatment. To maintain motivation, it is essential to carry out regular follow-ups and ask the owner to keep a record of aggressive incidents. This enables the owner to look back over weeks or months and make a realistic comparison between current and past behaviour.

Prognosis

Improvement depends on utter consistency from the owner and other family members. This is often difficult to obtain because one or more family members cannot accept that the lower-ranking dog, who is perceived to be the victim, must be given reduced privileges. It is best to discuss this in detail with owners so that they understand the situation they will be accepting if they do go ahead with treatment.

Poor prognosis is indicated if past fights have caused severe damage to one or both dogs, or if attacks continue after one dog has attempted submission, appeasement or escape. This may indicate that the intention is not merely to settle a disagreement but is being used by one dog as an opportunity to dispatch a rival. The despotic monopolisation of resources by the higher-ranking dog will leave nothing for the subordinate. This also cannot be an acceptable stable-status relationship.

If damaging fights continue then re-homing one dog is the best option. Failure is more likely when aggression exists between two females.

AGGRESSION TOWARD UNFAMILIAR DOGS

This form of aggression is extremely common, but underpresented. Owners often think that it is untreatable or they are embarrassed and never seek help. These become the dog-walkers who lurk in streets and deserted parks at times when no other dog is being walked.

Diagnosis

The main causes for the problem are:

- frustration
- social incompetence
- fear
- inter-male competition
- the effects of owner punishment and reinforcement.

Frustration is most common among young dogs that enjoy contact with their own species. They may get very excited when they see another dog and, if off leash, they will run over to play with it. On leash they will bark, jump up and down, and become highly aroused and frustrated. Repeated experiences of this kind often scare the owner who may not permit the dog to socialise off-leash because of a fear of fighting. The dog ends up becoming socially isolated and frustrated by a lack of contact with other dogs. Critically, this isolation often occurs from 4 months onward which means that the young dog never develops proper social competence with other dogs. Similar situations develop with dogs that have a poor response to recall; the owner keeps them on leash at all times because of a fear that they will not come back.

Full social competence is acquired through interaction with adult dogs as the juvenile dog proceeds to maturity. It is not enough for a dog to have been well socialised as a puppy; it has to learn how to deal with adult interactions too. Confidence in social situations enables interaction with unfamiliar dogs even when there is conflict. A lack of consistent social contact with unfamiliar conspecifics before maturity also predisposes to fear and anxiety around other dogs.

Fear of other dogs is quite common and stems from a lack of socialisation, lack of social experience with other dogs before maturity and the effect of aggressive attacks by other dogs. A dog that has inadequate experience with other dogs is more susceptible to developing a general fear of other dogs after an attack.

Inter-male competitive aggression is also common. Initial meetings between male dogs involve a lot of posturing, which is designed to determine the first elements of a working status relationship. After this is settled, many dogs will happily run off to play. If neither individual is willing to show deference, then the display becomes more physical with barging, body slamming and neck biting. Even then the amount of damage caused is usually minimal. The aim is to put on a good display rather than cause serious injury. Socially incompetent dogs or ones that have been attacked in the past may not feel secure enough to show deference, which leads to increasing aggression within the interaction. Due to a lack of confidence, these dogs may also launch a sudden and violent attack on the other dog, although the competition is relatively non-threatening.

The most reliable assessment of the motivation for the dog's behaviour comes from direct observation of a staged encounter with another dog. This should only be contemplated after discussing the dog's history and considering the risk involved. The dogs should be kept at a distance and under control throughout the exercise so that the behaviour of the patient may be assessed objectively (Box 11.30).

> ### Box 11.30   Preventions of aggression towards unfamiliar dogs
>
> - Good early socialisation with a wide range of different sizes and types of dog is essential.
> - Social contact must be continued throughout the dog's life if social competence is to be developed and maintained.
> - Owners should respond positively (happy and excited) whenever other dogs are encountered, to encourage the young dog to model the same behaviour. Young dogs should be trained to sit and wait before they are allowed to go and interact with other dogs, and also to come away from them on command. This reduces frustration when the young dog may not be able to go to another dog because it is leashed and enables owners to control their dogs well enough to give them more freedom with other dogs.
> - Early neutering may reduce competitive aggression between males.

Treatment

Frustration-related aggression and social incompetence can be avoided by proper socialisation and lots of contact with well-adjusted mature dogs during the first 18 months of life. Owners should try to take their young dogs to the park at busy times when other people with sociable and friendly dogs are there. They should avoid parks during times when they are relatively deserted because these are the times when cautious owners with aggressive dogs may be there. This increases the probability of the young dog being attacked. Owners must teach good recall and train their dog that it must wait to be let off the leash to interact with conspecifics.

Neutering males may prevent the development of inter-male competitive aggression and certainly reduces its severity in the majority of cases.

Fear-related intraspecific aggression towards unfamiliar dogs should be treated as other forms of fear-related aggression by using a desensitisation and counterconditioning programme with stooge dogs.

A complication is that many dogs with an intense fear of other dogs will show alarm and arousal at certain points on a walk where they anticipate seeing other dogs. These are usually dogs that are guarding their territory. A dog that shows this kind of anticipation should be counterconditioned to remain calm in such locations.

As with fear of people, the dog is rewarded for remaining calm when in the presence of a dog at a distance beyond that which evokes aggression or fear. The dog is brought closer over the course of a number of sessions. The aim is to condition the patient to remain calm throughout meetings with a range of different types of dogs, starting with them standing still and building up to them doing normal doggy things like fetching a ball or running about.

Owner reaction is very important and many people become tense when an unfamiliar dog appears. Instead, they should try to act happy and excited in the hope that their own dog will model the behaviour. At the very least, it will not get any indication that the owner finds the situations stressful or frightening.

In some cases the dog will react aggressively, even to the sounds of other dogs or the sight of an inflatable or toy dog. This offers a good opportunity to start counterconditioning without involving real dogs (Box 11.31).

Prognosis

Success is unpredictable for these cases because so much depends upon the behaviour of other dogs. Some owners may not be able to find any other dogs to practise with so they may benefit from joining a specific rehabilitation group for dogs with intraspecific aggression. A substantial number of dogs will remain aggressive, even after treatment. Consequently, good management is the only prospect for them.

Box 11.31 Treatment of aggression towards unfamiliar dogs

- Identify the type, gender and behaviour of the dogs that elicit a response and make a list grading the reaction.
- Identify the contexts and stimuli that cause arousal (park, places where dogs are encountered, sound of dogs barking, etc.).
- Desensitise and countercondition to contexts and simulated representations of other dogs (video recordings, recorded sounds, model dogs).
- Desensitise and countercondition to the presence of other real dogs, starting with those that have an appearance and behaviour that is least likely to produce a response.
- Build up to dogs at closer proximity and behaving in a manner that is more likely to evoke a response (playing, running, vocalising).
- The owner should try to remain relaxed and happy throughout training so that the dog does not become alerted or worried by their anxious or fearful behaviour.

The prognosis is best for dogs that have mild fear-related aggression, especially if it is specific to one particular type of dog. Prognosis is also good for dogs that have developed aggressive behaviour due to frustration because these dogs often react well once the owner has good control of them and they are able to begin to mix with other dogs.

ADVICE SHEETS THAT MAY BE RELEVANT TO THIS CHAPTER

In Appendix 2

1. Using a houseline
3. Reward and punishment
6. Muzzle training
7. Territorial triggers
9. The 'come away' command
10. The indoor kennel
14. Using training discs or a rattle can
16. Environmental enrichment for dogs
17. Using food rewards for training
18. Food for work
19. Introducing the clicker

Chapter 12

Canine training and miscellaneous problems

INTRODUCTION

The problems in this chapter are diverse in type and motivation. Many involve miscommunication between the owner and dog or a misunderstanding of the normal development, behaviour and needs of the companion dog. The fact that many of these problems appear minor in comparison to serious behavioural problems, like aggression or compulsion, should not be a reason to dismiss them as insignificant. Most of the dogs that are placed with re-homing charities have a behavioural problem, many of which are quite minor. However, the previous owners have not been able to cope and the dog has lost what might have been a good home. The relationship between a dog and the family it lives with is easily damaged by minor behavioural problems that do not fit with the owner's expectation of their perfect pet. Once the dog is perceived to be more of a nuisance than a companion, then the quality of its care may decline and if more serious behavioural or medical problems develop in the future, this dog may end up being given away or euthanised.

The problems in this chapter are all quite common, and the way that they are handled may determine the whole course of the dog's behavioural development. For example, a puppy that is punished severely for play-biting could become very aggressive as an adult.

TRAINING METHODS

Clicker-training will be mentioned frequently as part of the solution to these problems as it is a very efficient method. Advice sheet 19 in Appendix 2 introduces clicker-training but some discussion of the method will be provided here.

The noise of the clicker is a conditioned or secondary *reinforcer*. The simple explanation of this is that the click becomes representative of reward by repeated association with the delivery of food. So the click comes to produce the same mental effects of reward as the actual consumption of food. In fact, it is more complex than that. The click is the first signal that the animal is going to get food, so it is like the first sight of food when the dog sees a treat. The click is therefore conditioned to produce an expectation of food and, when the dog hears this noise, it enters a preparatory state ready to eat. This includes parasympathetic arousal (shift in blood flow to digestive organs, salivation, etc.) Most importantly, the animal will experience hunger and an anticipation of the arrival of food that will satiate that need to eat.

This may be why using secondary reinforcers is more successful in certain training situations when, otherwise, the dog is not particularly food-motivated. It has been conditioned to expect food and to eat after hearing each click noise.

The actual click is not special in any way and any non-aversive noise or visual stimulus may be conditioned in this way. For example, deaf dogs may be conditioned to associate a light flash from a torch with reward. Many dogs learn conditioned reinforcers from their owners by accident; verbal signals like 'good boy', for example. The problem is that verbal signals often get misused and misapplied so that they lose their meaning. Owners will often say 'good boy' to a misbehaving dog in the hope that it will become well-behaved. This means that they are actually unintentionally reinforcing the behaviour they do not want.

The sound of the clicker is novel and carries no previous associations, so it is much easier for a dog to learn the kind of association we want it to.

There can be problems with clicker-training: it requires good timing and owners frequently misunderstand when they should click and reward. The commonest error is to click to get the dog's attention; but all this does is to reward the dog for ignoring the person and continuing to go about its other activities. If you are going to use clicker-training to treat an animal, then you must be proficient with the method, be able to demonstrate it to the owner and then constructively criticise their performance without offending or patronising them. It takes at least 10–20 minutes to introduce clicker-training in a normal consultation.

Some dogs are very sound sensitive and, to begin with, are slightly alarmed by the sound of the click. In these cases, it is very important to mute the sound of the clicker during the initial period of introducing the sound.

In normal obedience training there is a definite benefit in increasing the dog's anticipation of reward so that it focuses its attention on the training. With the kind of clicker-training used in behavioural work, the emphasis is on reducing general anticipation and encouraging calmness. So the person doing the training must not move to pick up the food reward or give away any other signs of what they are doing. The click must be the only signal that tells the dog that it is about to get a reward. In this way, the dog must focus on what it is doing when it hears the click so that it can reproduce this behaviour for further rewards, rather than watching the trainer to look for tiny clues about when the next reward might be coming. This makes it possible to train the dog to adopt a very relaxed state on cue,

including deliberately reinforcing a reduction in muscle tension and heart rate.

In certain situations, dogs may be less than responsive to any form of training. There are many reasons for this, anxiety being the most important. Many dogs find the situation of being at the veterinary clinic unsettling so that they feel anxious. Anxiety produces sympathetic arousal and is associated with acute loss of appetite so that the food we are offering has absolutely no attraction at all. Indeed, acute loss of appetite of this kind may be used as a strong indicator of anxiety in training or real-life situations. Anxiety also reduces the selectivity of attention. The animal is unable to make sense of the things we are trying to teach because it is too distracted by other events and cannot concentrate.

If a dog shows typical signs of anxiety (hypervigilance, scanning, increased locomotor activity, sympathetic arousal) then this is not a good time to do training. If this pattern of behaviour is seen in the situations where training is essential, then it may be necessary to train the dog to become less aroused (on cue) in a range of situations that are similar to the one in which training will be carried out. An anxiolytic drug might be beneficial.

Another significant cause of slow learning is cognitive impairment. Senility is common in dogs over the age of 7 years and medical conditions such as hypothyroidism cause significant mental dullness, which impedes learning. Iatrogenic causes of cognitive impairment include the use of antiepileptic drugs and intraoperative cerebral hypoxia. It is quite useful to go through a standard pattern of training with every dog because this will soon indicate that the individual is learning impaired for some reason. In fact, this may the first or only indicator that serious disease is present.

Box 12.1   Benefits of clicker-training

- It requires little physical strength.
- No physical contact with the animal is required.
- The trainer does not need to make eye contact with or challenge the dog in any way.
- It is easy to train complex behaviours by building up from more basic training.
- The animal often learns to volunteer the behaviour we want so that it does not need to be constantly told what to do.
- The novelty value and high level of reinforcement encourages most dogs to take an interest.
- The animal can be trained to adopt a calm and relaxed posture on cue.
- Food-based training, by its nature, favours parasympathetic arousal, which conflicts with anxiety, fear, and aggression.
- The animal is forced to think during training, which is both mentally stimulating and uses up energy.

Box 12.2 **Box 12.2   Reasons for slow acquisition of clicker-training during a consultation**

- Cognitive impairment (dementia, hypothyroidism, intracranial disease, iatrogenic).
- Anxiety/fear (context, absence of attachment figure).
- Sensory abnormality (blindness, anosmia, etc.).

Not all cases are suitable for clicker-training. Some dogs are too sound sensitive to the clicker and will display apprehension when they hear it. Also, there are owners who are not capable of coordinating themselves well enough to do the training. In these cases, other methods of training should be used (Box 12.2).

ENERGY BALANCE AND ACTIVITY

In any day, wild dogs allot amounts of time and energy to different activities. They have a limited amount of time and energy which they must use wisely if they are to survive. Domestic dogs have far less control over their lives and the normal activities of finding food and eating it take up little or no time at all.

Some problems therefore relate to lack of stimulation in the environment and it is generally recommended that all dogs with behavioural problems are given a more stimulating environment, with more physical and mental exercise so that their time and energy budgets are used up. A basic Advice sheet (No. 16) on environmental enrichment using activity feeders is included in Appendix 2.

ATTENTION-SEEKING

All dogs seek attention from their owners to some extent and this only becomes a problem when:

- the frequency or style of attention seeking is undesirable for the owner
- attention seeking represents a symptom of an anxiety disorder, such that the dog is constantly and unnecessarily asking for reassurance from the owner.

Attention-seeking is often a factor in anxiety disorders and problems relating to training and control.

In many cases, it is hard to convince the owner to alter the way that they respond to demands for attention. This is often due to the owner's own motivations and is expressed in the dynamics of the relationship. The owner may enjoy the flattery of being the dog's constant source of reassurance and social contact and they may see any rejection of the dog's demands as cruelty or neglect. Being energy efficient, dogs will usually use the more moderate methods of attention-seeking first (licking, nudging, parading with toys). However, almost any kind of behaviour can become a method of seeking attention including barking, stealing, elimination, pica, biting and destructiveness. Some of these are very hard to ignore, and tend to be unwittingly reinforced due to reflexive responses such as eye contact, touch or even scolding.

Attention-seeking problems are often made worse by the fact that the dog has no reliable way of understanding when attention is and is not available because the owner's pattern of interaction is so haphazard. The owner never gives clear signals. Calm behaviour often gets ignored because the owner is anxious not to disturb the dog when it finally calms down. This creates a vicious cycle in which only the active behaviour is always reinforced with some kind of attention reward. This leads to the development of more extreme attention-seeking demands as the dog becomes increasingly frustrated by the lack of consistency in human response. As the dog discovers that extreme behaviour such as stealing or biting always get a response, it progressively abandons the lower level and more acceptable behaviours. This progression is most likely in anxious or dependent dogs that have an increased need for attention and reassurance. Punishment tends to increase the anxiety and hence maintains the attention-seeking.

Dogs are highly social animals and therefore require a lot of interaction and contact, particularly if they have been home alone all day. This means that, while the dog's human counterpart has been working, they have been waiting and sleeping. Instantly, this creates a conflict of interests between the returning owner's need for food and rest against the dog's need for activity and play. This intensifies attention-seeking and play-signalling.

For example, as modern life becomes more biased towards technology for entertainment, humans are shifting ever further from the dog's simple pleasures of social contact and interactive play. Where interactive play is not available, dogs may entertain themselves with destructive play such as chewing, shredding and tearing objects. These behaviours are derived from normal acts of prey handling and feeding behaviour; biting legs off prey, ripping its skin off and disembowelling it. It takes little imagination to see the connection between these behaviours and their domestic equivalents: chewing table legs or fixed objects, ripping fabric off a sofa or paper off a wall and pulling the stuffing out of cushions. It takes only one or two opportunities for the dog to learn that damaging things is not only pleasurable in itself but also guarantees that the dog will get some kind of attention from the owner.

Likewise, a dog that uses barking in a number of different circumstances may learn that this is also an effective way to demand attention. This kind of discovery is often made as a result of frustration.

Diagnosis

Attention-seeking is most easily assessed by observation of the dog in the presence of its owner. It is important to note not only how often the dog seeks a response but also how the owner responds and what kinds of behaviours the dog uses (Box 12.3).

The motivation for the attention seeking is also important. This will indicate what kind of therapy is going to be most effective. Is the dog seeking play because it is bored and under-stimulated? Is it seeking reassurance because it is frightened or anxious? Does it want contact?

It is important to compare the animal's expectations with the reality of its environment. Are the animal's demands for attention merely an attempt to gain a normal level of stimulation and social contact in an otherwise tedious environment?

Box 12.3   Characteristics of attention-seeking behaviour

- The behaviour only occurs in the presence of a person, usually the owner.
- The dog is being ignored when the behaviour starts.
- The owner often reacts immediately to the behaviour and the dog either stops or modifies its behaviour, such as with a play-bow or other enticement in an attempt to hold the owner's attention.
- If the owner does not respond, the dog may try a sequence of different methods of attention-seeking which rise in vehemence.
- More attention-seeking behaviour will follow if the dog is ignored again.

Treatment

Treatment of attention-seeking is difficult, because most of the time the owner is reinforcing the behaviour unwittingly. Owner education is therefore very important; the owner must understand that any eye contact, touching or talking to the dog, even scolding, all constitute attention. The owner must become highly self-conscious of their actions when responding to the dog.

It helps if the dog is taught a signal that tells it that its attention-seeking will fail, but this must be done through a training method or the dog will become frustrated (see Advice sheet 11 in Appendix 2). This signal, which usually involves turning the head away sharply and then saying 'no', is then used to show the dog that it is being actively ignored when attention-seeking. It also helps if someone else is present to then call the dog away and reward it with attention for sitting down quietly. If, after ignoring the attention-seeking they do not like, the owner still feels the need to give the dog attention then they may ask the dog to sit (while still avoiding eye contact) and then turn to give attention when the dog responds.

Dogs that are inclined to steal may also be rewarded with a moment of attention for bringing a particular object that the owner has designated as acceptable. This object must never be used to play games with the dog and the amount of attention given must be small.

To strengthen the association between calm behaviour and access to highly rewarding activities, the dog must always be made to sit in order to get food, play, have a leash put on or to go through a door into the garden. By giving it a guaranteed method of getting attention or getting what it wants, the dog is no longer forced to engage in a series of increasingly frustrated and irritating demands (Box 12.4).

Box 12.4   Treatment of attention-seeking

- Teach the dog a 'no' signal that may be used to indicate that attention-seeking is going to fail (Advice sheet 11). Use vivid body language; turn away, fold arms and say 'no' at the moment when the behaviour starts.
- Use this 'no' signal to actively ignore attention-seeking behaviour.
- Regularly seek the dog out to give it attention and play while it is resting or calm.
- All greetings and attention should be low-key.
- Increase the number of sessions of interactive and non-interactive play (activity feeding, etc.).
- Teach the dog a reliable way to get attention by sitting, or bringing a particular object; this action must always be rewarded with a moment of attention (looking at the dog and saying its name may be enough).
- Install dog appeasing pheromone diffuser.
- Never push the dog away as touch is a reinforcing gesture, but rather withdraw arms and legs from the dog or, in extreme cases, consider leaving the room if attention-seeking continues.

Prognosis

The prognosis for attention-seeking behaviour is good as long as the owner can be made sufficiently self-aware and consistent that inadvertent reinforcement is no longer given. The dog must be given an environment that satisfies its normal needs so that the motivation to make demands is reduced.

Use of human analogy is also useful to improve owner understanding; 'It would not be acceptable for a child to demand attention so relentlessly', or 'Show me how you would use body language to shrug off someone you did not like'. Owners must be prepared for a backlash at the start of treatment; the dog may become more provocative for a few days until it becomes obvious that the new rules are permanent and attention is still available but on different terms.

As with other behaviour problems, the dog may retry old methods of attention-seeking occasionally until they are fully extinguished through lack of reward. The best way to show owners how to thwart attention-seeking is to demonstrate the method from the moment the consultation begins. Many owners will notice that the dog is not pestering the clinician in the way that it does with other guests, which creates a good opportunity to explain what is being done. This will make it easier for them to go on and demonstrate the techniques to other family members and friends.

PLAY-BITING

Biting is part of normal play in young dogs, both to develop skill and to learn about how to moderate the power of the bite. If a puppy bites too hard during play, then the play partner will protest, yelp in pain and stop the play. It is essential that a puppy learns about the social consequences of hard biting because this enables moderation in play and self-defence biting in adulthood.

Play-biting is very frequently misinterpreted by owners, especially those with small children. They fail to understand the communication that is going on around play and assume that the biting is an act of aggression. This usually leads to punishment of the dog. A worrying and recognisable trend has recently developed, in which owners are recommended to 'hang' (hold dogs off the ground by their collars) or 'alpha roll' (flip dogs onto their backs and restrain them there while punishing). These are very violent acts which the dog will find extremely alarming.

These methods are also ethologically inappropriate and will lead to immense distrust from the dog which was intending to evoke play and not a fight. As discussed in the section on inappropriate punishment, these methods constitute abuse.

Diagnosis

Play-biting can become quite ferocious and cause nasty injuries. When dogs play they will hurt each other. Within play, biting is accompanied by play meta-communication. This differentiates play from genuine aggression. Play is characterised by a loose-limbed and springy posture, frequent play-bowing, darting about and a 'play face'. The play face involves snorting and mock growling behaviour with the mouth open and teeth shielded. The front lip may be pulled up to show the incisors and canine teeth, while the head is swung from side to side. Some of these behaviours may appear threatening in some way, but observation reveals that the dog is actually making itself vulnerable because these 'mock threats' are not functional as aggressive behaviours.

Any withdrawal, freezing or expression of fear resulting from misinterpreted rough play is countered with further play meta-communication in order to re-establish confidence in the game.

Treatment

Individual people have differing pain thresholds and it is important for an owner not to allow a dog to play-bite hard simply because they can tolerate it. It is best to stop play

after any kind of bite against human flesh and to concentrate all physical play on toys.

Owners who get bitten during play should emit a hurt cry, look away from the pup and terminate all contact for a period of several minutes.

Problems can arise when a puppy uses biting as a means of getting attention and play. This should be dealt with in the same way as other methods of attention-seeking and overactivity.

Certain other signals are play invitations between dogs, a common one being a paw placed on the shoulder, neck or chest, followed by a small darting play-bow or a 'play face'. Unfortunately, young dogs frequently misinterpret hand contact with this play gesture and will start to play-bite a person's hand as they stroke.

This misunderstanding starts because people play physical rough-and-tumble games that involve pushing with hands. Confusion over the meaning of hand gestures gets even worse if hands are used for smacking and other kinds of physical punishment. In non-aggressive dogs this can be countered by response-substitution; the dog is taught to stay calm when stroked. A protocol for this is included in Appendix 2 (Advice sheet 12).

Another occasion when play-biting is common is at the end of a game when the dog is frustrated and wants play to continue. This can be helped by teaching better signals between owner and dog and by teaching the dog to modulate its play behaviour according to the owner's posture and signals. Protocols for this are also in Appendix 2 (Advice sheets 8 and 11).

Play can become overenthusiastic or frustrated. This is often the case when owners play games with a young dog too infrequently and for too long at a time. Play increases a dog's level of arousal and it also uses up reserves of readily accessible energy (e.g., blood glucose). Once aroused, some dogs find it hard to stop play and may become bullying and excessively physical during play. The best way to deal with this is to direct all play through toys, over which the person retains ultimate control. When a toy is brought out, the dog understands that play may begin and, when it is put away, the play stops.

It is best to keep bouts of play well-structured, alternating between actual play and command-based training. The aim is to keep calming the dog down before it gets overexcited. Games should end before the dog becomes hysterical, tired or fractious and are best ended with a brief session of training and an edible chew or scatter feeding game (Advice sheet 8, Appendix 2)

Regular training with food during play keeps control in the hands of the person, prevents excessive arousal and maintains blood glucose levels so that the dog does not become irritable and fractious at the end of, or after, play.

Owners should also be encouraged to use human equivalents of meta-communications to ensure that both parties are aware that play is still going on. For example, a puppy may be pushed on the shoulder with a toy (not with a hand) or the owner may squat down and imitate a play-bow (Box 12.5).

> ### Box 12.5   Treatment: play problems
>
> - Avoid play that involves pushing, shoving, or wrestling.
> - The focus of play should be a toy, not hands or feet.
> - Toys should be taken out at the beginning of play and put away afterwards.
> - During a session of play, the game should be broken up with short bouts of food-reward based training so that the dog's level of arousal is controlled.
> - Click-touch training should be used to condition the dog to associate hand contact with calmness and food rewards, rather than punishment or an invitation to play.
> - Games should begin and end with a session of training.
> - The dog may be given a small chew to eat after the game is over to reduce frustration and divert demands for additional play.
> - Dogs should be encouraged to join in group play involving several people. If the dog runs away with the toy then it is ignored. The people immediately bring out an identical spare toy and continue the game so that the dog has to ask to join in again. This helps to reduce competitiveness.
> - If the dog bites during play, then the person should emit a quiet 'yelp' of pain and freeze. Play stops for at least 5 minutes. If play-biting continues, then play stops until the next session and the dog is ignored.

BARKING AND EXCESSIVE VOCALISATION

Barking is one of many forms of vocal communicative behaviour that has a variety of functions depending upon the circumstances and the pattern and type of barking.

The first associations between man and dog depended upon the dog's utility as a guard and selective breeding has been used to increase barking and make dogs into better guards.

Following biting, excessive vocalisation is the next most likely reason for a dog to become the source of an official complaint. Before commencing any sort of investigation and treatment programme, it is vital to establish the kind of problem the dog is creating for the owner and others. If the owner has been threatened with imminent eviction or prosecution, it is better to seek referral at once rather than become involved in what may be an impending disaster.

To make an accurate assessment of why barking occurs, the following obvious points must be addressed:

- When and where does the barking occur?
- Who or what is the target of the barking?
- What stimuli trigger the barking?
- What is the dog seeking to achieve through barking? (What is the motivation?)
- Does the dog bark in any situations other than that which is the source of the problem?
- What are the dog's posture and other behaviours around the time of the barking?

Once these questions have been answered, it should be clear what the cause of the problem barking might be.

If there is any indication that excessive vocalisation is part of separation anxiety, then this should be investigated. Likewise, many older dogs with cognitive deficits or deafness will bark more often and for longer, often in the absence of a perceptible triggering event or stimulus. These problems need to be addressed, especially when treatment is to employ any form of punishment regime to control or curb the behaviour. Automated anti-barking collars should not be used to suppress barking until the motivation for it has been determined and this form of treatment judged to be safe and likely to be effective. Electric shock collars should not be used for the treatment of excessive barking problems.

Territorial barking is very highly motivated and dogs will often ignore adverse events, including powerful shocks, because the need to defend territory has such a high priority. Even if barking is suppressed, the dog will still be motivated to control territoriality in another way, perhaps by attacking silently instead. Often territorial behaviour is supported by both fear and anticipation of the perceived threat. A dog may therefore associate the experience of a shock with the presence of the intruder, leading to increased aggression in the future. Shock collars have been proven to be less effective than other forms of remote training device and represent a potential welfare problem. **They should not be supplied for use by the general public.**

Remember that each type of barking has some innate meaning but, being adaptable, the dog can learn to use barking through repeated reinforcement. For example, dogs that successfully bark for attention often go on to bark to get other things, such as food, play and walks. Once barking becomes a successful strategy for taking control, it can become the overriding communicative behaviour that the dog uses. For this reason, it is important to train a dog to bark and become silent on command so that the behaviour is under control. Then demand-related barking can be terminated and the dog asked to perform another behaviour to get what it wants. Once trained in this way, a dog is usually easier to control when barking in territorial or other situations.

Example treatments

Territorial barking

The motivation and opportunity to defend territory should be reduced; for example, by moving deliveries to a box away and out of view from the house. Removable, plastic film or spray-based glass coatings can help to obscure the view of areas that the dog observes and guards from within the house. Secure, opaque fencing should surround areas to which the dog has access, whether supervised or unsupervised. The dog should not be involved in greeting people at the front door or boundary but, instead, be shut in a quiet place until the person has been admitted.

Table 12.1   Typical observations in vocalisation problems

Type of vocalisation	Context	Target	Triggering event	Objective/motivation	Posture/behaviour
Territorial barking	Dog on familiar territory (home, car) with or without owner	Potential intruder (human or other species)	Target approaches territory	To repel potential intruder, alert group, and call for assistance from others	Tense body posture, possible hackles raised, fast movement to projected place of entry, rising frequency and ferocity of bark as intruder approaches boundary. Ends once threat gone.
Attention-seeking vocalisation (e.g. barking)	Anywhere person is present	Human owner (usually)	Loss of human attention or to gain an immediate reward (such as when begging for food)	To gain attention or some other favour from the owner	Frequency of barking fixed, dog may stare at owner or pace while barking. May continue for many minutes.
Howling/barking when left alone (different from separation anxiety)	Any	None	Owner has been away for some time. A sound or other stimulus causes false expectation that owner is approaching or nearby	To reunite with owner/ group	Barking or howling is brief, infrequent and episodic (unlike separation anxiety). The dog rests normally between bouts.
Fear related/ self-defensive	Any	Unfamiliar person or object	Person/object approaches	To defend against perceived threat	Body tense, frequent lunges toward threat and backtracking from it.

The dog can then be taught to bark and become silent on command.

When the dog barks, the owner should resist the urge to run to it to stop the barking because this satisfies one of the functions of the vocalisation (to alert the group and call for assistance). Instead, the dog should be called away from where it is barking and rewarded for sitting calmly.

Repeated planned provocations using a 'stooge' person will enable the dog to learn to ignore people at the boundary of the territory. Such stooges are only allowed to walk away from the boundary once the dog has been silent for 1 to 2 minutes and should hurry back if the dog barks as they leave.

Attention vocalisation

The dog should be taught to bark and become silent on command and then treated as for other forms of attention-seeking behaviour.

Fear-induced/self-defensive barking

The main objective is to reduce the animal's fear through desensitisation and counterconditioning procedures. Punitive methods are not likely to succeed until fear of the target is reduced, and there is the potential for other more aggressive behaviours to develop if the barking is suppressed. For some dogs, barking has become an almost 'superstitious' action; they are not willing to take a risk that barking is not necessary. By rewarding quietness in the presence of the target, the dog often learns quite quickly that quietness is a more successful and less demanding strategy.

DESTRUCTIVENESS

Destructiveness is seen both in the presence and absence of people.

Destructiveness in the owner's presence

Where people are present somewhere in the household, although not necessarily in the same room as the dog, the motivations are likely to be attention-seeking (or another similar kind of display, perhaps designed to attract the attention of another animal or as an invitation to play), or exploratory behaviour. Dogs do not have hands so they will tend to investigate things with their mouths. If the texture of the object is appealing, then the dog may start to chew or tear at it.

Most owners will punish dogs when they see this sort of behaviour but this can have serious consequences, dependent upon the exact nature of the owner's response:

- Young dogs may be very intimidated by shouting, smacking and other physical punishment. This may sensitise them to eye contact, certain hand gestures and raised voices so that, in the future, these stimuli evoke fearfulness or even self-defensive aggression.
- The dog may learn that destructiveness is a successful means of getting attention.

Diagnosis

The attention seeking or exploratory nature of the destructiveness should be clarified. Attention-seeking destructiveness will follow the same pattern as all other forms of attention-seeking behaviour. Where destructiveness is not due to attention-seeking, then the dog usually shows a range of preferences for the kinds of thing it destroys. The material and construction of the object is important because the dog is getting some positive experience from destroying it.

Treatment

It is far better to divert the animal onto a more suitable target for chewing, such as a nylon chew toy, chew or uncooked bone. The dog is mildly rebuked as soon as it shows an interest in something it is not permitted to have and given something else to investigate. It should then be heavily praised when it shows an interest in the substitute object. If the dog is repeatedly given small amounts of attention whenever it is seen with one of its legitimate chews, then these will become the main things that it destroys.

Owners must be prepared to provide young dogs with a seemingly endless series of things to chew and destroy, which goes against the natural inclination to take away anything that the dog damages, or at least not replace it. To do this risks giving the puppy a reason to investigate other things. For example, an owner may take away a puppy's bed because it gets chewed. The pup could then move on to chew selected soft furnishings, rugs, couches and chairs that it is attracted to and may sleep on. This presents the owner with an increased scale of damage that financially far outstrips the cost of the pet bed. It is far better to accept that young dogs experiment with a range of potentially destructive behaviours and to provide opportunities for them to do this in safety. Chews, rags, special places to dig and activity feeding are all obvious substitutes but it sometimes requires a little imagination to come up with something that will appeal to the dog. Care must always be taken to ensure that toys cannot cause intestinal obstruc-

tion. Valueless items such as cardboard boxes provide endless entertainment.

Destructiveness when people are absent

'Separation anxiety' is the condition commonly presumed to be the cause of dogs being destructive in the absence of the owner; however, this condition is not common and most destructiveness is not related to separation anxiety. Nevertheless, given the serious welfare implications of separation anxiety, it is vital to rule out this problem using detailed history-taking and video observation. Separation anxiety is covered in Chapter 8.

A number of other problems of destructiveness are often confused with separation anxiety:

- Phobia problems (in which the dog has a fear of being trapped because it cannot access an escape route).
- Opportunistic destruction (bored, often young, dogs that experiment with stealing and chewing as a pastime).
- Anxiety about owner return (dogs that have become conditioned to anticipate punishment by returning angry owners).
- Poor habituation to solitude.

Noise phobia problems are quite common in the general canine population and dogs can easily develop a fear of being trapped if they experience a series of loud noises from which they cannot escape. Typically, this happens with dogs that are familiar with using a particular place at home and either this escape route becomes inaccessible or the owners move to a home where there is no comparable hiding place. We also see cases where the dog comes to view the owner as its 'hiding place' so that, if the owner is away, the animal panics when it hears a loud noise. This is engendered by owners trying to soothe and comfort noise-phobic dogs. Dogs deprived of their natural hiding place within the home may try to get out of the house in order to get away from the noise. The simple change of context from indoors to outdoors is sometimes enough for the fear to subside, but many of these dogs continue to panic. The dog will only calm down after the noises have gone away, whereupon it may revert to normal and be found happily wandering in a local park looking for something to do.

Opportunistic destruction is very common. Chewing, digging, ripping and shredding of objects are all quite normal in young dogs who will experiment with a range of activities during their development. Once again, it is the context and target of the behaviour that is the source of the problem. Such dogs will raid bins and cupboards searching for food and things to destroy. These dogs often benefit simply from having some activities to do while the owner is away. Activity feeding with a Buster Cube®, activity ball or similar puzzle feeder is very useful, as is providing the dog with a number of things to destroy which are only available when the owner is out and which closely match the things that the dog has already shown a predilection for chewing or tearing up. There is little point in giving these dogs indestructible rubber bones because part of the reinforcement they get is from actually destroying something.

In some cases, opportunistic destruction is converted into anxiety about the owner's return. These dogs are repeatedly punished by the returning owner for some misdemeanor but the dog has no idea what the punishment is for. Dogs are not able to make associations between events that are separated by even a few minutes so they are unable to connect past misbehaviour with current events. It has to be remembered that the owner's return is of great significance to all dogs and it takes only a few occasions on which the owner has been verbally or physically aggressive for the dog to come dread the owner's return. Anxious dogs will often resort to self-appeasing oral displacement behaviour, such as chewing, because this makes them feel comfortable and more relaxed. The increasing destruction makes the problem worse. These dogs will often attempt to appease the returning owner by acts of vivid submission, such as rolling over or hunching and averting their gaze. Unfortunately, the owner usually misinterprets this as guilt or an 'apology' but, being furious, then continues to corner and physically punish the dog.

Being social animals, dogs are dependent upon having the security of a group. A single house-dog may feel highly isolated if it is left alone all day and this should be a welfare concern. Some dogs do not habituate to solitude because, during puppyhood, they were never away from people or their mother. This becomes a problem when the dog starts to be left while the owner is at work.

All of the above problems can be complicated by mild anxiety that is common in dogs that are not fully used to being left alone or who have had some kind of disruptive life event (like the death of an owner or re-homing), so dogs from rescue kennels are at increased risk of showing separation problems of one kind or another.

There is no reliable data on the exact proportion of animals that have each of these problems, as opposed to separation anxiety, but true separation anxiety is probably rather rare.

Separation anxiety is a very specific condition characterised by over-attachment usually, but not always, to an individual person. The absence of that person causes the dog great distress even if the separation is brief. Anxiety can be defined as the 'apprehensive anticipation of threat or harm' and, since dogs with separation anxiety are concerned with the absence of the person to whom they are attached, we would expect signs of anxiety as that person prepares to depart (Box 12.6).

Treatment

Separation anxiety and anxiety about owner return are discussed in Chapter 8.

Box 12.6 Typical signs of separation anxiety

- The dog shows intense anxiety as the owner prepares to leave.
- The dog is anxious or distressed, even if left with another familiar person.
- The owner will find physical signs of sustained activity and anxiety when they return (hypersalivation, an increase in body temperature, physical exhaustion).
- The dog refuses to spend any time away from the owner; for example it will not sleep in another room overnight.
- Destructiveness, where present, is geared towards escape.
- The pattern of behaviour is always the same; every day sees a repetition of the same destructiveness, elimination or vocalisation.
- When the owner returns the dog is always overwhelmingly excited, even if the separation has been very brief.

Opportunistic destruction is treated by confining the dog in an environment in which there are few opportunities to cause damage other than the range of activities that have been provided by the owner. The dog must be given a wide range of things to rip, shred and chew which provide the same sensory stimulation that the dog has gained from damaging the owner's property. These activities will become less appealing as the dog matures because they are intrinsically unrewarding. The dog should also be given feeding-related activities, such as food-finding games and activity feeding. Since these activities *are* intrinsically rewarding they will come to replace the other more destructive ones.

As always, punishment must not be used because the dog may become anxious if it is punished when the owner returns to find damaged property. An indoor kennel may be used to isolate the dog from things it may destroy.

Dogs that are not habituated to solitude benefit from being given a wider range of stimulating activities that do not involve human participation. They need to be left for short periods of a few minutes (just long enough so that there are no signs of distress) many times each day throughout the week. Quite quickly they will get used to these short times alone and the owner can then begin to extend the time the dog is left on its own.

Prognosis

The prognosis is good for these dogs as long as they are given opportunities to express normal behaviour as they grow up. Most destructive behaviour diminishes before maturity and normal dogs can cope with periods of 3 to 4 hours alone without suffering from stress.

PREDATORY BEHAVIOUR

Predatory behaviour directed at people is uncommon in dogs. It usually results from failure to properly recognise the target as part of the same social group, which is in turn a potential result of inadequate socialisation.

Small children are most commonly the victims of predatory behaviour because of their size and their tendency to emit high-pitched screams and dart about in a manner that, to some dogs, simulates the behaviour of prey.

Diagnosis

It is important to distinguish predatory behaviour from play and true aggression.

The main distinctions are of intent and communication. Aggressive dogs use postural and vocal communication to convey their attitude and conviction prior to taking action. Their aim is to avoid direct conflict. Predatory animals, on the other hand, need the advantage of stealth and surprise to catch their prey and so do not attempt to communicate with the target in any way. Predatory behaviour is extremely dangerous so it is vital to describe accurately all the attributes of the target or prey. For example, the age or size of children at risk, specific clothing, backpacks or other triggers.

Treatment

People, children and other animals that are the potential victims of a predatory dog are at great risk and must be protected. It is essential to keep such dogs leashed and muzzled in any public place or where there is even the slightest chance of encountering a prey target.

Remote punishment may be used to suppress the behaviour, combined with reward for leaving the target of predatory behaviour alone or coming away from it.

Prognosis

Predatory behaviour has a poor prognosis unless owners can predict and control the circumstances in which predation occurs; training methods are not sufficiently reliable to completely stop this highly motivated behaviour. If the predatory target is a child, then the only certain way to protect it is to avoid contact with the dog.

OVERACTIVITY

Overactivity is common and represents an abundance of normally motivated behaviour that is perhaps misdirected or problematic to the owner. Because people are familiar with the term 'hyperactivity' in children, they often will describe the dog's behaviour as such. However, true hyperactivity is a rare and discrete behavioural abnormality that probably has a neurophysiological origin.

The pattern, timing and involvement of the owner are important indicators in deciding the nature of an activity problem.

Hyperactivity shows many common features with other medical conditions and a dog suspected of this problem should be thoroughly investigated to rule out conditions including endocrine, neurological and liver disease.

Overactivity, on the other hand, relates to lack of exercise, excess calorie intake and a lack of owner control over the initiation and termination of activity. It is often associated with play-biting, barking and destruction in order to demand attention (Table 12.2).

Treatment

Dogs with a lack of available stimulation in their environment will seek to find alternative opportunities to occupy themselves. They will find outlets for their energy in ripping fabric, chewing and digging. Young dogs should therefore be provided with a range of activities to serve as outlets for their energy. It is important that some of these activities are solitary; they do not need the participation of a person or another dog. This prevents the dog from becoming dependent on interaction with other individuals to relieve boredom.

Much the same as in small children, some young dogs experience increased frustration and irritability when tired, as their blood glucose level falls during the few hours before a meal. It is therefore sensible to give young dogs proper rest periods in a place where they will not be disturbed and food-rewarded obedience training between bouts of play.

As mentioned elsewhere, food-reward-based training of this kind has the dual benefit of rewarding a calm behaviour and providing the dog with small amounts of food

Table 12.2 Differentiation between hyperactivity and overactivity

Hyperactivity/hyperkinesis	Overactivity
Unable to relax, even in the absence of stimulation	Shows normal ability to sleep and rest
Baseline heart rate, respiratory rate and temperature may be raised when dog is 'at rest', and remain similar when active	Heart rate and other parameters vary normally with activity level
Paradoxical calming effect of dosing with stimulants	Normal stimulant effect
Attention-seeking uncommon; the dog may behave independently of the owner and environment	Attention-seeking is frequent
Videotape will show activity is spontaneous, even in the absence of stimulation or the owner	Periods of activity usually related to stimuli and events

between meals to maintain blood glucose levels. A general plan for the management of overactive dogs should balance the dog's diet with both age and anticipated activity level. Activity feeding balls also contribute to both exercise and easing the active animal's levels of frustration by improving and enriching the animal's environment through self-play.

Playtime itself should be focused onto toys the owner keeps out of reach of the dog at other times so that the owner still remains in control of play.

Clear signals should be given by the owner, using both vocal demands and hand gestures; for example, touching the dog's shoulder with a toy or performing a mock play-bow to start play and turning the head away and giving a pretrained stop signal at the end of play.

Play must be kept brief and punctuated with short bouts of obedience training so that the dog does not become overwhelmingly excited. Frustration and opposition become most apparent when intense play is ended suddenly at the peak of excitement for the dog. Chews can be a useful diversion and pacifier as the young dog learns to wind down and relax at the end of play.

As we have discussed, frequency of activity is important and young dogs need short but frequent periods of activity followed by rest periods; these can gradually be lengthened as the young dog matures. Activities should also take place in a suitable environment and owners need to clearly define the communal areas of the house as active areas (e.g., the garden) and calm areas (e.g., the kitchen, bathroom, stairs and lounge).

If an element of attention-seeking behaviour is suspected, then those rules should be used in conjunction with those described above. The prognosis for curbing overactivity depends on the management of the dog. Normal dogs will mature and calm with age but, until that time, they will seek out a wide range of activities that may displease the owner.

CONSUMPTIVE PROBLEMS

Coprophagia

To most owners coprophagia is simply one of the more revolting aspects of typical dog behaviour. Indeed, it is normal for bitches to eat faeces in order to clean the nest environment.

Some dogs will consume large amounts of their own faeces or those of other animals and then suffer vomiting, diarrhoea and other illnesses as a result. Thus, in some cases, there are genuine health concerns for the pet.

Diagnosis

Coprophagia can occur in normal dogs with no apparent gastrointestinal disease, but it is sensible to check exocrine pancreatic function, occult blood and for evidence of bacterial overgrowth. These are all conditions that can encour-

age a dog to become interested in its own faeces. Although dietary deficiency is rarely a cause of coprophagia or pica, it is worth checking that the animal's diet is balanced and complete. Likewise, check any animals in the household whose faeces have been exclusively selected for consumption. Coprophagia can develop in a number of ways and an understanding of the motivation will assist in finding the solution:

- Attention-seeking behaviour.
- As part of play in a barren environment, either during puppyhood or later when kennelled for a long period.
- Observation of the dam cleaning up a perpetually soiled environment.
- Exploratory behaviour.
- Hunger.

An accurate history, including age of onset and context in which coprophagia occurs, is therefore important. Attention-getting forms of the behaviour should be treated in the same way as other attention-seeking but, because there may still be an appetitive aspect, it is best to give food and attention rewards to the dog for ignoring its faeces immediately after passing them.

Treatment

This problem is made worse when dogs realise they are being followed and observed by their owners who rush and try to stop the dog from eating faeces whenever it investigates them. This actually encourages the dog to swallow the material because this is a way of carrying the 'food' away so that it can be investigated later. These dogs will regurgitate the faeces later on, often in the owner's home.

First, owners must be educated to leave the dog alone when it is investigating its own faeces or those of another animal because then it will not be in 'competition' with the owners for the faeces and is not getting attention for eating them.

Taste aversion methods have long been recommended for discouraging coprophagia but they rarely work. Dogs have a relatively poor sense of taste combined with a heightened sense of smell. This enables them to find and consume food that is in a state of decay. Since vomiting and regurgitation are a part of daily life for a dog, 'taste aversion' is fairly meaningless.

Methods that discourage a dog from sniffing and investigating stools will work much more effectively. Crushed pineapple and grated courgette added to the diet have been successful in some cases, but this may be the result of an odour rather than flavour change.

The best deterrent is to discourage the dog from sniffing faeces, which is a normal precursor to eating it. Most dogs will not eat what they cannot smell first. Finely ground pepper will cause sneezing and irritation whenever it is inhaled. If, for a number of weeks, the dog is only allowed access to faeces that have been sprinkled with fine pepper then the urge to investigate faeces will gradually pass (Box 12.7).

Box 12.7   A summary of alternative ways to reduce coprophagia

- Teach the dog a leave command, which is then used to discourage any investigation of faeces. Fake faeces from a joke shop can be used for practice.
- An activity ball can be given as a reward for ignoring faeces immediately after elimination or for obeying a 'leave' command.
- Provide environmental enrichment and activity feeders for dogs that have developed coprophagia due to poor husbandry.
- Try pineapple or grated courgette as an odour/taste repellent.
- Use peppered faeces to discourage sniffing.
- Finally, in both pica and coprophagia, the use of a remotely operated gas collar (not a shock collar) can be an effective treatment in the last resort.

Pica

Ingestion of plastic, stones and other non-food items is common amongst young dogs and puppies. Pica is part of normal experimental behaviour in young dogs and so it is best to provide a varied enriched environment that satisfies the need for *safe* investigation.

Once again, this can develop into attention-seeking or an invitation to play chase when the dog refuses to relinquish the object. Some dogs will aggressively defend such objects and need to be taught not to be possessive by using exchange games, as described in Advice sheet 5, Appendix 2. They may also learn to swallow objects in order to avoid giving them to the owner.

Some authors have suggested that the specific selection of objects by some adult dogs represents a form of compulsive disorder, especially when the dog disregards other activities in favour of 'stone chewing' or a similar activity.

Treatment

Attention-seeking and compulsive causes should be treated accordingly. If pica is seen as part of a pattern of exploratory and destructive behaviour, then it may be resolved through provision of an enriched environment with things for the dog to damage and investigate safely.

Dogs that swallow objects in order to avoid surrendering them should be treated as for other possession-related problems.

Anorexia

In this context the term 'anorexia' is applied to healthy dogs that refuse to eat.

Sudden onset anorexia is a common sign of discomfort and illness, so medical causes and dental pain should be ruled out first.

Diagnosis

Typical behavioural causes of anorexia include:

- Fussy eating borne out of attention-seeking behaviour or learned 'negotiation' for better food.
- Fear of some event or stimulus associated with feeding, such as the noise of a boiler that switches on while the dog eats or the sound of metal food dishes.
- Fear of conspecifics within the household, especially when learned through aggressive competition for food.
- Competitiveness in bitches may be worse during oestrus, pregnancy and pseudopregnancy.

The image of dogs is as 'walking dustbins' but plenty learn to hold their owners to ransom by refusing to eat regular meals. Dogs that have become fussy in this way are often difficult to train or treat for behaviour problems because food is no longer a motivation for them. Frequently, this fussiness develops as a result of the owner's preoccupation with the dog's nutrition, as is common with new puppies, re-homed and ill dogs. As the animal refuses each meal, it is replaced with a tastier one and the dog becomes the focus of much attention. The dog begins to hold out for better food and more attention so that being fed dog food from a bowl is definitely second best!

These dogs rarely starve and, in many cases, will become obese because they shift the balance of their intake from dog food to scraps begged from the owner.

Treatment

Fear, pain and socially related causes should be treated accordingly. Stimuli associated with fear or pain are counterconditioned. In some cases, it is possible to train dogs to consume food in order to gain access to other more rewarding activities.

Where attention-seeking and negotiation are the cause, the following regime is usually effective:

- Restrict food to mealtimes and training.
- Increase the dog's level of activity and stimulation. Lots of imaginatively designed short games each day will provide more stimulation and increase hunger.
- Scraps can be given, but only when thoroughly mixed into a meal or as a reward during training.
- Access to food at each meal should be no more than 20 minutes.
- Attention should be focused on the dog while it is eating or accepting a treat; attention must be abruptly withdrawn if the dog refuses a meal or stops feeding.

- Activity feeding can be a good way to encourage eating because there is the additional motivation of play.
- Lots of small meals may be better than a single large one, especially for very bored or obese dogs.

Obesity

Diagnosis

Encroaching obesity is not just an indication that a dog is being over fed. It may also be under-stimulated and under-active, a situation that could lead to other problems such as destructiveness, separation problems and frustration. Weight gain is common in older dogs that have become debilitated, depressed or senile.

The same dogs that are apparently fussy eaters are also often obese. This is because the food they are given is rarely measured out into a bowl and is often higher in calorific content than normal dog food. The owner is so grateful that the dog has eaten that they become unaware that the dog is actually gaining weight. Since there can be medical reasons for excessive weight gain, for instance hypothyroidism, these need to be ruled out.

Treatment

The dog's daily ration is divided into several smaller meals, each of which is provided in an activity feeder of some kind. The amount consumed is decreased gradually and more energy is expended to get food. Short, regular bouts of play are easier to fit in with the daily routine than a long walk and yet owners are rarely aware that the two are equally valuable to maintain fitness and health.

Owners are often concerned about the animal's weight and health so regular planned weighing and health checks will give the owner the confidence to proceed. Low-load exercise, such as swimming or walking on soft sand, is a good way to increase exertion without injury.

Excessive water consumption

Polydipsia can be a sign of disease, so medical factors should be ruled out in advance of the behavioural consultation.

Diagnosis

Potential behavioural causes of excess water consumption include:

- play behaviour
- compulsion/stereotypy
- stress/anxiety.

Water play is more common if the water bowl or dispenser is placed in a brightly illuminated area where light can reflect from the water surface, especially if the environment is otherwise barren. So, while water play is not usually a problem, it could be evidence of under stimulation.

Anxious or stressed dogs may drink more water, either because drinking acts as a form of oral displacement behaviour or because stress increases endogenous cortisol, which leads to increased thirst. Causes of anxiety must be investigated and treated.

Treatment

Diversion with increased play and activity feeding will definitely help, as will moving the water bowl to a very dark corner. In some cases, access to water must be restricted but this is safe only as long as water balance and urine specific gravity are monitored. Like many other behaviours, water play and consumption can become compulsive. This is evident when water play substitutes for a range of other previously important activities and the animal becomes progressively more difficult to distract. As with other assumed compulsive or stereotypical behaviour, all factors leading to the behaviour must be addressed, including management, environment and owner attention.

DIGGING

Digging is a normally motivated behaviour in many dogs and is something that young dogs will experiment with as part of their behavioural development. Whether it becomes a problem largely depends upon the motivation to dig and choice of digging location.

Diagnosis

In many cases, digging is an exploratory and food-finding activity, but some dogs dig to escape. Normal motivations to escape include access to a mate, to find food, to repel a potential intruder (neighbour's dog or cat, person), to engage in exploratory behaviour or to gain social contact with conspecifics. Digging to escape is dealt with under roaming. Digging can also become compulsive in some individuals.

Treatment

It is not acceptable to use punishment to suppress unwanted normal behaviour unless the dog has another outlet for the same activity. Punishment will simply divert the dog's activities away from one activity to another that may be even less desirable. In any case, punishment will not completely suppress motivated exploratory behaviour like digging. Young dogs often grow out of random digging as long as they have some opportunity to carry out the behaviour.

It is very useful to train the dog to dig on command because this enables the owner to redirect the digging to specific places in the garden or on walks. This is easily achieved by finding some loose earth in a dog-recreation area and hiding several small pieces of chew just under the soil. The dog is taken to this location and, before it has had a chance to investigate the spot where the chews are hidden, the owner should start to say the dig command excitedly, point at the ground and possibly paw at it in a way that simulates digging. Most dogs will immediately join in unless they have been severely punished for digging in the past. In some cases, the owner may simply have to point at the ground and say 'dig' for the dog to start investigating the spot. Clicker reinforcement may be used to repeatedly reward the action of digging; either with additional treats thrown into the disturbed soil for the dog to root out or no reward being thrown and simply depending on the dog finding the treats and chews that have already been buried. After a number of training sessions of this kind, the dog will respond to the dig command and may be rewarded for digging in any location where it is more desirable for the owner, either at home or on walks.

If possible, the dog should be given a digging spot in the garden which is trained using the same method as above. A large, deep hole is dug and then filled with a mixture of sifted topsoil and sand so that it drains easily and is safe and pleasant for the dog to dig in. Small chews are then regularly hidden in this spot so that the dog can find them. Other digging places will become less rewarding and digging will focus on this special area. It also gives the owner the opportunity to scold the dog for digging in less desirable places and then command it to dig in the right place.

For owners who really don't want any digging in the garden, one potential solution is to heavily reward digging on command in places off-territory and provide other kinds of food-finding games at home using hidden food and activity feeders (see Advice sheet 16 in Appendix 2).

Areas that the dog must not dig may be protected by removing a layer of topsoil (6 inches), covering the under soil with a 1 inch plastic mesh and then replacing the sifted overlying soil. The soil now contains nothing worth finding and the dog soon comes to a barrier that prevents further digging. The sheets of mesh must be large so that the weight of soil over them prevents the dog from dragging or pulling the mesh out.

ROAMING

When animals are allowed to roam they are at risk of loss, injury or even death due to road traffic accidents. They can become involved in fights with other animals over territory and food. When startled or frightened, they can bolt across roads, injure strangers trying to come to their aid or cause others to have an accident. All these incidents can lead to a legal claim and resulting prosecution being made against the owner. It is therefore advisable for pet owners to have third party liability insurance as well as the animal's normal health insurance.

Diagnosis

The precise reason for the roaming must be understood if treatment is to be effective. Is the dog escaping from a boring environment in search of something to do or is there a specific attraction to escape? Male dogs will break out of almost any enclosure to get to a bitch on heat.

Treatment

The motivation to roam can be reduced in a number of ways. If the home and garden environment is made interesting enough and the dog is properly exercised both mentally and physically, then the motivation to wander will be reduced. The dog's own garden should provide as much mental stimulation as possible with activity feeders, scatter feeding, places to dig and raised platforms so that it can adopt a central vantage point in the garden. Often the garden is just a place where the dog is put out to go to the toilet so it is not associated with any enjoyable activity. Owners should try to concentrate periods of play and attention in the garden so that the dog does not merely see it as a toilet and escape route. Regular off-territory social contact with other people and dogs can also inhibit a dog's desire to roam as it helps to fulfil the dog's social needs. However, it is vital to train a proper recall for walks in public places. A dog that is still learning proper recall can still be safely and easily exercised by a fit and enthusiastic owner who is willing to run about with a dog on an extendible leash. In fact, this often builds a really good relationship.

Fences and gates must be properly designed. Most dogs can jump even a high fence and can climb up chain link. They are more than capable of digging several feet under a fence.

Shock-collar-based containment systems are not a substitute for proper conventional fencing because they cannot provide absolute security. Animals may still escape and, once off-territory, they will be shocked for trying to return. Also, if the power fails the dog is free to roam.

Dogs may also roam to seek out reproductive opportunities. This is especially true for entire males who have exhibited a previous sexual interest whenever a female is in oestrus within the neighbourhood. In 75% of this group neutering reduces roaming.

CAR TRAVEL

Problems of car travel mainly relate to:

- aversive experiences (motion sickness, journey to the veterinary surgery or kennels)
- overexcitement, with hysterical vocalisation (excited anticipation of the journey's end at a favourite location). These dogs are frequently worse on the outward leg of a journey.

- movement chasing (often collie type dogs follow and bark at cars and people as they pass by). These dogs settle better when they cannot see moving objects around the car, such as when in a constant flow of fast moving traffic on a motorway.

The dog's response will begin with anticipatory and preparatory behaviour as the time for car travel approaches, becoming anxious or overexcited. Hypersalivation and other signs of nausea may be seen before the dog even gets in the car. The treatment of all of these problems uses essentially the same methods, but with slight variations according to the individual problem.

Treatment

A typical plan for training dogs to tolerate car travel:

Associate time spent in the motionless vehicle with a calming and positive experience, such as feeding, so that the dog shows signs of calm but positive anticipation when taken to the car.

Train the dog to adopt a calm behaviour (sit or lie down) on cue and then reward the dog for remaining in this state in the motionless vehicle.

Once the dog is resting calmly, other key features of car travel are introduced individually over a number of sessions (seatbelts on, engine on, trickling movement down the drive, short journeys), only moving on to the next stage when the dog is not showing anxiety or overexcitement at the current stage.

DAP® spray (CEVA Animal Health) may be applied in the car before training sessions or travel, in accordance with the manufacturer's instructions, to make this location feel safer and less stressful. DAP® spray has been shown to significantly reduce the severity of car travel problems involving stress and nausea.

Other actions should be taken for specific problems:

- *Motion sickness:* Do not feed the dog before car travel, consider use of non-sedative medication that has proven efficacy against motion sickness.
- *Overexcitement*: To begin with, introduce car travel only on return legs of walks, and take the dog on many short journeys that go nowhere in particular.
- *Movement chasing*: Tether the dog into a rear compartment foot well so that it cannot see and track the movement of objects outside the car. Positively reinforce non-attendance to stimuli to which the dog would normally react.

For dogs that experience intense anxiety or fear, perhaps as the result of car accidents and other trauma associated with vehicles, it may be necessary to use other methods for treating specific fear, perhaps including psychoactive medication.

Dogs should always be secured in a harness during travel to prevent them from interfering with control of the vehicle and attacking service personnel or passengers after an accident.

SEXUAL BEHAVIOUR DIRECTED AT PEOPLE (MOUNTING)

Mounting behaviour is not always sexually motivated and starts to be displayed from only a few months of age, well before puberty. In young dogs, this is normal experimental behaviour and will not necessarily respond to castration. Neutering is only effective for behaviour that is genuinely sexually motivated and, even then, there is a significant learned component.

Rather than being purely sexual, mounting often starts as a response to overexcitement and frustration. Where this occurs in young dogs, it is essential not to shake or move the body part that the dog has attached itself to because this will make the experience more stimulating and rewarding. Instead, the dog should be distracted at the first moment when it is about to mount and rewarded for doing something else. The dog may be called away and rewarded for compliance. If the dog does latch on, it should be removed impassively without giving any attention.

Mounting may be a signal of a failure of communication between the owner and the dog so a general plan of remedial training of communication signals should be instituted according to the handouts in Appendix 2.

GETTING DOGS ON AND OFF FURNITURE

Dogs that refuse to get off furniture are often seen as dominant, even if they show submissive behaviours and are not aggressive. This is because any kind of opposition may be interpreted as a challenge to authority.

Before making assumptions of this kind, it is very important to investigate pain and other medical factors that may cause a dog to be reluctant to step off the couch. Back pain, for example, is a common reason for dogs to growl or refuse to get down.

In most cases, the dog refuses to get off and shows submissive behaviour because it interprets the owner's approach as a threat. The reason for this is easily understood if we look at the situation from the dog's point of view:

- In the past, the owner has approached and told the dog to get off the couch in an angry voice.
- The dog has not understood and has remained where it is.
- The owner has become progressively more annoyed and has finally forcefully dragged the dog from the couch and scolded, smacked or socially excluded it.
- Repeat this sequence of events a few times and the dog sitting on the couch will automatically see the owner's approach as potentially aversive.

- If the owner continues to punish the dog after it has repeatedly submitted then it may start to become aggressive.

The solution is to begin training before the dog starts to become aggressive and to train getting on and off the couch as a kind of game. A clicker-training method can be used:

Basic clicker-training is used to associate clicks and rewards with cued behaviour.

- A piece of food is used to lure the dog to get onto the piece of furniture.
- As the dog gets on, the command cue is spoken (after the dog's name).
- Once the dog is on the furniture, a click is delivered and the food treat follows.
- The same process is used to lure the dog off the furniture.
- This cycle is repeated, getting the dog on and off the furniture until it will get on and off on cue.

Gradually, the lure is phased out and the dog is asked to perform several acts of obedience before getting the click and reward (random reinforcement schedule).

This command can then be used in genuine situations where the owner wants to get the dog off furniture, but the owner must always give clicks and rewards each time until it is clear that the dog is responding without posing a challenge. Then food rewards can be phased out and replaced with praise.

JUMPING UP

Jumping up represents an attempt to get closer to the facial area of the person and to get attention. It is very common among dogs but should be absolutely discouraged because it can easily cause injury. Elderly people and small children are at serious risk of injury if jumped at and pushed. This has resulted in legal action against dog owners.

The traditional advice to prevent jumping up has usually been to use extinction; the dog gets no reinforcement and is supposed to learn that jumping up is no longer rewarded. The problem with this approach is that jumping up tends to be worse at times when the dog is already very excited and, if ignored, the dog is very likely to increase the intensity of its behaviour to a level that cannot be ignored. In any case, it is beyond belief that anyone can really manage to ignore a large heavy dog that is jumping up at them. Even if the owner can do this, what about visitors to the home?

Treatment

It is far better to use a method of response substitution in combination with some clear communication and extinction:

- Train the dog to sit, on cue.
- Teach the 'no' signal (see Advice sheet 11, Appendix 2).
- Reproduce the situation that normally provokes jumping up, but at times when it is less emotionally significant and the dog can concentrate better. For example, the person goes in and out of the house repeatedly, staying out for only a few seconds at a time. When they come in, they ask the dog to sit and then give a series of clicks and food rewards while the dog stays calm.
- If the dog jumps up, the person uses the 'no' signal and asks for a sit instead.
- After a number of repetitions, the person may try coming in without giving a cue and simply wait to allow the dog to choose what it is going to do. If it jumps up, then the 'no' signal is given. If it sits then it gets clicks and food.
- In this way, the dog learns what it should do in a relatively unchallenging situation and the same training can be generalised to times when the person is coming home after longer periods away.

If jumping up is seen during play, then the protocol for controlling play behaviour should be used (Advice sheet 8, Appendix 2) and the 'no' signal used to inhibit jumping up. To make the 'no' signal even more significant in these situations, it is often helpful to use a tiny sideways or backwards step so as to avoid the dog being able to put his feet against the person.

It is generally not a good idea for a person to turn their back on a large dog that is jumping up because these dogs may get frustrated and are big enough to get hold of and damage clothing or nip the person on the neck or face. This is hard to ignore and, when the person turns around to scold the dog, it rapidly learns that this new behaviour is an even more reliable means of demanding a response, albeit a negative one.

It is also inadvisable to use punishment methods such as pushing the dog away, shouting at or hitting it because, at best, the dog may think the person is acting playfully and, at worst, they may see punishment as a threat.

For very boisterous dogs, the additional control of a muzzle, halter and leash can make training safer, especially for visitors, because this limits the dog's ability to make the mistake of jumping up. At the start of training, a trailing leash can be useful because the person who enters the home can stand on the end while doing training, thus preventing the dog from jumping up.

LEASH CONTROL, PULLING, ETC.

As with any behaviour, understanding the motivation is the first step:

- Pulling to get to a place (e.g., the park).
- Pulling to get home (sign of fear or anxiety).
- Lunging at cats, other dogs, moving cars, bikes, people, children, etc.

If there is some specific motivation, such as fear of traffic, people or other dogs, this has to be dealt with. Basic methods such as reward-based training and omission training work well.

With reward-based training, the dog might be given a series of highly valued food treats while it is walking alongside the owner, perhaps in combination with clicker-training. This response is best taught in a quiet and non-distracting location, such as the garden, and then generalised to other more challenging situations.

Omission training is very powerful for dogs that are motivated to pull toward the park but walk nicely on the way home. If the dog walks next to the person, leaving the leash slack, the person continues walking. If the dog walks ahead of the person or pulls on the leash, the person stops and starts to walk backwards until the dog is alongside them again. In this way the dog's pulling has the opposite effect to that which is anticipated. Instead of hurrying the person along, it actually delays getting to the park. The most important feature of this training is that the person stops moving forward as soon as the dog is ahead of them, not just when the leash goes tight. The aim is to have a dog that understands that it should walk alongside the person, not that it should pull more gently.

Choke collars are not suitable for any dog that continues to pull and should not be used to jerk dogs back or apply pressure to the throat. Laryngeal fractures or paralysis and retinal haemorrhage can result from inappropriate use of choke chains or conventional collars if force is applied too often or for long periods. Dogs have very little sensation in the throat area and will disregard the pain and discomfort from pulling, so it is very easy for the throat to be damaged just as a result of the dog's own pulling.

Body harnesses are not appropriate for training and should only be used if there is some need to protect the dog's throat. The attachment point to such harnesses is above the dog's centre of rotation, which means that they provide no control whatsoever. They also allow the dog to pull harder.

Special body harnesses are available which apply pressure to the dog's axilla when it pulls. These harnesses are also of limited usefulness. If used harshly they have the potential to cause damage to the brachial plexus, often cause localised soreness and skin damage around the axilla in shorter-haired breeds and are not entirely secure. A dog may learn to allow the harness to go slack and then step out of it, unless there is a specific design or adjustment to prevent this.

It is best to use a face halter (Halti®, Gentle Leader®, etc.) because this allows greater leverage against the dog's pulling and avoids injury to the animal's throat. The dog should not be jerked back on this kind of harness either, because harsh use can still cause neck injury through twisting. It is generally recommended that these harnesses be used in combination with a double-ended leash so that the other end of the leash can be clipped to the dog's conventional collar. This provides extra security if the dog breaks the harness. Alternatively, a single-ended leash may be clipped to the muzzle harness and the ring of a correctly fitted half-check collar. This provides a similar level of security without interfering with the function of the muzzle harness.

NON-AGGRESSIVE OBJECT POSSESSION

Possession is a normal part of play and many dogs will enjoy playing a game in which they are chased while running around with a toy. This can become more serious as the dog matures and possession becomes a more important issue for the dog. The pattern of growling may change to become more aggressive and the dog will not let the person take the toy away. Play ends up being stifled.

It is best to tackle these problems before they are so severe that there is genuine aggression and a risk of biting. The dog needs to be taught to drop objects on command, as part of a play routine, so that giving up objects is not seen as a challenge by either party.

Dogs tend to have certain favourite types of toy that they are most keen to withhold or guard. Owners should make a list of the objects the dog plays with and then allot a value to each according to the level of guarding the dog displays. Training should start with objects that the dog does not guard and gradually build up to things that it does want to possess. Free access to toys should be withdrawn so that the dog retains 'ownership' of nothing.

A typical clicker-training procedure might be as follows:

- Owner sits with a food pot and clicker
- Get out a toy and play a short game with it (throw–fetch or tug, whichever is most appropriate).
- Ask the dog to drop the toy.
- As the toy drops from its mouth give a click and then a reward.
- Hand the toy back or recommence play as before.
- If the dog does not drop it, withdraw attention and use the 'no' signal.
- Repeat the drop command.
- Give the dog three chances to drop and then stop the game if it fails to comply (go away and ignore the dog for 10 minutes)
- Repeat this cycle of play and requests for a drop command.
- At the end of the game, ask the dog to drop. Take away the toy and give the dog a favourite food chew to occupy it for a few minutes.

In this way, the dog gets a reward and ends up with the return of the toy for continued play. At the end of the game, it has the benefit of a chew but if it fails to comply with the training it gets ignored. If the owner can commit to several short bouts of this training each day then there will be evidence of success within 2–3 weeks.

There is also an Advice sheet (No. 5) in Appendix 2, which offers a play-based method for helping to resolve the problem.

FOOD STEALING

Dogs are opportunists and their survival in the wild depends upon an ability to find and make use of all available food resources. Food left in bins, unlocked cupboards and on unattended plates is 'fair game' for an animal that has evolved to scavenge and whose bargain with mankind was to eat whatever was leftover after we had eaten.

However, owners can become very angry when they return to the kitchen to find that their roast dinner has disappeared. This is a problem of owner education. The more opportunities the dog has to 'steal' food, the greater the chance it will learn to find this rewarding and will continue to look for opportunities to do so in the future. Punishing a dog after it has finished eating the food will have the same negative effect as any other kind of delayed punishment. If the owners catch the dog while it is still eating what it has stolen, it may become aggressive if they try to punish it, especially if the dog is going through the food hierarchisation phase of development (around 6 months of age). The perceived competition with owners over food can make these dogs aggressive around their food bowls or in other situations where food is present. This may spill over into guarding areas where food is consumed which can become a serious problem.

The best solution is for owners to avoid leaving opportunities for the dog to scavenge in an undesirable manner by using child locks to protect cupboards, fridges, etc. They must then give the dog legitimate scavenging opportunities by using activity feeders, scatter feeding and food-finding games.

FAILURE TO RESPOND TO RECALL COMMANDS

Young dogs should not be allowed off leash until they have been trained in some basic commands such as sit and recall, at home. The reason is that quite a number of dogs run away and will not come back on their first time at the park. The owner may punish the dog, which damages any possibility of being able to train recall in that context in the future. The owner then refuses to allow the dog to run free, which sets the scene for developing social problems and frustration which may ultimately result in aggression.

A recall can be strengthened during play and training sessions involving groups of people using the methods in Advice sheet 11, Appendix 2 and the various games. Young dogs should be called at dinner time and regularly during the day to be given food treats or to play. Interactive play and training should be performed several times each day at home and in the garden. Most puppies are effectively housebound until their vaccinations are complete, which allows for a month of training during which the pup can learn basic signals and how to interact with friendly dogs to which it is introduced.

Training should then be extended to the park with the puppy on an extending leash and the owner regularly calling the puppy and then giving food or play as a reward for coming. The aim is to make the owner the centre of the dog's attention so that the owner's signals can overcome the dog's enthusiasm for investigating what is around it. This interaction between dog and owner during walks should continue throughout the dog's life, otherwise the dog will learn to ignore them and find its own entertainment.

Older dogs that do not perform a reliable recall have often learned to ignore the owner because that person is of no interest during walks. The first step to correcting this is to increase the amount of play and training the owner carries out so that their presence begins to matter to the dog. The dog should be kept on an extending leash on walks and the owner should continue to play and interact with the dog.

Basic recall is trained at home in the same way as with an immature dog and then practised with the adult dog still on an extending leash. The dog must not be allowed off leash until the recall has been perfected.

Clicker-training may be used to improve recall in dogs. First, the dog is taught to understand the meaning of the click and then clicker-trained to do a few basic commands. Recall is then trained on an extending leash for safety. The dog is given the recall signal and, as soon as it looks around and starts to move toward the owner, a series of closely spaced clicks and plenty of encouragement should be given. The clicks continue as long as the dog is coming toward the person who recalled it. If the dog turns away or gives up then the clicks stop immediately. The recall command is repeated and clicks begin again when the dog starts to obey again. A large food or play reward is given when the dog arrives at the owner. The idea of giving repeated clicks is that this increases the dog's anticipation of reward and helps it to understand that continuing to run back to the owner is what gets the reward. Turning away or stopping is harder for the dog because this means potentially losing the reward that it has already begun to expect. Loss of anticipated reward is a form of punishment. Once the dog is behaving well on an extending leash, the same training may be continued with a 50 foot long trailing rope or line attached to the dog's collar. The rope must be very fine and slippery, such as plastic coated washing line, so that it does not snag or tangle in vegetation. This is used as a safety precaution so that, if the dog does attempt to run away, the owner can put a foot on the line to stop it. The line must not be picked up while the dog is moving, because severe skin burns can result. Once recall is perfected the line is gradually shortened a few inches per day until none is left.

ADVICE SHEETS THAT MAY BE RELEVANT TO THIS CHAPTER

In Appendix 2

1. Using a houseline
2. Jumping up
3. Reward and punishment
5. Reducing possessiveness through play
6. Muzzle training
7. Territorial triggers
8. Play and calm signals
9. The 'come away' command
10. The indoor kennel
11. Attention-seeking and the 'no' signal
12. Click-touch training
13. Preparations for phobic events
14. Using training discs or a rattle can
16. Environmental enrichment for dogs
17. Using food rewards for training
18. Food for work
19. Introducing the clicker

PART 4

Feline behavioural problems

PART CONTENTS

Chapter **13**

Feline fear, anxiety and phobia problems

INTRODUCTION

Although fears and phobias are perhaps more closely associated with dogs, it is true that feline fear is a real issue in behavioural medicine and the behavioural consequences can be many and varied. Cats that are fearful may become more dependent on the owner, while others may lack confidence in dealing with family members. In extreme cases, fearful cats can go on to form abnormal attachments with their owners and may display separation-related behaviours. Cats can also become agoraphobic and may show reactions to sounds, people and other animals which are indicative of a fearful motivation. The most commonly documented fear-inducing stimuli in cats include other animals (both cats and other species), strangers (human), noises and unusual experiences such as travelling or visiting the vet. (A general discussion of fear and anxiety is included in Chapter 8.)

Cats who are reacting in a fearful manner to stimuli which are not innately fear-inducing may do so for a variety of reasons.

Potential causes of feline fears, phobias and anxiety-related problems include:

- a lack of appropriate socialisation and habituation
- genetic influence on timidity
- one-off traumatic incidents
- anticipation of unpleasant experiences, e.g., anticipation of attack by neighbouring cats can lead to cases of agoraphobia
- old age – loss of competence and an increase in general fearfulness in geriatric cats is well-recognised
- unintentional owner reinforcement of fearful responses.

The most obvious response to fear is self-defence when there is some prospect of driving the fear-eliciting stimulus away, or when escape is not possible. However, responses to fear are complex and may produce long-lasting changes in behaviour.

In fearful situations cats can therefore either:

1. Withdraw from the environment, both social and physical, or
2. Show a decreased threshold of reactivity to stimuli, leading to reactive behavioural manifestations of the fear.

Withdrawal from the environment can lead to:

- an increase in withdrawn and secretive behaviour, including hiding
- reluctance to go outdoors or to enter open spaces within the home
- a desire to get up high onto inaccessible resting places within the home
- a decrease in desire for interactive behaviour with familiar humans
- a decrease in interest in social and object play.

More obviously reactive signs of fear in cats can include:

- indoor marking behaviours, such as urine spraying
- loss of house-training, owing to some fearful association with the latrine location
- low-threshold flight reaction
- defensive aggression
- wool-eating and other pica
- over-grooming and even self-mutilation.

Somatic signs of fear may also be evident including:

- tachycardia (bradycardia in chronic situations)
- pupillary dilatation
- tachypnoea
- piloerection
- inappetence
- vomiting.

Normal fear and phobia are different from one another, both behaviourally and clinically. Normal fear protects the individual without interfering with normal behaviour that is important for survival and self-maintenance. Normal fear has only temporary effects while the object of fear is present or perceived to be a threat. A normally fearful animal will naturally habituate to any static stimulus that is presented at relatively low intensity. For example, a cat might initially show fear of a carrier bag but, as the fear subsides, this turns to approach and investigation. Ultimately, the bag is accepted as non-threatening. This process of habituation will be slower if the object is moving and slower still if it shows signs of intent (i.e., if it is animate). Movement delays habituation because the threat posed by the object is constantly changing. Although definitions of phobia are controversial, one definition is that phobic fear limits or interferes with normal behaviour and persists after the object of fear has gone away. Phobic fear does not naturally lessen with the kind of exposure to a stimulus that would otherwise produce habituation. The treatment of phobic fear and normal fear are intrinsically similar, although the duration of treatment of phobia is likely to be longer and there is a greater possibility of the need for psychoactive drug therapy.

PREVENTION

As with fear in any species, the rule of prevention being better than cure certainly applies. It is essential to remember that cats need to be taught to live in human society and to accept that all the signs of human activity are, in fact, normal. To this end, it is paramount that breeders understand the importance of the socialisation period and ensure that there is sufficient and appropriate socialisation and habituation of very small kittens. In cats, the primary sensitive period of socialisation is very early, running from approximately 2 to 7 weeks of age. During this time, the majority of cats, especially pedigree ones, are with the breeder on their premises and therefore the duty for ensuring that kittens come into society as acceptable companion animals rests largely on the breeder's shoulders. The potential genetic influence on feline temperament through the boldness trait of the tom-cat is a topic that has received a lot of attention in recent years and it is now generally accepted that the temperament of both the queen and the tom are important when deciding on breeding programmes. The fact that kittens can be reliably identified on the basis of the behavioural reactions of the father is evidence for a genetic factor, and the boldness trait is believed to be important in enabling kittens to cope with interaction with their environment, both social and physical (Box 13.1).

Puppy parties are now a relatively common feature of general practice but rather less provision is offered to kittens. It is possible to organise kitten parties, although the risks of infectious disease are greater than for puppy parties, and the kittens will almost certainly have finished their socialisation period at the time of the party. What may be easier, more practical and equally worthwhile is to offer clients an educational evening on cat behaviour, to cover aspects of environmental enrichment, handling and social

---

Box 13.1   Prevention of feline fear, anxiety and phobia problems

- Select kittens that come from bold, sociable parents.
- Avoid kittens that have been reared in isolation from normal domestic activities.
- Properly reared kittens should meet a wide variety of people and other animals.
- They should be exposed to a wide range of noises and other everyday events.
- Confident behaviour can be shaped by a reinforcing approach and other bold behaviours using food rewards and play.
- To encourage confidence, it is important not to pick up and hold cats, but rather to allow them to approach voluntarily.
- Owners should be taught to understand and appropriately reciprocate normal feline greeting behaviour.

interaction so that kitten owners can properly understand and mould their cat's behaviour.

Many of the principles of the origins of feline fears are the same as those that apply to canine fears, but the influence of the individual cat, the owner and the environment need to be considered. Once kittens are living in their new home, there are a variety of potential factors which can contribute to the establishing of feline fears and new owners need to be advised on how to minimise the risk factors. Owners need to be aware of the risks of unintentional reinforcement of fear-related responses and they should ensure that, when the cat is showing signs of fear, they do not react in a way which could be misinterpreted.

It is important to:

- cease untimely reassurance
- avoid all confrontation and physical punishment
- minimise upheaval in the core territory during major renovation or redecoration
- prevent over-attachment by encouraging access to outdoors and enabling the cat to express its full range of natural behaviours.

When dealing with cats who are exhibiting fear-related behaviour problems, it is essential for owners to realise that the cat needs to feel in control of the situation and that forcing the cat to confront its fear is unlikely to be effective. Flight is a primary defence strategy for the cat and, therefore, in some cases it may be necessary to block the flight route while desensitisation and counterconditioning techniques are applied. Obviously, one of the most important factors in the success of any behavioural treatment for feline fears is the correct application of reinforcement and an understanding of the relative value of resources is essential.

INTRODUCING A CAT TO ITS NEW HOME OR ENVIRONMENT

The importance of properly introducing new cats to a home where there are existing cats is well-known (see Chapter 16). If introduction is not managed correctly, there is a greater probability of fear and anxiety problems in the future. It is also important to introduce cats correctly to households where there are no other cats but where animals, children and the general routine in the household may be unfamiliar and stressful. The same is true when moving cats from one home to another (Box 13.2).

GENERAL PRINCIPLES OF THE TREATMENT OF FELINE FEAR PROBLEMS

Behavioural modification techniques which can be used in the management of feline fears are the same as those used in the canine field, but the way in which they are applied will be modified to take into account differences between cats and dogs in terms of natural behaviour and perception of reward (see Chapter 8).

> **Box 13.2   Introducing a cat to a new home/environment**
>
> - Before moving the cat to its new home, try to harvest some of the cat's flank and facial odours onto a clean cloth. Place this cloth into a sealed bag ready to use in the new home.
> - When transferring the cat, bring items that will carry some of the cat's facial and flank odour marks (bedding, resting places).
> - Prepare a quiet room in the new home with food, water, a latrine and familiar items from the cat's previous home. This will be the room into which the cat will be initially introduced so it is best if this place has not recently been occupied by other cats.
> - Use the cloth to transfer facial and flank odours to furniture in this room of the new home.
> - Install a F3 diffuser (Feliway®, CEVA Animal Health) in this room 1 to 2 hours before the cat arrives.
> - Install additional diffusers throughout the home at a rate of 1 per 50–70 m^2.
> - Allow the cat to explore the new room by opening the cat basket. The cat should be able to return to the basket if it desires. The cat should not be pulled out of the basket or coaxed.
> - Do not allow access to the rest of the house until the cat is completely relaxed in this first room. This may take several hours or even a few days. The cat should be relaxed, playful and approachable.
> - The cat should then be allowed free access to one or two additional rooms in the house every couple of hours until it has explored the whole house. The cat should be allowed to do this in peace, not with people rushing around or trying to distract it.

The role of the environment

The normal feline coping strategy in fearful situations is highly dependent upon familiarity with the environment and the opportunities it provides for escape and avoidance behaviour. In this way, the cat is highly attached and dependent upon its territory for security which also means that success in treating fear-based problems is substantially dependent upon the cat's environment.

The core zone of the cat's territory is where it expects to be safest. This is where it may meet familiar conspecifics. Recognition of the core territory is partially dependent upon pheromone odour signals. The cat expends a lot of time and energy placing face and flank marks within the core territory area, not only to identify elements of the environment as familiar but also to create an appeasing environment for itself. From the cat's perspective, marking of this kind is very efficient. It enables the cat to recognise a safe location from a set of scent mark 'mementos' without having to remember details about its appearance and the events that have happened there. This reduces the cognitive burden of processing and memorising the information. In a new home, these personalised signals will be absent and may even be replaced by the odours of other cats that were previously resident. The anxiety caused creates the conditions for establishing problem behaviour.

It is possible, by using synthetic pheromone analogues such as F3 (Feliway®, CEVA Animal Health), to recreate or enhance core territory odours. This can increase perceived safety and familiarity in an existing environment or make a new environment appear familiar and safe.

This attachment to environmental familiarity makes cats very vulnerable to stress when they are relocated through re-homing or when the owners move house. Proper introduction to a new 'core territory' reduces stress and the likelihood of fear problems. Creating attachment to a new core territory also reduces the risk of the cat straying or trying to return to its original territory after a house move.

Normal exploration of a new environment follows a star-shaped pattern. The animal makes forays into the environment away from an initial safe place. Any fearful event will cause the animal to return briefly to its place of safety. Indeed, successfully learning about a new environment depends upon already having somewhere safe to return to. Without this, the animal will experience considerable anxiety and fear which may create long-term aversions to the stimuli the cat encounters during the first few hours in a new location. For example, a well-socialised cat might enjoy the company of children when they are in an environment that it understands but the same cat may react fearfully to boisterous children when in a new environment. This kind of encounter can condition fear reactions that continue to plague the cat's relationship with the children, even once it has settled into the new home.

It is therefore essential that the cat accepts and feels safe in the new environment before encountering any potential stressors.

Examples of behavioural modification techniques

- Habituation
- Desensitisation
- Counterconditioning
- Controlled exposure

Selecting rewards which are of sufficient value to override the fear response can be difficult and, with a high priority for flight as a defence strategy in cats, it can be difficult to keep cats in the vicinity of the fear-inducing stimulus during processes such as habituation. Flooding is also a risky approach since the panic induced by the lack of opportunity to escape can potentiate rather than ameliorate the condition. Controlled exposure, desensitisation and counterconditioning can be useful techniques and, pro-

vided that the fear stimulus is diluted sufficiently, it should be possible to override the flight response. Introducing a cat to an environment for desensitisation may require leading it in on a body harness and extending lead. The cat should be fully acclimatised to the harness and leash for several weeks before using it in a training situation. For further information on practical aspects of behavioural therapy for fear problems, see the problem-specific information below.

Pharmacological intervention

There are a number of reasons why medication may be indicated in cases of feline fear. Cases involving central nervous system pathology, in relation to neurotransmitters, may require medication on a long-term basis and, in situations where the fear-inducing stimuli are either unidentifiable or uncontrollable, long-term or recurring medication may also be indicated. In other cases where medication is necessary as an adjunct to behavioural therapy owing to the severity of the fear response and the adverse effect that it has on the learning process, the usual aim is to have short-term drug support.

As with behavioural therapy, it is important not to simply transfer treatment regimes from the canine world but to consider the differences between cats and dogs in terms of metabolism and potential side-effects.

Modifying the owner's reaction

The final part of the equation when dealing with feline fears is to modify the owner's reaction to the cat's behaviour. Unintentional reinforcement of fears is most likely to occur in cats when they flee and escape the stimulus but owner interaction, both vocal and tactile, may be seen by some cats as reward for their response. Punishment is always going to be counterproductive and techniques designed to make the animal 'confront its fear', such as flooding, have limitations which have already been discussed.

FEAR–BASED PROBLEMS

Fear of species other than humans (e.g., dogs)

Prevention

When introducing cats to unfamiliar dogs, it is important to allow the cat an escape route which allows it to get away from the dog without triggering a chase behaviour. High shelves or a baby-gate are ideal because they allow the cat to get away but still remain in sight of the dog. Once dogs have learned how rewarding it is to chase a cat, it may be very difficult to get the animals to co-exist without further stress. Critical to this is the cat's initial response. Remembering that cats recognise familiarity through

The immediate aims are to prevent progression from escape–avoidance behaviour to aggression, and to reduce stress.

- Avoid any uncontrolled exposure to fear-eliciting stimuli, especially in the home.
- Stop all punishment of fearful behaviour. Do not use restraint or coercion to force the cat to remain in the presence of the thing it fears.
- Do not hold the cat while it is in the presence of the object of its fear, as this can produce outbursts of very aggressive and dangerous behaviour.
- Stop attempts to soothe the cat by giving it attention as this may reward fearful behaviour.
- The cat must be supervised at all times when in contact with dogs.
- The dog must be properly controlled when in the presence of the fearful cat.
- Provide the cat with one or more safe and readily accessible places to which it can escape. These should contain food, water, resting places and latrines.
- If the cat needs to leave a situation where a dog is present, provide it with an escape route through an open door, whilst restraining and controlling the dog to prevent chasing. DO NOT PICK THE CAT UP TO CARRY IT AWAY FROM THE DOG.

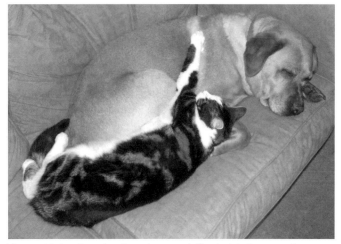

Figure 13.1   Cats that have been socialised with dogs can form very strong relationships with them.

Diagnosis

Diagnosis is based on observation of the behaviour of the cat: its facial expressions, postures and initial attempts at avoidance when in the presence of the fear-eliciting stimulus (Fig. 13.2). However, given that the emphasis should be on prevention, it should be assumed that a cat that has not been reared or previously socialised with a particular species is likely to experience fear when meeting members of that species (Box 13.4). For example, cats with outdoor access will already have a substantial number of aversive experiences resulting from interactions with dogs. It is important to remember that experienced cats, or cats that

odour signals, it is sometimes very effective to use F4 (Felifriend®, CEVA Animal Health) to mark the unfamiliar dog around the head and flank areas. To the cat, the dog appears to be marked as 'familiar', which may inhibit escape behaviour by the cat so that the dog's desire to chase is not reinforced. Obviously, this is only safe when the dog has no history of harming or attempting to harm cats. It is also important to remember that cats that have already had experience of being chased or injured by dogs may be greatly confused by the dissonance between the visual recognition of threat combined with an odour cue that implies safe familiarity. This can induce panic.

The cat should be allowed times when it is able to watch the dog and approach from a position of security. It needs to have food, water, resting places and latrines that are freely accessible without having to approach close to the dog. If the dog has any tendency to chase or approach the cat too boldly, it should be trained to sit and then be kept under control using a leash during initial encounters (Box 13.3).

Cats that have been well-socialised with dogs during kittenhood often form very close attachments to them (Fig. 13.1).

- Cats that are expected to live alongside dogs should be well-socialised with them during kittenhood.
- Provide the cat with a number of easily-accessible escape routes: baby-gates, high perches etc. These enable the cat to avoid contact with the dog.
- The cat should have several locations where there is food, water and a latrine so that it at no time feels confined and vulnerable because it cannot access resources.
- Pheromone products such as F3 diffusers (Feliway®, CEVA Animal Health) may be used to reduce overall anxiety or stress. F4 (Felifriend®) applied to the dog's head and flanks in order to convince the cat that the dog is familiar and non-threatening may be useful if the animals are meeting for the first time. (Not to be used if the dog has a history of aggression or of chasing cats.)
- Manage the introduction carefully.
- During all initial encounters, the dog should be restrained. It should also be reliably trained to come to the owner and sit on command.

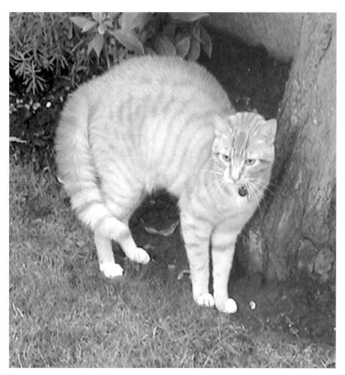

Figure 13.2   Fearful feline body posture.

feel cornered, may immediately resort to offensive aggression. This is usually a strategy for regaining access to an escape route so that, once successful, the cat will flee.

Treatment

Fear-related aggression to dogs or other animals outside the home is unlikely to be reported as a problem because the cat is able to avoid these situations and the owner may not even be aware that there is a problem. However, fear of other animals resident on the owner's property is a common issue.

The first step is to re-establish the cat's confidence in its environment, especially if the animal it is fearful of is sharing the same dwelling. The cat should be allowed to explore, face/flank mark and utilise resources in the area that it will share with the cohabiting dog while that animal is not present. This also allows a gradual desensitisation to the odours of the dog. If the cat is insecure in the environment, perhaps because of a series of previous encounters with the dog, then the use of F3 diffusers (Feliway®, CEVA Animal Health) may help. Client advice sheets on improving the indoor and outdoor environment for cats are included in Appendix 3 (sheets 1 & 2).

Good indicators that the cat is relaxed and confident in the environment include:

- restoration of normal levels of facial- and flank-marking of objects
- resumption of normal affiliative and play behaviour

- relaxed resting posture (front feet folded under the body whilst laying down)
- confident movement around the environment without hesitation
- low tendency to startle at sudden noises or movements.

Specific treatment of the fear problem involves desensitisation and counterconditioning methods. Since the cat is fearful of the compound stimulus of the sound, sight, smell and movement of the dog, it is sensible to break down this composite of stimuli and treat each component individually. Although this may appear to make treatment more laborious, it will probably make it quicker and produce a better outcome.

As with the introduction of a new cat, it is beneficial to try to associate the odour of the dog with activities that the cat enjoys, such as feeding or play. This is a counterconditioning-based procedure. Initial reactions to presentation of the dog's odour, on a cloth or pair of clean gloves, may cause alarm. After a number of presentations the cat may begin to rub against the cloth. At this point, the dog's odour may be rubbed onto the owner's clothing (such as trousers) so that, when the cat sniffs and face/flank marks against the owner, the scent of the dog will be picked up. It is very important that the cat does not encounter the dog during this introduction process as this may cause aversive associations that delay success of behavioural therapy or may make it hazardous.

Once the dog's odour has been introduced, it may be appropriate to desensitise the cat to dog vocalisations, especially if the dog is likely to bark at it. This may be achieved using commercially-available recordings of dog barking and growling played at low levels. Sound volume is increased over a number of sessions until the cat is tolerant of playback levels that are close to real levels. Some dogs will bark at a cat in order to intimidate it into running. A cat that has been thoroughly habituated to canine vocalisation is less likely to be startled and so the dog's behaviour does not gain the reinforcement of a chase. Desensitisation is likely to be slower if the cat has already learned that dog barking precedes a chase or attack.

Finally, the dog should be introduced as a visual signal. This depends upon the dog being relaxed, quiet and well-trained. At no time should the dog be allowed to lunge or bark at the cat, so it must be easily controllable. This also follows a desensitisation process, with the dog being introduced initially at a distance that produces little or no fear in the cat. In a domestic environment this may be difficult, which is why the cat must first feel completely secure in the introduction environment. An alternative to keeping the dog at a distance is to provide a partial visual barrier, such as a screen. For example, a child gate or glass door may be adapted by applying strips of tracing paper. Glass etch spray can be applied to a glass door to produce the same effect. This enables gradual exposure to the dog as a visual stimulus. In some cases, it may even be necessary to use a realistic stuffed toy dog as an initial stimulus because the cat is too frightened of the real thing. The cat may be introduced into the room on a harness and extending leash or in a carry box, or the dog may be brought in quietly on a leash.

Initially these introductory sessions should be brief, not longer than 10 to 15 minutes, to avoid undue stress to the cat. This also avoids the dog becoming bored and disruptive during training. The owner should always try to terminate the session before the cat reaches a point of high arousal and fear.

Sessions should become longer and progress to include movement and activity on the part of the dog. This should take the form of controlled activities, such as obedience training, and then short bouts of calm play. The aim is to make these activities controlled and repeatable so that the cat's response can be monitored and the range of activities expanded without triggering fear. This assumes that the dog is being actively trained to participate in the sessions. As stated earlier, F4 may be used to enhance introduction to a new dog, but should be used with caution where the cat already has an existing intense fear of a specific dog.

In some cases, the cat will continue to mount an escape response because this has become habitual rather than motivated by intense fear. The escape response of these cats may be slowed or delayed using a harness and trailing line, with the cat being rewarded for non-escape or when it returns after having attempted to move away. Pressure is placed on the line as it drags along the floor so that the cat's escape is slowed down. Methods like this are not routinely required and should only be used if escape or avoidance behaviour superstitiously persists after desensitisation, psychoactive drug therapy and counterconditioning have all been used (Box 13.5).

Prognosis

The outcome does not depend solely upon the cat's response which makes prognostication impossible without a complete behavioural history, including details of the dog's (or other animal's) behaviour toward the cat.

Placid dogs that have no interest in chasing or persecuting cats are much more likely to contribute to a good prognosis. Unless the dog (or other animal) can be relied upon not to antagonise the cat, then they may never be able to be left alone safely and there is a significant probability that the cat's welfare will be impaired or the situation may progress to overt aggression. Clients who expect to be able to leave their pets together alone without consequences will be disappointed.

Likewise, cats that show intensely fearful and avoidant behaviour may never develop sufficient confidence to utilise space and resources in the way that is a necessity for them. These cats also suffer a reduction in welfare and may be better re-homed away from the animals they fear. Part of the judgment when investigating a case has to be whether the client's demands can realistically be met whilst preserving the animal's quality of life.

Fear of people

Fear of people is considered separately from fear of other species because the client's expectations are different and the range of situations that the cat may be expected to tolerate are more demanding. The owner is also at greater risk if aggression results from mishandling. Clients always hope that the love they and other people radiate toward the cat will be reciprocated, so there is a need to educate the cat owner about the cat's own needs and expectations of interaction with people. Owner appreciation of the cat's perspective of the relationship always improves the prognosis (Box 13.6).

Box 13.5   Treatment: Fear of species other than humans (e.g., dogs)

- Provide the cat with a safe environment with readily-accessible resources.
- Consider the use of F3 to increase familiarity and security of the environment.
- Allow the cat to feel secure in the environment so that it can make use of all resources and escape routes before introducing specific therapy for the fear problem.
- Desensitise or countercondition the cat to elements of the stimuli it fears separately: sight, sound, smell and movement of the animal.
- DO NOT CARRY THE CAT INTO A SITUATION WHERE A DOG IS PRESENT FOR TRAINING AS THIS MAY TRIGGER AGGRESSION. Instead, bring it in in a carry box or allow it to enter from another room on a harness and flexi-leash.

Box 13.6   Immediate action: fear of people

The intention of this advice is to prevent fear of people progressing to aggression.

- The cat must be given opportunities to escape from situations it finds alarming.
- Provide the cat with a safe area that includes all necessary resources within easy access. The cat should always have access to this location.
- Identify the types of person of which the cat is most fearful.
- Identify items of clothing and patterns of behaviour that elicit most fear.
- Prevent exposure to these stimuli wherever possible.
- Do not handle, restrain or otherwise force the cat to remain in proximity to people who induce a fearful reaction.

Fear of people can have a number of manifestations and underlying factors. Cats may have a general fear of all people, causing avoidance behaviour and potential aggressiveness if the cat is cornered. This is most likely in poorly socialised cats or those that have been threatened or harmed by people in the past. Cats that are feral and have had no early rearing experience with people are a major challenge. The basic framework of positive associations with human contact is missing and has to be trained from scratch. This can be extremely time-consuming but rewarding. Cats that have a good early socialisation history but which have developed fear as a result of one or two aversive events may be easier to treat initially, but they often present a greater challenge later on as the full extent of the range of human-related stimuli they react to (clothing, size, vocal tone) becomes apparent over time.

Fear of people may be confined to certain situations, such as in a particular context, during handling or when approached or touched. These cats may be relatively relaxed around people until a specific event or situation of this kind arises. These cats ought to be the easiest to deal with as long as clients can be effectively counselled to approach the problem systematically. However, the cat's generally relaxed demeanour often leads people to try to initiate contact that alarms the cat and further teaches it to dislike human contact.

With the wrong approach and enough perseverance, any one of these types of fear-related problems can progress to aggression. Once actual aggression is seen, the whole style of treatment must change and some cat owners will be reluctant to proceed at all, so it is vital that the cat is not unintentionally provoked (Box 13.7).

Box 13.7   Prevention: fear of people

The 'socialisation' period of the cat is shorter than in the dog, ending at around 7 weeks. The breeder is therefore responsible for exposing the kittens to a wide range of people and other species before homing.

- Do not pick kittens that are the progeny of aggressive or fearful parents.
- Avoid choosing kittens that have been reared in impoverished or barren environments.
- When introducing new cats to an environment, provide them with a secure space that includes all major resources and a number of hiding places.
- Allow the cat to become confident in its environment before introducing it to new people.

Diagnosis

Fear of people is apparent from the pattern of avoidance behaviour and the cat's body postures. The specific nature of the fear problem should be thoroughly investigated including:

- rearing history
- early responses to unfamiliar people
- responses to handling by familiar people
- types of human appearance and activity the cat most fears
- details of the owner's previous attempts to treat or manage the problem, including their reactions to the cat's fearful behaviour.

This information is essential to understanding the full nature of the problem so that all aspects of the cat's fear can be dealt with.

Treatment

Essential steps in reducing fearfulness of people are a mixture of the techniques used for treating fear of other species and fear of inanimate objects. The process described for the treatment of fear of people will be considered from the perspective of treating a cat with a severe general fear of people. Less severe cases might require fewer steps and could then go on to the kind of handling techniques described in the section discussing aggression related to handling and human interaction in Chapter 16.

The benefit of using desensitisation and counterconditioning procedures for cats with a fear of people is that, with some cooperation, we can control many aspects of the person's behaviour whilst in the presence of the cat. The cat can be desensitised or habituated to a variety of different human appearances using different clothes and other paraphernalia, such as walking sticks, hats and glasses. This means that only a relatively small number of volunteers are needed.

If the cat has already shown different levels of fear according to the appearance of the people it has encountered, then a list should be made of the features of appearance the cat tolerates least. Typically, animals least like tall people wearing dark clothing, hats or hoods because these make them seem more threatening. This enables therapy to start with people who dress and behave in the ways that the cat is most likely to accept. A good starting point is to start with female volunteers sitting down and wearing light coloured casual clothing. Cats that show signs of fear when they hear unfamiliar voices may be desensitised to these noises using recordings or radio programmes.

Desensitisation to the presence of a person will be most rapid if that person can remain as still as possible without watching the cat at all. This effectively makes the person inanimate and without any intention towards the cat.

As the cat becomes confident with several different people dressed on different occasions in a wide selection of clothes, the next stage is for the cat to encounter these same people while they are standing up. This will make them appear larger and therefore more dangerous. In successive stages, the volunteers should begin to move about slowly, then more rapidly, but always remaining disinterested in the cat.

The process may be speeded up if F4 (Felifriend®) is applied to the person acting as the stooge and the environment is one in which an F3 diffuser (Feliway®) is operating. However, F4 should be used with care as it can induce panic in cats that already have memories of specific aversive events involving people. These cats experience a dissonance between the visual stimulus associated with threat and danger and the pheromone cue that signals familiarity (Box 13.8).

Box 13.8   Treatment: fear of people

- Make a list of the types and appearances of people of which the cat is fearful, placing them in order of the degree of fear elicited.
- Prepare a quiet and familiar environment for training, allowing the cat to get used to this in advance of training. Provision of F3 diffusers in this environment will increase the perceived sense of security. The cat should have resting places and bolt-holes where it can avoid contact if it wishes.
- Desensitise or countercondition the cat to elements of the stimuli it fears separately: sight, sound, smell and movement of the animal.
- Psychoactive medication may help behaviourally inhibited cats or those that are too apprehensive to commence training (selegiline).
  DO NOT CARRY THE CAT INTO A TRAINING SITUATION WHERE A DOG IS PRESENT, AS THIS MAY TRIGGER AGGRESSION. Instead, bring it in in a carry box, or allow it to enter from another room on a harness and extending leash.

Prognosis

The prognosis depends very much upon the client's ultimate expectations for the cat. If they intend to have a reasonably sociable house pet but are willing to accept that the cat may hide occasionally when visitors come to the home, then they may be very happy with the results of behavioural therapy.

Fear of inanimate objects and stimuli

The extent of this problem is relatively unknown in cats, probably because its effects are hard to observe or are misunderstood (Box 13.9). There are a number of reasons for this. Cats that have a fear of fireworks or thunder may hide in a variety of places, some of which are outside the home so that the client may never see signs of fear. When the cat is at home, the facial and flank marks it has left create a sense of increased security that may be sufficient to coun-

---

Box 13.9   Immediate action: fear of inanimate objects and sounds

- List all stimuli that evoke fear.
- Wherever possible, prevent exposure to fear-eliciting stimuli, especially in the home.
- Stop all punishment of fearful behaviour. Do not use restraint or coercion to keep the cat in the presence of the fear-eliciting stimulus.
- Do not hold or restrain the cat while it is in the presence of the object of its fear as this can produce outbursts of very aggressive and dangerous behaviour.
- Stop attempts to soothe the cat by giving it attention as this may reward fearful behaviour.
- Provide the cat with one or more safe and readily-accessible places to escape to. These should contain food, water, resting places and latrines.
- If the cat needs to get away from the fear-eliciting stimulus. then the owner should open a door and allow the cat to go into another room. THE CAT MUST NOT BE PICKED UP OR CARRIED.

---

teract the apprehension it is experiencing. Loud, low-frequency noises are very hard for cats to localise which means that an effective escape response is impossible. So a genuinely fearful cat may enter a state of behavioural inhibition, staying very still until the threat has gone away. Clients often misinterpret this passivity as a lack of fear, especially when the cat engages in increased self-maintenance behaviour such as grooming. In fact, the increased grooming is a form of displacement activity or an attempt at self-appeasement. Often cats will groom their flank area and it has been hypothesised that the cat is deliberately taking in a quantity of its own pheromones to alter its emotional state.

Fear of inanimate visual stimuli may develop as a result of associations with noise stimuli; for example, light flashes that resemble lightning before the sound of thunder. A minority of cats, usually coming from an inappropriate rearing environment, do suffer from specific fears and phobias of visual stimuli. Cases include fear of flapping or flying objects such as kites, paragliders and polythene bags. Cats will also show increased fear of visual stimuli that startle the cat while it is in the presence of another stimulus that it fears, or when it is in an unfamiliar environment. This can create negative associations with almost any kind of stimulus so that it evokes fear in the future.

Fear responses of cats appear to be relatively context specific. Cats will often react fearfully to otherwise familiar stimuli when they are encountered in an unfamiliar context or when the cat encounters the stimulus when it is outside of its own familiar territorial boundaries. This may be because a significant part of the cat's emotional self-control is based on its ability to rapidly engage avoidance behaviour and also to discriminate the level of threat likely in a given environment according to the scent marks that have previously been left there (Box 13.10).

Box 13.10   Prevention: fear of inanimate objects or sounds

- Good rearing practice is essential, with exposure to a wide range of normal domestic sounds and activities during the period before 7 weeks of age.
- Exposure to sound stimuli may be provided using recordings. Unlike puppies, kittens should not be habituated to traffic sounds.
- Novel or potentially fear-evoking stimuli should be introduced carefully so that fear is not increased.
- Use of F3 pheromone diffusers help to enable cats to adjust to a new environment after re-homing. This reduces the risk of the development of specific fear problems.
- Do not pick kittens that are the progeny of aggressive or fearful parents.
- Avoid choosing kittens that have been reared in impoverished or barren environments.

Diagnosis

Again this depends upon observing the cat's typical avoidance behaviour and body language in the presence of the stimulus. With animate objects it is usually obvious what the cat is reacting to but with inanimate objects or sounds it may not be so clear-cut unless the client has closely observed the cat. Fear of inanimate objects or sounds may be an underlying factor in other behavioural problems so it is important to take a detailed history. Given that cats tend to become inhibited in situations where they cannot mount a proper escape response, the owner may not be aware of low-level fear reactions. Direct observation or video recording of the cat's behaviour is necessary.

Treatment

The treatment of fear of inanimate objects or sounds is similar in cats and dogs. The basis is to use desensitisation and counterconditioning to alter the emotional response to the stimulus. This may be augmented with pheromone or drug therapy.

The situation is complicated by the fact that some of the treatments available for dogs are not useable in the cat. For example, no appeasement pheromone product is available for the cat, so the basis for the use of pheromonotherapy will be different. The F3 pheromone fraction (Feliway®) can be used to increase the familiarity and security of the home environment, which will indirectly alter the cat's reaction to stimuli. Individual spots of F3 might be sprayed onto *static* environmental stimuli of which the cat is otherwise mildly fearful.

Benzodiazepine drugs, such as diazepam, are extensively used to manage and treat fear and phobia problems in the dog but these drugs have limited use in the cat because of the risk of serious adverse reactions. Diazepam impairs the judgment of distance and should not be used for cats that have outdoor access as they may fall or become involved in a road traffic accident. This drug is also associated with potentially fatal liver damage if given by mouth. The safety of other benzodiazepines, such as alprazolam, is believed to be more favourable for cats but there is a lack of scientific data to support that.

Before beginning specific behavioural therapy for the fear problem, it is important to make sure that the cat's home environment closely satisfies the cat's needs. Increasing the range and availability of resources such as feeding places, rest sites and latrines will reduce the cat's general level of arousal and anxiety (see Advice sheets 1 and 2, Appendix 3).

Desensitisation and counterconditioning procedures are similar to those in the dog:

- All stimuli or elements of compound stimuli that evoke fear must be identified.
- Some means to present these stimuli at lower intensity must be found.

Desensitisation:

- The stimulus is repeatedly presented below the threshold that evokes fear. The intensity of the stimulus is gradually raised over a number of sessions until the animal is fully habituated to it.

Counterconditioning:

- The stimulus is presented in association with something that the cat unconditionally enjoys (play, food, etc.) After repeated presentations, the previously fear-eliciting stimulus begins to elicit the same emotional state as the pleasant event now associated with it.

The process is complicated by the cat's unique reliance on its environment for security and safety. This makes it absolutely vital that sounds or other stimuli must be presented systematically while the cat is relaxed, so that fear is never elicited. Otherwise, the cat may associate the context of its own core territory with memories of fear. This undermines the cat's general security and could cause it to refuse to enter the home. It is also important to exclude children and other animals from the environment during training. This reduces any possibility that a cat may use aggression to regain access to an escape route or learn negative associations with the presence of those individuals.

Specific protocols for desensitisation are included in the section on canine fears and phobias, and these can be adapted for use with feline problems (see Chapter 8).

Choice of reward is an essential component for success in counterconditioning. The 'reward' used must be something that the cat unconditionally enjoys. The previously fear-eliciting stimulus is presented at an intensity at which the reward is more pleasurable than the fearful stimulus is aversive; otherwise the cat may become fearful of eating or play because these have come to be associated with an unpleasant emotional state. Clients should experiment with a wide range of toys and food before beginning counterconditioning. For cats, play is often a better counterconditioning stimulus because it produces an immediate emotional response. Most cats are rather circumspect regarding food treats and it may be hard to use meals for counterconditioning when many cats share a household and need to be fed ad-lib. It is also important to remember that cats habituate to toys very rapidly, which means that counterconditioning exercises that use play must be kept brief (less than 5–10 minutes) to maintain interest and the toys used at each session must be varied. Effectively, part of the counterconditioning stimulus is the novelty of the toy and the play. If toys are swapped during play, then the sessions may be extended beyond 5 to 10 minutes but they must end before the cat becomes bored.

Training sessions of this kind should be undertaken when the cat is already voluntarily in the environment where training is to take place. Cats should not be carried to the place where training is to take place because any accidental negative associations made in that situation may also affect the cat's attitude toward handling, resulting in fear of or aggression toward the owner.

Treatment of specific fears of inanimate objects may be augmented with psychoactive drug therapy, although no drug is specifically licensed for this use in the cat. Extreme care must be taken in using these drugs when the cat also has a number of other fear or aggression problems involving people or other animals because anxiolytic psychoactive drugs carry a risk of producing disinhibition. Selegiline (Selgian®) is the first choice for specific fears as it is licensed for the treatment of this condition in the dog. It can be used in cats if the client's informed consent is obtained, the dose rate being 1.0 mg/kg once daily. The onset of efficacy may be 4 to 6 weeks or more and it is important to warn owners not to try to progress too quickly with behavioural therapy during the induction period with this drug as the cat's increase in confidence and reduction in apprehension are relatively fragile until the drug is in full effect. Attempts to take advantage of the cat's growing confidence during the induction period can backfire, with the cat becoming even more uncertain of human contact. This is temporary but very disheartening for owners when it happens. Selegiline is most appropriate for fearful cats that also show a high degree of inhibition of normal behaviour, such as:

- reduced self-maintenance behaviour (grooming, eating)
- failure to utilise resources

- perpetual hiding and avoidance
- frequent freezing behaviour in even mildly fear-eliciting situations.

Apart from increasing exploratory behaviour and confidence and reducing apprehension, selegiline also increases the rewarding nature of reinforcers and improves cognitive function so that it may be of benefit in improving responses to counterconditioning procedures.

Box 13.11   Treatment: fear of inanimate objects or sounds

- Before starting therapy, the cat's domestic environment should be optimised so that it can perform normal avoidance and hiding behaviour. Social and other problems should be treated.
- Identify the full range of stimulus types and variations of which the cat is fearful.
- These may be grouped into general categories as an indication of other potential stimulus types that may evoke fear.
- If more than one stimulus evokes fear, the stimuli should be listed in order of the level of reaction they create, based on the owner's experience (do not set up challenge tests).
- Consider methods for presenting each of these stimuli at a reduced and controllable intensity, e.g., using recorded sounds.
- Begin desensitisation with low-ranking stimuli that evoke the least amount of fear and which conveniently lend themselves to behavioural therapy. This allows the client to build up experience of the behaviour modification methods with minimal risk of making them worse through flooding.
- Training should be done in an environment where the cat feels safe. F3 diffusers (Feliway®) can help to accomplish this, in conjunction with environmental enrichment.
- Desensitisation: The stimulus is presented at below the intensity threshold that would normally trigger a fear response. Sounds are played at low volume. Visual stimuli are presented at a distance or behind a partial screen. Once the cat becomes fully habituated to one level of intensity, the stimulus is then made a little more intense. Gradually the intensity is raised over a number of sessions until it reaches a realistic intensity.
- Counterconditioning: The stimulus is associated with an activity or event that the cat enjoys. For example, the sound of dogs barking might be played at low volume, starting just before the cat is enticed into a game. Over successive training sessions, the sound level is gradually increased until it reaches realistic levels.
- Psychoactive medication, such as selegiline, may be used to support behavioural therapy if the animal shows intense fear.

Serotonergic drugs like clomipramine (Clomicalm®, Novartis) or fluoxetine are more suited to cases in which the cat shows chronic and generalised signs of anxiety in an environment that is generally devoid of specific fear-eliciting stimuli. These are cats that anticipate harm although no threat is actually present. They may also be appropriate if there are signs of excessive self-appeasement or displacement behaviour such as over-grooming (Box 13.12).

Box 13.12   Deciding when to use psychoactive medication for fears of inanimate objects or sounds

Possible indications:

- Widely-generalised fears and phobias, especially when the range of fear-eliciting stimuli is expanding.
- Longstanding cases where many fear-related associations have already formed.
- When welfare has been impacted: cats with significantly inhibited patterns of behaviour.
- Cats with cognitive impairment, such as due to senile dementia.

Prognosis

For stimuli that may be presented according to a strict plan of desensitisation and counterconditioning, the prognosis is good. The prognosis is guarded if the stimulus is regularly encountered at fear-eliciting intensity during behavioural therapy because memory-blocking drugs are more limited in their use in the cat than they are in the dog. Drugs that reduce apprehension, such as selegiline, may be useful in these cases and can also speed up therapy in intensely fearful individuals. Drug therapy is also useful for individuals that have a wide range of fears, with a pattern of generalisation.

Problems of attachment

Normal primary attachment in felines is to location and territory, rather than to other individuals. This is because cats are solitary hunters and do not require other cats to help them to gain the resources that they need to survive. Cats that are anxious or fearful may come to depend on their owner(s) for security and reassurance, either because their environment does not offer them sufficient opportunities to regulate their own emotional state or because the owner has repeatedly reinforced dependent behaviour. Keeping cats indoors is observed to increase the level of interaction between cats and their owners and it might be expected that attachment problems would be more common in these individuals.

Diagnosis

Cats with attachment problems may follow their owners, vocalise, and demand attention continuously. They may become anxious as the owner prepares to depart. When alone they may spray or eliminate on the owner's property.

There are a number of underlying reasons for attachment problems in cats:

- Lack of environmental stimulation and novelty.
- Lack of opportunities to exert control over resource access.
- Owner reinforcement of attention-seeking behaviour by the cat.
- Owner comforting of the cat or offering it security when it is fearful or anxious.

Owners are likely to be inconsistent in their responses to the cat, sometimes reinforcing attention-seeking behaviour and at other times admonishing the cat for being a pest. This only serves to make the cat more anxious, especially if the owner is responsible for controlling access to resources such as outdoor access or food. Cats have a uniquely direct relationship with their environment, being able to utilise resources on demand. They therefore find waiting for human intervention to be frustrating and stressful. Attachment problems in cats are therefore often accompanied by frustration-related aggression and protest urine spraying.

Cats are also likely to show increased dependence on their owners if the presence of that person guarantees safety in an otherwise stressful environment. For example, the cat may be safe from attack by other cats in the household only when the owner is present, so the cat cannot eat, drink or eliminate in safety when the owner is absent. A similar situation is seen in cats that are terrorised by local despots and refuse to enter the garden unless the owner is present. Specific underlying fear or anxiety problems must therefore be identified and addressed.

Treatment

The aim of treatment is to return the cat to a normal relationship with its environment and reduce the importance

---

Box 13.13   Prevention: feline attachment problems

- Provide indoor cats with a wide range of environmental enrichments: activity feeders, opportunities to hide and climb and opportunities to play.
- Provide indoor-outdoor access: to a garden enclosure if freedom must be curtailed for some reason.
- Continually change toys and add novelty to the environment to prevent boredom.
- Do not reinforce attention-seeking behaviour.

> **Box 13.14   Treatment: attachment problems in cats**
>
> - Provide an enriched environment.
> - Return complete control of resource access to the cat (adlib activity feeding, etc.)
> - Give the cat outdoor access or a range of distracting activities in the home.
> - Reduce reinforcement of attention-seeking behaviour.
> - Stop soothing of the cat when it is anxious or fearful.
> - Resolve underlying fear and anxiety problems.

of the owner. The cat should be given back control over feeding and outdoor access. Activity feeders help to use up the cat's time and activity budgets in useful work. In long-standing cases, or in cats that show generalised anxiety, then this may be treated with a suitable anxiolytic drug such as clomipramine (Clomicalm, Novartis). Care must be taken if there is any possibility of disinhibiting an already frustrated aggressive pattern of behaviour.

Specific fear and phobia problems should be treated according to diagnosis.

ADVICE SHEETS THAT MAY BE RELEVANT TO THIS CHAPTER

In Appendix 3

1. Improving the outdoor environment for cats
2. Improving the indoor environment for cats
3. Multi-cat households
6. Introducing new cats to the household

Chapter 14

Feline compulsive disorders

INTRODUCTION

There are many similarities between canine and feline compulsive disorders and the neurochemical basis for these conditions is thought to be similar across a range of species, including man. For a discussion of this, please see Chapter 9.

The character of the more commonly-presented feline compulsive disorders appears slightly different from those in the dog and reflects the way in which the underlying motivation of arousal and anxiety reduction, thought to be common in all compulsion, is expressed in behaviour that is specific to the species or breed.

Feline compulsive behaviours are generally associated with repetitious or exaggerated self-maintenance behaviour such as grooming, sucking or self-mutilation. The exception is hyperaesthesia syndrome in which the cat responds aggressively to what may be tactile hallucinations. The behaviour in hyperaesthesia syndrome is variable between cats and it is probable that a range of different aetiologies will become apparent as this condition is better understood. Indeed, it may be found to share greater aetiological similarities with orofacial pain syndrome (seen primarily in Burmese) and feline idiopathic cystitis.

Apart from these common compulsive disorders, cats may develop compulsive behaviour that originates in a range of other activities: for example, light spot or shadow chasing, psychogenic polydipsia or polyphagia (Box 14.1).

Underlying factors

The factors that underlie compulsive disorders in the cat are different from those in the dog. The cat is highly self-reliant and depends on its own ability to control and utilise resources in its environment. It experiences strong drives to hunt, feed and carry out self-maintenance behaviours at set intervals. Hunting, for example, is not primarily regulated by appetite or satiation so that cats will continue to hunt regardless of their earlier successes or failures. The cat's normal behaviour is therefore highly-structured and self-disciplined. This reflects the fact that, in a given area, the territories of several cats may partially overlap so that each

---

Box 14.1   Common feline compulsive disorders

- Hyperaesthesia
- Psychogenic alopecia (over-grooming)
- Self-mutilation
- Pica
- Wool-sucking

---

individual can gain access to certain common resources, or traverse corners of each other's territory in order to get from place to place. The temporal structure of the cat's behaviour, combined with its system of marking, allows each cat to exist in isolation from others thus minimising conflict and maximising the cat's ability to utilise resources on demand. Great reliance is placed on the reliability of access to resources.

Environment

Environmental factors are therefore extraordinarily important in all feline behavioural problems, especially compulsive disorders. For the cat to live in an environment that places it in close proximity with potential competitors, inside or outside the home, and with limited control over access to resources and territory, can have a very damaging effect (Box 14.2).

Canine compulsive disorder is frequently rooted in social deprivation, isolation and the stress of broken psychological attachment (as seen in compulsive disorders linked to attachment disorders and long periods of barren kennelling). Feline compulsive disorder is more commonly associated with a lack of ability to carry out normal behaviour, combined with the social stress of perpetual competition and conflict. Improvement of the physical and social environment is therefore critically important for cats with compulsive disorders. Even without a compulsive element, the cat is likely to increase the amount of self-maintenance behaviour it performs as a substitute for thwarted hunting behaviour and territory maintenance.

Predisposition

There is some breed predisposition in the incidence of compulsive disorder with Burmese, Siamese and other pure-bred oriental cats showing higher than normal rates of wool-sucking and self-mutilation. This may reflect a genetic component to the disorder but it also has to be remembered that these cats are often reared and housed differently from ordinary house-cats. Concerns over disease transmission mean that they are often reared in a 'non-domestic' situation such as a cattery. This limits the exposure these animals have to social interaction and common domestic stimuli and events, which would seem to predispose them to a range of fear and anxiety problems.

As adults, their financial value means that they are less likely to have outdoor access which places even greater pressure on the cats if the indoor environment is unsuitable for them. The same breeds also have a higher predisposition to urine marking, inter-cat aggression and attachment disorders. Whilst these cats may have some genetic predisposition towards a range of problems, their rearing and husbandry is probably a significant factor. Client information about improving the indoor and outdoor environment is included in Advice sheets 1 and 2 in Appendix 3.

Treatment

Early intervention is very important in compulsive disorder. As discussed in the canine compulsions chapter, compulsive behaviour becomes more pervasive over time as the animal 'learns' that performing compulsive behaviour provides reliable relief from negative emotional situations. Compulsive behaviour can ultimately become a substitute for a wide range of normal behaviour so that, even when presented with a substantially improved environment, the cat continues to behave compulsively.

The use of medication for these conditions is sometimes controversial because it may be regarded as merely reducing the incidence of unsightly behaviour that is an expression of the animal's attempts to cope with wholly-unsatisfactory living conditions. This criticism could fairly be levelled at the medication of wild felids that continue to be poorly maintained in some zoos or circuses. However, the use of medication is absolutely justifiable if it enables the animal to engage in normal behaviour in an enriched environment, when otherwise it might continue to stereotype. In this situation, the drug is being used to facilitate rehabilitation. This is the model we should adopt for domestic cats: drugs are most useful where their use will enhance the animal's response to environmental improvement.

Punishment of compulsive behaviour, or attempts to physically prevent it, are misguided. Compulsive behaviour forms part of the animal's coping strategy so that preventing one expression of compulsion just forces the

---

Box 14.2   Preventing feline compulsive disorders

- Kittens should be exposed to a wide range of stimuli during the sensitive period (people, domestic activities, interaction with other species).
- The domestic environment should provide security, mental stimulation and free access to resources. This is particularly important for indoor-only cats.
- Avoid overpopulation, especially with oriental breeds of cat.
- If establishing a multi-cat household, choose kittens from parents that already live in successful multi-cat households.

animal to find other opportunities. For example, using flavour or odour aversion to deter pica related to one type of material, such as wool, will merely encourage the cat to find something else to suck or chew instead. The motivation to carry out some kind of related compulsive behaviour remains. Punishment may also increase stress that contributes to the problem.

FELINE HYPERAESTHESIA SYNDROME

The incidence of hyperaesthesia is not known but it may be more common than once thought and could play a significant part in other behaviour problems such as inter-cat aggression.

Age of onset varies but, if the condition starts in early adulthood, it can cause the breakdown of previously excellent relationships between cats sharing a household. Historically, affected cats will begin to resent play or contact with conspecifics, becoming progressively more irritable and aloof from them. The cat may also begin to resent human contact. Analysis of specific incidents will show that play or grooming began to initiate bouts of hyperaesthesia, which then lead to aggression (often by the other cat).

The behaviour is highly bizarre but is often overlooked by the owner as a quirk of the cat's personality. They may consider it to be playful or amusing, unless it becomes frequent or involves self-trauma. The fact that the cat suffers from hyperaesthesia may only come to light as a result of investigating some other behavioural problem. It is unknown whether hyperaesthesia occurs in discrete bouts or, in fact, produces an ongoing altered perception of touch contact. The fact that bouts may be triggered by contact implies that touch sensation is persistently altered in some way (Box 14.3).

Diagnosis

Feline hyperaesthesia is relatively poorly understood and there are a number of medical differentials that should be excluded before a behavioural investigation.

Box 14.3   Immediate action: feline hyperaesthesia syndrome

- Stop the owner from interacting with the cat in a way that may cause hyperaesthetic attacks (stroking along the cat's back, etc.)
- The owner must not attempt to sooth or punish the cat during an attack.
- The cat must not be physically restrained to stop it from showing hyperaesthetic behaviour.
- Children and animals should be kept away from the cat during an attack in case their presence causes the cat greater stress.
- THE CAT MUST NOT BE PICKED UP DURING AN ATTACK.

Box 14.4   Prevention: feline hyperaesthesia syndrome

- Kittens should be reared in an environment that provides experience of social interaction with people, cats and other species, as well as exposure to a wide range of normal domestic noises and events.
- Cats from breeds or lines that have a known increased risk of feline hyperaesthesia (such as littermates of an already hyperaesthetic cat living in the same household) should be kept clear of ectoparasites and treated systematically for other pruritic skin diseases. If hyperaesthesia causes general changes in tactile sensation, then pruritic skin disease may be a risk factor for increasing hyperaesthetic signs in at-risk individuals.
- At-risk cats should be sensitively managed to provide a low-stress social and physical environment.

Differentials include:

- allergic skin disease (atopy, food allergy)
- ectoparasites
- epilepsy (petit mal type – limbic location)
- local or referred pain (spinal lesion, intermittently luxating patella, etc.)
- hyperthyroidism
- central nervous system (CNS) pathology.

Signs indicative of hyperaesthesia are very variable, but include:

- skin or muscle twitching or rippling (commonly thoracolumbar or at the tail base)
- sudden bouts of intense grooming, self-mutilation or attacks on rear quarters, feet or tail
- freezing, with tail swishing, and then sudden turning or darting movements
- ear twitching (often as if the cat is alert to a sound behind it)
- sudden bouts of increased arousal, with the cat dashing about and jumping as if pursued or pursuing an invisible opponent
- bouts are often accompanied by vocalisation.

During these attacks, the cat's behaviour is generally indicative of a state of alarm and as if it is reacting to hallucinatory visual, auditory or tactile stimuli. The bouts may occur without any obvious trigger, in which case the first sign may be skin twitching. Bouts also occur during handling or stroking by the owner or grooming and play by other cats.

When deciding on treatment it is important to examine situations in which the attacks are most likely to occur. Specific triggers should be identified, such as:

- human contact
   –stroking certain places (usually the back)

–grooming
–play
- contact with other cats
–play
–allogrooming.

Treatment

The number and character of attacks should be recorded during the 7 to 14 days before treatment begins to give a baseline of frequency and severity. The cat's environment should be improved in accordance with general recommendations, especially if social stress in a multi-cat household is thought to be an underlying factor. The aim should be to introduce activities that use up the cat's time and energy budget and give it greater control over access to resources. For example, introduce activity feeding using toys that dispense portions of the cat's daily food allowance as they are played with. Making these changes in multi-cat households will help to reduce overall competition and social stress, which can only be beneficial to all of the cats.

Specific triggers of the behaviour should be identified and prevented, for example:

- Stop stroking the cat along its back or in other areas that trigger an attack of hyperaesthesia.
- Avoid grooming.
- Redirect play between cats using fishing toys or laser pointers so that the hyperaesthetic cat is not pushed or pounced on during play.
- Keep other cats amused using activity feeders and play so that the hyperaesthetic cat does not become the victim of predatory play.

If the attacks usually require some kind of triggering event, these first steps may substantially reduce their frequency. These cats will also possess a number of conditioned associations between normal activities and the initiation of a hyperaesthetic attack. For example, the approach of a person or another cat may predict when a bout is likely to occur. This kind of negative association heightens stress and anxiety which may, in turn, contribute to the worsening of the condition. Reducing factors that trigger hyperaesthetic attacks will therefore have direct and indirect effects on the frequency of attacks.

It is sometimes possible to redirect the cat onto an alternative behaviour once an attack has started by calling the cat and engaging it in play or some other non-tactile distraction. A 'recall' type response can be easily conditioned by calling the cat before offering a food treat or playing a game. This strengthens the response during distraction.

Drug therapy is frequently beneficial for hyperaesthetic cats which respond well to serotonin re-uptake inhibitor drugs like clomipramine (Clomicalm®, Novartis) and the more serotonin selective drug fluoxetine (Prozac®). These drugs are commonly used to treat compulsive disorders and do appear to provide considerable relief for hyper-

aesthetic cats. Onset of action is 4 or more weeks. The dose of clomipramine may need to be increased from an initial dose rate of 0.25 mg/kg once daily, to 0.5 mg/kg once daily or greater if initial response is insufficient after 6 to 8 weeks. Higher doses are associated with increased adverse effects, such as sedation, and it is important that genuine response to therapy is not confused with undesirable profound sedative effects which will suppress all sorts of behaviour including the reaction to hyperaesthetic sensations. SRI drugs like clomipramine reduce the threshold for seizures, which makes it particularly important to rule out petit mal type epilepsy as a differential.

The effect of serotonergic drugs is to reduce the severity and frequency of the hyperaesthetic attacks and it may become easier to distract the cat from the behaviour. Response to normal touch should be diminished so that the cat may then be desensitised and counterconditioned to the stimuli and events that previously triggered an attack, such as stroking and grooming. Care must be taken if there is any risk that disinhibition may release aggressive behaviour during handling.

Drug treatment should continue until there has been a period of at least 2 months without hyperaesthetic attacks and until the cat is able to tolerate normal tactile contact with people and conspecifics. The drug may then be phased out gradually over at least 4 weeks. Recidivism during dose reduction indicates that drug therapy should be reintroduced at the lowest dose that produced complete relief from symptoms. Another attempt to wean the cat off medication may be attempted after a further month at this dose. In some cases, medication will need to be permanent.

Once long-term drug therapy is producing a stable improvement, there should be a regular 6-monthly case review to make sure that beneficial environmental changes remain in place and drug therapy is still effective. Otherwise, there is a significant chance of relapse. If permanent therapy is required, then drug dose and type may need to be changed more than once during the cat's lifetime in order to maintain effectiveness (Box 14.5).

Box 14.5   Treatment: feline hyperaesthesia syndrome

- Record baseline rate and severity of hyperaesthetic attacks as a comparison for future reassessment.
- Provide an enriched environment.
- Identify and minimise exposure to events or stimuli that trigger hyperaesthetic attacks.
- Consider use of an SRI (clomipramine) or SSRI (fluoxetine) drug.
- Desensitise and counter-condition responses to approach, touch, grooming and other activities that may be associated with hyperaesthetic attacks.

Prognosis

The prognosis is best if the cat is treated thoroughly early in the course of the condition. The use of medication, environmental enrichment and other treatments should all be introduced as soon as a diagnosis is reached. There is usually some progression unless environmental and social underlying factors can be addressed successfully. Clients must be made aware that behavioural and/or drug treatment will need to be continued throughout the cat's life.

GROOMING DISORDERS: COMPULSIVE GROOMING AND SELF-MUTILATION

Cats frequently fall back on introverted self-maintenance behaviour as a means of self-appeasement during times of stress, anxiety or emotional conflict. This can become compulsive when the cat carries out the behaviour to the detriment of its own health and in place of normal behaviour or in inappropriate contexts (Box 14.6).

Diagnosis

In true alopecia, hairs are easily epilated in the areas that are becoming bald but the hairs remain normal to touch. When the hairs are being removed by deliberate grooming, barbering or hair-pulling, then the hairs will feel spiky and sharp because the tips have been taken off. Microscopic examination of a hair pluck will confirm the state of the hair tips. Hair loss is restricted to parts of the body that may be reached while grooming with the tongue. These signs are an immediate indication that the cat is not suffering from a true alopecia. Parasitism and allergic skin disease are major differentials for over-grooming. Localised or referred pain, or deep pruritic conditions such as notoedric mange may be a cause of over-grooming that progresses into self-harm. Feline idiopathic cystitis (FIC) has recently been found to account for the vast majority of feline lower urinary tract disease. Cats with this condition, which has behavioural and medical components, will often barber and over-groom the perineal area to create a bald groin and abdomen. They may also bite and chew the skin in this area. Cats with over-grooming and hair loss that is chiefly restricted to this area should be investigated as potential

cases of FIC. Feline hyperaesthesia can cause frantic bouts of self-biting and hair pulling but this is accompanied by other signs that differentiate the condition from compulsive over-grooming or self-mutilation.

Target areas for over-grooming include the flanks and abdomen but it must be remembered that barbering of groin fur can be a sign of lower urinary tract disease (Fig. 14.1).

Feline orofacial pain syndrome is a condition involving gross self-mutilation which is especially prevalent in Burmese cats, although occasional cases have been seen in the domestic shorthair, Burmilla and Siamese. There may be a slight male predisposition and all ages can be affected (Box 14.7).

> **Box 14.6 Immediate action: grooming disorders: compulsive grooming and self-mutilation**
>
> - Treat non-behavioural causes of hair loss and over-grooming such as parasitism, allergic skin disease and feline idiopathic cystitis.
> - Do not punish or attempt to soothe the cat when it is over-grooming as this may cause distress or reinforce the behaviour.

> **Box 14.7 Prevention: grooming disorders: compulsive grooming and self-mutilation**
>
> - Kittens should be reared in an environment that provides experience of social interaction with people, cats and other species, as well as exposure to a wide range of normal domestic noises and events.
> - If increased grooming is seen, then aspects of the social and physical environment may be causing stress. This situation should be rectified before grooming becomes excessive or habitual.

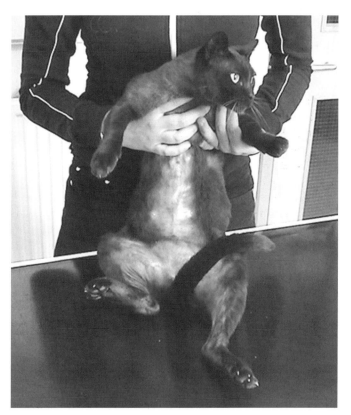

Figure 14.1 Stress related over-grooming.

The clinical signs are characterised by exaggerated licking and chewing movements, with pawing at the mouth. Typically the discomfort is unilateral or worse on one side and can be episodic or continuous. In the episodic version, the distress usually occurs after eating and lasts between 5 minutes and 2 hours. There is a short prodromal period of anxiety preceding the episode. The cat will claw at its face, attempting to claw at, catch and pull at its own tongue. The aetiology of this condition is being investigated but several separate causes have been identified. Some cases appear to be associated with oral disease, which can be divided into four groups:

1. Mouth ulceration, especially as a consequence of Calici virus infection or primary vaccination.
2. Cutting permanent teeth.
3. Dental disease, most commonly periodontal disease and dental resorptive lesions.
4. Recent routine dental treatment, including extraction.

Treatment of, and natural resolution of the lesions can result in improvement; however, many cases have recurrences which prove more difficult to treat successfully.

Removal of retained dental roots left after feline erosive neck lesions have caused teeth to break off, or when teeth have been inexpertly extracted, has benefited some cats. Cats with this pattern of self-mutilation can cause themselves great harm and demand the most thorough medical investigation.

Psychogenic causes for hair loss and self-injury should only be considered once all medical causes have been eliminated. However, stress is known to alter immune function, either exacerbating auto-immune disease or allergy or causing immune suppression. The precise effect appears to depend upon the type of stress the individual experiences. Living in a stressful social or physical environment will therefore contribute to the worsening of many of the medical conditions that are differentials for compulsive over-grooming. Success in the treatment of these conditions will improve if the cat's living conditions are improved.

Treatment

Given that stress and anxiety are significant factors in over-grooming, it is vital to improve the cat's living environment. Increasing the range of activities available to the cat will use up a greater proportion of its time and energy budget, leaving less time for introverted self-appeasement. A proper assessment of inter-cat relationships within the home should be made so that underlying psychosocial stress may be alleviated. More information is available in the chapters on feline house-soiling and feline aggression.

Medical therapy with psychoactive medication is indicated in cases of compulsive self-mutilation or severe self-grooming. The SRI drug clomipramine (Clomicalm®, Novartis) may be given at a rate of 0.25–0.5 mg/kg, once daily. Initially, the lower dose rate may be used, with an increase if there is limited improvement after 4 to 6 weeks. As with other compulsive problems, it is useful for clients to make an assessment of the number and severity of self-grooming bouts seen during the 7 to 14-day period before treatment, as a baseline. Drug therapy should be gradually phased out over approximately 4 to 8 weeks, once the cat's full coat has been restored and a period of 6 to 8 weeks without further over-grooming has elapsed. Successful drug therapy should produce around 70% reduction in the behaviour and an increase in normal activity as a substitute.

If specific events or stimuli are associated with signs of anxiety, fear or directly with bouts of excessive grooming, then these may be desensitised and counterconditioned. Relapses are common but may be managed effectively using the same methods as for initial treatment. Response to successive courses of the same SRI or SSRI drug may diminish so it is sometimes better to treat relapses with a different psychoactive drug from the same class. Any additional underlying factors that may have initiated another period of self-mutilation should then be identified and resolved.

> **Box 14.8   Treatment: grooming disorders, compulsive over-grooming and self-mutilation**
>
> - Rule out all other medical and behavioural causes.
> - Record baseline rate and severity of bouts of over-grooming or self-mutilation attacks as a comparison for future reassessment.
> - Investigate and rectify underlying environmental and social factors that may be the cause of anxiety or stress.
> - Consider drug therapy for refractory cases.

In cases of feline orofacial pain syndrome medical treatment is dependent on the underlying disease, if there is one. In a recent study, some cases with gingivitis appeared to respond to antibiotics although spontaneous remission could not be ruled out. NSAIDs provided effective analgesia for some mildly affected cases. Opioids proved to be very useful for hospitalised cases; but antiepileptic drugs (diazepam or phenobarbitone) gave more sustained and consistent relief. Phenobarbitone is the preferred drug because of the greater risk of idiosyncratic hepatic failure with diazepam. Occasionally, life-long therapy is required. Some cases, especially those with chronic dental disease, responded to steroid therapy. Finally, selegiline is effective for some cases and is probably more appropriate for those with a behavioural component or contributing stressful environment. For these cases alterations to the environment and application of behavioural modification are also essential (Box 14.8).

PICA (INCLUDING WOOL–SUCKING)

Some reports indicate that the chewing or sucking of woolly items is most common in early-weaned oriental breed cats that continue to display suckling behaviour but transfer it to clothing and bedding. Typically, the first sign is that the cat chews the owner's clothes while being held. These cats usually stop 'wool-sucking' before the age of 6 months. The precise reason for this delay in weaning from oral suckling behaviour is not understood but such juvenile behaviour is *not* considered to be compulsive and does not necessarily lead into adult 'compulsion'.

Genuinely compulsive pica in adult cats usually begins at maturity and can involve various different materials, including fabric, wool, rubber and cardboard. Usually the cats show a specific preference for a material but this may generalise or change over time, especially if the owner attempts to stop the cat from chewing the items that it currently favours. Wool is often the first target with progression from that to cotton and synthetics over time.

The behaviour may be restricted to chewing or mouthing the material but can involve ingestion. The risk this presents depends upon the type of material being swallowed. The motivation to swallow objects is different from that in the dog. Dogs swallow food items as a means of carrying them between locations. They will then regurgitate the undigested food to eat or bury. Dogs often learn to swallow non-food items that they have stolen when the owner approaches to try to take them away. Cats do not do this and are also less inclined to steal and retain objects as a means of gaining attention. However, cats with existing attachment problems, especially oriental breeds, may steal and chew objects to get attention.

Diagnosis

Wool-sucking is characterised by rhythmic repetitive mouthing and sucking of woolly objects and has therefore been classed by many authors as a compulsive disorder. Other possible explanations for the behaviour include a possible mis-wiring within the hypothalamic region of the brain which leads to errors in the detection of potential prey items and the redirection of hunting responses onto unsuitable items such as fabric. Cats with pica consistently choose to chew and swallow the same kind of non-food items rather than simply engaging in oral investigation of a range of different items and materials, which is relatively normal in immature cats.

There are a number of differentials for compulsive pica or wool-sucking, including:

- repetitive chewing to relieve oral pain
- consumption of non-food items to induce vomiting (which can also occur repeatedly if a previous foreign body remains lodged in the stomach)
- stealing and chewing objects as a means of getting attention from the owner
- cats with severe CNS pathology or senility may sometimes attempt to eat non-food items because they may perceive them as food
- conditions causing polyphagia may encourage cats to investigate and consume borderline non-food items.

Cats with pica should be thoroughly medically investigated before commencing a behavioural investigation.

Treatment

Young cats that wool-suck before the age of 6 months will probably stop spontaneously but should be given alternative safe objects to chew. Food that is chewy may help to redirect the behaviour. Hide-based dog chews tend to be too hard for cats and have little flavour but they can be adapted by soaking them in hot water until the hide becomes softer. It may then be flavoured to make it appealing using a few drops of fish sauce used in oriental cooking. The pieces must be sufficiently large that they cannot be swallowed whole. Other alternatives include dental hygiene dried cat food, which comes in large pieces, or meat jerky sold for human consumption.

The same diversionary tactic can be tried with adult-onset cases of pica, and the texture of the chewing substitute should be matched to the cat's existing preference. These cats should also be provided with general environmental enrichment and any specific underlying environmental or social stressors should be dealt with. Psychoactive medication may be used, with SRI and SSRI drugs producing significant improvement in both juvenile post-weaning and adult-onset cases of pica, although the mode of action of the drug in the two conditions may be different. Clomipramine should be given at an initial dose of 0.25 mg/kg, once daily, rising in dosage to 0.5 mg/kg, once daily, if there is insufficient response after 4 to 6 weeks.

Drug therapy should be continued until a period of 6 to 8 weeks without pica has elapsed and the cat is chewing the alternatives provided.

Prognosis

Cats with pica represent a serious risk to themselves as ingested material may cause gastrointestinal obstruction.

Withdrawal of successful therapy may cause further potentially life-threatening bouts of pica, so the aim is to maintain a stable and low-stress environment compatible with producing the minimum amount of abnormal behaviour. In some cases long-term medication may be needed.

ADVICE SHEETS THAT MAY BE RELEVANT TO THIS CHAPTER

In Appendix 3

1. Improving the outdoor environment for cats
2. Improving the indoor environment for cats
3. Multi-cat households

Chapter 15

Feline house-soiling and marking problems

INTRODUCTION

Enquiries relating to house-soiling problems in domestic cats are common in veterinary practice and the potential negative effects on the cat–owner relationship make them some of the most important issues in feline behavioural medicine. This does not mean that they are necessarily the most common behavioural issue in the domestic cat but they are certainly one of the most frequently quoted reasons for relinquishing cats at rescue centres and even requesting euthanasia in an otherwise healthy pet. One possible reason for the strength of reaction to these problems is the high expectation that owners have in relation to cleanliness in their feline companions and the resulting lack of tolerance when urine or faeces are deposited in any location other than the facilities provided for that purpose. Indeed, cat owners may have chosen the cat as a pet specifically because of expectations of cleanliness. However, a breakdown in house-training is just one potential reason for depositing urine or faeces in inappropriate places and it is important to take time to differentiate these true elimination problems from cases of unwanted marking behaviour and also from behavioural consequences of organic disease.

House-training

Although most owners do not play a very active role in the house-training process for cats, the development of associations between certain substrates and locations and the act of elimination is still achieved through a process of learning. When kittens are first born, the act of elimination is dependent on abdominal stimulation from the queen and this enables the queen to ensure that the nest site is kept clean and free from potential sources of infection. However, as the kittens get older, their movement away from the nest begins to stimulate the act of elimination and it is at this stage that the formation of an association between toileting and substrate begins. The availability of suitable latrine substrates is therefore essential at this young age, and kittens whose mothers are reliable in their own use of litter facilities will benefit from increased exposure to suitable sites as they follow their mother away from the nest. The fact that the act of toileting is in itself rewarding means that the presence of external reward for the selection of an appropriate latrine site is not necessary and, provided suitable toileting facilities are available, most kittens will establish a classically conditioned association between the presence of cat litter and the act of elimination within the first few weeks of life. Maintaining this association into adulthood will depend on ensuring the continued availability of suitable latrines and, in many cases of inappropriate elimination, it is important to consider the domestic environment from a feline perspective and to be aware of the shortcomings of many litter facilities.

Box 15.1   Characteristics of indoor elimination behaviour

Behaviour and posture:

- The location may be sniffed and investigated before elimination.
- Urine or faeces are deposited while the cat is in a crouched position with back slightly arching.
- Abnormal postures may be seen during elimination: urination while standing up, or when crouched with a greatly arched or flattened back is indicative of pain or dysuria. In extreme cases, cats may cry or run away from the area where they have eliminated, as if in pain.
- Unlike marking behaviour, there is no visual 'display' element to normal elimination.

Deposit:

- Relatively large volumes of normal urine or faeces.

Location:

- Unless a particular location is excessively soiled and becomes objectionable to use, the cat will tend to use only a small number of latrine sites for elimination: one for urine and one for faeces.
- Latrines are usually in quiet locations where the cat will have some privacy when eliminating.

Marking behaviour

Deposition of urine and faeces is most readily associated with the act of evacuating the bladder and bowels during elimination but in the feline world, these deposits may also be made in the process of communication. Urine and faeces can both be used to convey messages from one cat to another or indeed to provide a reassuring scent message for the perpetrators themselves. When deposits are used in this way, there are certain characteristics, both in terms of the nature and location of the deposits and the history

of the cat that is making them, which should help to differentiate marking problems from cases of inappropriate elimination(Boxes 15.1, 15.2).

Organic disease

In any case of house-soiling it is important to consider medical differentials before embarking on a purely behavioural assessment of the problem. Any condition which affects gastrointestinal or urinary tract function is a potential candidate for involvement in cases of inappropriate elimination and a full medical examination is therefore essential. Conditions which result in polydipsia and polyuria may also be implicated when urine deposits are found in unusual locations and endocrine disorders should be considered when investigating these cases. Any medical condition which alters the cat's mobility may limit its ability to gain access to latrines and conditions which alter the animal's cognitive ability or sensory perception may also contribute to a breakdown in previously well-established house-training. Organic disease may also be a factor in cases of undesirable marking behaviour.

Box 15.2   Characteristics of marking behaviour

Behaviour and posture:

- Cat approaches and sniffs the location.
- It then turns around and reverses up to the spray site.
- Whilst spraying the cat will paddle its feet.
- The tail will twitch and vibrate.
- The cat may have a glazed and vacant look on its face.

Deposit:

- Small to medium volumes of urine, perhaps with a greasy or oily appearance.
- Intense odour, often musty.
- Dries to a yellow-brown colour, with a greasy appearance and occasionally containing crystals.
- Faeces (middening) are of normal appearance.

Location:

- Usually highly visible locations, where marks will be easily noticed.
- Most often urine is placed on vertical surfaces, but occasionally on horizontal ones.
- Urine may be placed high up on the vertical object.
- Objects that heat up and cool down may attract spray marks (heaters, toasters, TV and audio equipment).
- Bags, shoes and other objects that may carry foreign odours into the home may be targeted.
- Faeces (middening) are deposited, unburied, in open spaces where they will be most visible.

Immediate intervention

Clients who present cats with house-soiling problems are often in a state of desperation and may be close to requesting euthanasia. Many of these clients may have known about a problem for months or years but some change of circumstance has provoked an urgent need to prevent the house-soiling.

Specific reasons for an increase in the urgency include:

- arrival of a new baby
- new partner moving into the home
- forthcoming redecoration
- recently completed redecoration
- owner is about to sell their home
- damage to property causing conflict with landlord.

In each situation the client has an immediate short-term problem that needs to be dealt with in order to buy enough time to treat the house-soiling problem properly. It is therefore important to ask clients about any such circumstances.

Underlying these situations are some basic concerns:

- odour
- hygiene
- damage.

Immediate action should include giving advice on how to protect property from urine damage and how to improve hygiene. Areas should be cleaned with a biological cleaner that contains no ammonia compounds, strong odours or bleach. A good choice is a 10% solution of biological clothes washing powder in water. Only odour-free disinfectants should be used. Urine that soaks into woodwork can cause a great deal of damage and can be very difficult to remove.

Furniture and floors should be protected from urine contamination so that cleaning becomes easier and further damage is limited. Residual urine odour will encourage cats to re-visit and use latrines or spraying sites so removing urine odour is an essential element of preventing house-soiling as well as helping to reduce the immediate problem of urine contamination. Information for clients is provided in a handout in Advice sheet 4, Appendix 3 (Boxes 15.3, 15.4).

GENERAL ASPECTS OF INVESTIGATING HOUSE-SOILING CASES

Medical assessment

Medical factors are very important in house-soiling and marking problems. Certain conditions are directly involved in the generation and maintenance of behavioural problems, while others are contributory in an indirect sense (Box 15.5).

The medical workup must include:

- medical history
- clinical examination, including abdominal palpation
- urinalysis

Box 15.3   Removing urine contamination

1. Make up and label three plant sprayer bottles containing:
   A: 10% solution of biological washing powder/liquid in water*
   B: Plain water
   C: Surgical spirit*
2. Mop up excess urine and dry the surface using paper towels. Do not soak up urine using the cloth you intend to use for cleaning or wring a urine-soaked cloth into the cleaning bucket as this will spread urine odours.
3. Spray the surface with bottle A (biological detergent solution). Mop the surface with paper towels.
4. Spray the surface with bottle B (plain water). Mop the surface dry with paper towels.
5. Mist the surface with bottle C and allow it to dry naturally. Do not allow the cat access to the area for at least 30 minutes to allow the alcohol to dry.
6. Dispose of paper towels to a dustbin *outside* the house.

*Test these cleaning products on an inconspicuous area of cloth or carpet before using them more widely to make sure that no discolouration or loss of colour is likely to occur.

- assessment of mobility, cognitive function and sensory perception
- further investigation through haematology, biochemistry or imaging techniques.

If a case is to be referred to a non-veterinary behaviourist, it is essential to rule out any potential underlying or contributory medical factor (Box 15.5).

Behavioural assessment

House-soiling and indoor marking behaviour may be difficult to differentiate in some cases and in many they occur together. It is important to collect all of the information needed to make a judgment which comprises:

- age of onset
- previous record of house-training
- present reaction to litter facilities
- pattern of deposits – location, frequency, volume
- orientation of deposits – onto vertical or horizontal surfaces
- posture of cat during deposition
- relationships between animals in the household
- presence or absence of the owner or other animals around the time of soiling (including other cats seen outside).
- owner's reaction to the deposits
- events in the household or the neighbourhood coinciding with the onset of the behaviour
- assessment of the cat's emotional reactions to novelty in the environment and to strangers.

Box 15.4   Protecting property from urine damage

Wooden floors:

- Seal joints and junctions between flooring and skirting boards or fitted furniture (kitchen units) with a silicone or appropriate waterproof sealant to prevent urine from getting into cracks.
- Carefully seal joints between the panels of laminated flooring (urine ingress will cause panels to expand and pop up).
- Paint wooden floors with two or more coats of a heavy varnish (matt or gloss according to choice) or damp-sealant paint. If possible, extend the painted or varnished area to over-paint the sealant and thus create a complete barrier.

Concrete floors:

- Clean the floor and allow it to dry.
- Seal cracks as above.
- Paint it with several coats of a waterproofing paint.

Vinyl floors:

- Some vinyl floors are porous, especially if they are old.
- They may be sealed using specialist paints and coatings available from DIY centres.
- Cracked vinyl flooring should be removed and replaced.

Tiled floors:

- Glazed tiles are generally nonporous but grout between the tiles may absorb urine.
- Terracotta tiles are porous unless regularly sealed with a specialist coating (available from DIY stores).
- Use a specialist sealant on grout.
- Consider scraping out old grout in heavily urine-contaminated areas and replacing it with new waterproof grout.

Carpets:

- When fitting new carpet, clean and seal the flooring underneath (as above).
- Consider applying a layer of heavy plastic sheeting beneath the carpet or underlay to prevent urine from seeping into the floor.
- Protect existing carpets by covering them with heavy plastic sheeting and then cleaning the carpet underneath at least 2 to 3 times weekly until no further urine odour persists.

Wooden furniture:

- Where possible, apply 2+ coats of varnish, especially under wooden feet of furniture (to stop urine absorption into wood grain).
- Otherwise, use regular applications of a heavy wax furniture polish.

Computers and electronic equipment:

- Urine marking or soiling on electrical equipment is a serious health hazard: it can cause fires and electrical failures.
- Disconnect the equipment from the electricity outlet and clean carefully in accordance with the manufacturer's instructions.
- Allow to dry thoroughly.
- Dispose of any cooking equipment that is impossible to clean thoroughly (e.g., old toasters), because these represent a health hazard.
- Keep the equipment in a cupboard where it cannot be further soiled, or cover it in plastic sheeting when you are not using it (remembering the need for some equipment to be properly ventilated).

Electrical outlets:

- Urine entering a wall socket can cause a fire or shock hazard, so access to the location should be restricted.
- As an additional protection, cover the outlet with cling-film or a large flap of polythene hanging down over the socket, taped to the wall above it or alternatively use child proof plug guards.

- Conditions causing PU/PD: renal insufficiency, diabetes mellitus.
- Feline lower urinary tract disease.
- Diseases causing debilitation: osteoarthritis, senile dementia, sensory loss.
- Diseases affecting cognition: senile dementia, CNS pathology (primary or secondary to systemic disease).

Using a house plan

One of the most useful tools when investigating a problem of feline house-soiling is a plan of the house in which the cat lives. This does not need to be a detailed scale drawing but, rather, a basic plan indicating the layout of rooms in the house, the position of windows, doors and major furniture and the location of major resources such as feeding and watering stations, sleeping locations and play areas. Each individual cat's favourite resting places and rooms they prefer to inhabit should be noted on the diagram. The client should then mark onto this diagram the location of urine and faeces that they have found (Fig. 15.1).

To give a better indication of the development of the problem, the client should note the current frequency of urine or faecal deposition at a particular site, as well as how early in the development of the problem urine or faeces were first found there. A convenient way to do this is to label each location on the diagram with a number of stars to indicate current frequency and a number that indicates whether that spot was one of the first or last places to be soiled, or somewhere between. The clinician may use this diagram (see example) as a basis for recording additional information about each mark, such as the volume of urine at a site, where precisely on furniture or decorations it is located and whether any particular event appears connected to it.

The pattern of urine and faecal deposits can point to the source of the problem. For example, if the first deposits were found close to doors and windows, it is suggestive that the perceived threat was coming from outside the home; whereas initial deposits in the centre of rooms or onto new pieces of furniture would suggest that the disruption to the cat's security was coming from within the household.

Once all of this information has been collected, it is then possible to make judgments about the nature of the problem, whether it is a matter of indoor marking or elimination and what the motivation may be.

DIFFERENTIATING BETWEEN ELIMINATION AND MARKING

Once full information has been collected about the location and characteristics of each urine or faecal deposit, it is possible to differentiate between its causes.

Positioning of deposits and reaction to the litter tray

In the case of marking, the areas that the cat uses to deposit urine or faeces will often be of behavioural significance; for example, areas that smell of the owner or of the new cat in the household or locations which are associated with potential threat from the outside world. There is often a provoking stimulus for this inappropriate behaviour, such as some disruption to the home environment or competition within the local neighbourhood, and the location of the marking deposits will reflect this. Urine or faecal marks are placed strategically in order to provide a signal to other cats, which means that they must be placed in locations that are likely to be noticed. The act of spraying itself also involves an element of visual display. It should be remembered that odour marks are not merely of use to the 'sender' of the signal who is trying to maintain distance from other cats; they are also of use to the 'receiver' who is equally keen to avoid direct physical conflict. The location of scent marks therefore follows conventions that allow other cats to find and investigate them easily. Such places might include door frames, doors, or pieces of furniture that face doors or windows (Fig. 15.2).

Inappropriate indoor elimination, on the other hand, will usually take place in quiet secluded locations which reflect the sort of places cats would naturally choose to use

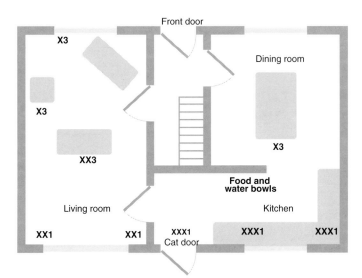

Figure 15.1   House plan showing location of resources and sites where urine and faeces have been found. X = Frequency of urine deposits (the more Xs, the higher the frequency). 1, 2, 3 = Order of locations where urine was found (1 for first location, 2 for second and 3 for most recent).

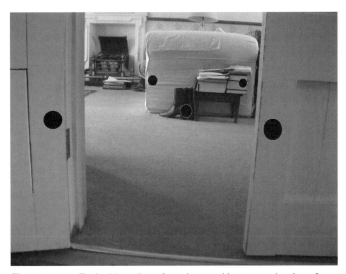

Figure 15.2 Typical locations for urine marking around point of entry into a room.

as latrines. It is also likely that elimination sites will have certain common characteristics in terms of the substrate that is used and cats will often develop preferences for the inappropriate substrate, such as carpet or linen, and return to similar surfaces repeatedly. These inappropriate substrates may be similar to those the cat was forced to use as a kitten, through an inadequate provision of proper latrines in the rearing environment.

One useful difference between indoor 'markers' and 'toileters' is their reaction to the indoor latrine facilities, with 'markers' often continuing to use the litter tray and 'toileters' actively avoiding the facilities provided. Indeed, in cases of a lack of or a breakdown of house-training, signs of aversion to the litter tray may be the first thing that the owner notices.

Cats with feline lower urinary tract disease (FLUTD) will often use several different sites in the house during the same period, breaking the usual pattern of the cat using only one or two latrines. This is because pain associated with micturition in each of the latrine sites discourages repeated use of the same locations. The cat associates eliminating in that place with pain or dysuria and chooses somewhere else next time. Amounts of urine found at each site may be smaller then normal and have a strong odour or contain blood. This pattern of urination is often cyclical with cats eliminating normally for a few weeks and then suffering another bout of generalised house-soiling. This fits with the cyclical nature of the severity of FLUTD which may wax and wane.

Frequency of deposits

If a cat is depositing urine and faeces as part of the normal function of elimination, the frequency will reflect this and deposits will be limited in their number. However, when cats are using the deposits as a form of marking there is no limit on the frequency of deposition and it is not unusual for a urine-spraying cat to leave in excess of thirty marks within the home in a 24-hour period.

Volume of deposits

The amount of urine that is deposited can also help to determine the motivation for the behaviour with toileting problems usually involving larger quantities than marking problems. However, this can be confusing since a small amount of urine can be absorbed by carpets and other fabrics and the size of the moist patch on the floor can be misleading! Cats with FLUTD will pass many small quantities of urine in several sites, causing confusion with a marking problem. Likewise, cats with chronic diarrhoea. However, the choice of location will still fit with normal defecation or urination.

Posture of cat and orientation of deposits

The posture of the cat can help in the differentiation process since indoor urine spraying is usually associated with a characteristic stance. This is related to the function of the marking behaviour since a standing posture allows the cat to deposit urine on a vertical surface at just the correct height for another cat to sniff at it and take in the important information.

However, urine marking does not exclusively occur from a standing posture and it can be performed from a squatting position which closely resembles the posture adopted during the act of elimination. This fact must be borne in mind when attempting to differentiate between motivations; it is easy to dismiss squatting urination on horizontal surfaces as always being eliminative and yet there are occasions when the cat is actually using that sort of urination as a marking behaviour.

Pattern of urine and faeces deposition (identified using a house plan)

Certain patterns are classic indicators of a specific underlying motivation (Box 15.6). For example, if the first urine marking deposits were found close to external doors and windows, it is suggestive that the perceived threat was coming from outside the home, whilst initial deposits in the centre of rooms, corridors or staircases, or onto new pieces of furniture would suggest that the disruption to the cat's security was coming from within the household. As a situation progresses, the pattern becomes more confusing so that it becomes very difficult to identify the originating cause unless the historical development of the pattern of the marking or elimination is known. For example, urine marking may progress from door and window areas to

Box 15.6   Characteristic patterns in urine and faeces deposition

Indoor marking

- *Initial locations are around cat flap, external doors and windows*: external threat.
- *Initial locations are entry points to internal rooms, on landings and in corridors*: internal conflict within home.
- *Spread of marking sites into the home from around cat flap*: potential intruder cat.
- *Random locations throughout the home*: emotional disturbance within the household.
- *Initial deposits on new items in the household, shoes or shopping bags*: insecurity and reaction to potential threat.

Indoor elimination

- *Single indoor toilet location or substrate (litter box available):* location or substrate of litter tray is unsuitable or cat may be afraid to use the litter tray.
- *Single indoor toilet location or substrate (no litter box, cat previously used garden latrine):* cat is unable to use outdoor latrine because it is unusable (e.g., waterlogged, frozen or paved over), or inaccessible (e.g., cat is unwell or a dog now inhabits garden where the latrine is sited), or it is defended by other cats as part of their territory (e.g., despotism).
- *Multiple indoor toilet locations and substrates:* cat is unable to use a regular latrine due to conflict with other cats, aversive experiences during elimination (e.g., pain associated with FLUTD, or owner punishment).

hallways and rooms if a neighbourhood despot begins to invade the resident cat's home.

ASSESSING EMOTIONAL FACTORS IN CASES OF FELINE HOUSE–SOILING

In situations of both marking and elimination behaviour within the home, it is important to assess the cat's emotional status and to attempt to identify any triggers for alteration in that status. Perception of threat, either from within or outside the home, is commonly associated with the onset of marking behaviour but it is also important to remember that cats that are feeling threatened and insecure may be reluctant to use litter facilities that are positioned in vulnerable locations or that pose difficulties for the cat in terms of competition with other feline household members. In general, it is the insecure and timid feline that is more likely to present with problems of marking behaviour and

individuals that do not cope well with change in their environment are going to be predisposed to the use of urine deposits that are designed to increase home security. In addition, cats that are living in a hostile social environment where there is underlying tension between feline housemates, may use marking behaviour in an attempt to increase distance between them and to avoid overt physical confrontation. Therefore, an assessment of the compatibility between cats in the household is an important part of the investigation process. Likewise, the relationship between the cat and the owner should be considered and questions about the owner's reaction to the discovery of deposits within the home should be included in the consultation. It is perfectly understandable for people to find it unacceptable that their pet is depositing urine or faeces within their home but the use of punitive techniques may be a factor in perpetuating the behaviour and confirming the cat's perception that the house is no longer a secure core territory.

Owners often misinterpret relationships between cats in multi-cat households because they are unaware of the significance of certain behaviours. For example, cats will often be described as 'getting on well' because they eat and rest in proximity to one another on the owner's bed or couch. Unfortunately, this apparent tolerance may exist only because the cats are forced to be close to each other when they are feeding or resting. They have no other choice because there are no other feeding stations or equivalent resting places. The cats may be very wary and hesitant while feeding and the owner will report that there are frequent bouts of hissing or spitting around the food bowl. Likewise, as one cat leaves a resting place or feeding area, it may be pursued or attacked and cats may attempt long distance intimidations, such as staring eye contact, to frighten each other away from resting places or latrines. Some cats can try to pull food out of a dish with their paws so that they can take it to eat in private. The same desire for privacy can drive them to make a toilet of their own somewhere in the house.

It is important to make a formal assessment of the relationships between cats in the household. A diagram should be constructed to illustrate the relationships. The social function of cats that have died or been re-homed may be important so it may be necessary to draw more than one diagram to illustrate the changing relationships as cats have departed or been added to the group.

Positive affiliative reactions that should be noted include allorubbing and allogrooming, tail up and trilled greeting between cats. Aggressive behaviours include active threats such as chasing, hissing or spitting and physical attacks, as well as the more passive or distant threats made by staring eye contact, threatening body or facial posture or spraying in front of other cats.

These classes of behaviour and their direction should be noted on a diagram of interactions as illustrated in Figure 15.3.

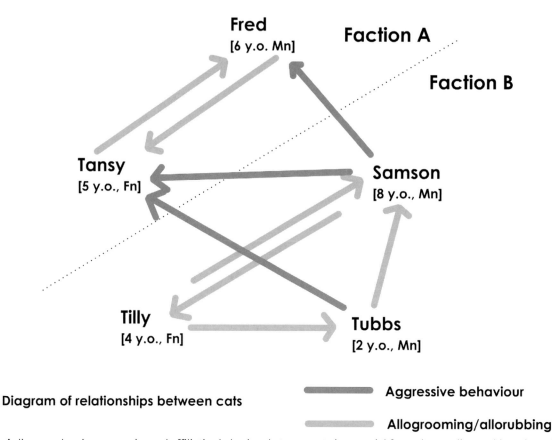

Figure 15.3   A diagram showing aggressive and affiliative behaviour between cats is essential for understanding problems in multi-cat households.

This may enable certain factions to be identified within the household. Combined with the information already obtained about where cats spend most of their time in the household, this makes the allocation of resources easier during treatment. It may also help to identify feline despots. Making an assessment of this kind is important, even when looking at a multi-cat household with what appears to be reactionary spraying due to conflict with outside cats. If resources in the home are sparse, then certain cats may perceive there to be a local overpopulation problem which is made worse by competition with outside cats. Sorting out internal conflict is likely to improve the cats' general welfare as well as help to resolve elimination and marking problems.

INAPPROPRIATE ELIMINATION

Once the initial history taking has been completed and the case has been categorised as one of elimination, it is important to spend time investigating the potential trigger factors which lead to the onset of the behaviour. Only once the underlying reasons for the alteration in toileting behaviour have been identified can effective behavioural therapy be instituted and the cat taught to return to more acceptable patterns of elimination.

In some cases, the cat may never have achieved a state of successful house-training, although this is relatively uncommon. In the past, a belief that kittens needed to observe their mother's eliminatory behaviour in order to learn how to toilet appropriately was thought to be supported by the over-representation of pure-bred cats, such as Persians, and the occurrence of house-soiling issues within familial lines in those breeds. However, research suggests that observational learning is not involved in this process and that a lack of opportunity to explore and experiment with suitable substrates early in life is more likely to influence a failure to house-train successfully. Obviously this access to suitable litter is going to be influenced by the mother's behaviour since kittens will follow her when she goes to use the tray and will thereby come into contact with an acceptable substrate. Kittens from mothers with poor toileting skills are therefore likely to have less interaction with a suitable substrate and may develop problems as a result but, even when the mother is a very clean individual, lack of suitable facilities near to the nest will have a similar effect. Failure to provide a suitable substrate can also lead to the development of undesirable substrate associations (Box 15.7).

Box 15.7 Immediate action: inappropriate elimination

- Start medical investigation of possible causes for elimination problems.
- Stop punishment of the cat as this may make it more secretive and fearful.
- Use appropriate cleaning methods to remove urine or faeces and protect furniture and household items (see text and Advice sheet 4, Appendix 3).
- If the cat does not have an indoor litter tray, then provide at least one deep-filled litter box with a mineral-based or clumping litter in a quiet and secluded location, possibly close to where the cat has previously been soiling.
- If the problem is in a multi-cat household, then provide two or more trays according to the number of cats (general rule of one tray per cat and one spare).

Box 15.8 Using fluorescein to identify urine marking or soiling cats

- Fluorescein is available as sterile paper strips for ophthalmic examination. These contain approximately 1 mg of fluorescein per tip, but this should be checked with the manufacturer.
- The tips should be torn off and rolled to fit into gelatin capsules, giving approximately 5 per capsule (5 mg).
- This dose is given once daily for 3 to 4 days.
- Urine sites are checked daily.
- Lightly spray each site with a solution of sodium bicarbonate (baking powder), mixed in water (1 tablespoonful in 125 ml water).
- A UV lamp is then used to check the site for fluorescence.
- It is vital to start by testing the least probable culprits first, working up to the most probable. Otherwise fluorescence marks left by one cat will obscure those of another. If it is certain that the culprit is a resident cat, then the culprit may be identified by a process of elimination, which minimises the risk of leaving lots of fluorescent stains for the client to clean up.
- A 5-day washout is left between testing of each cat to make sure that each individual has excreted all of the dye before testing the next.
- Although fluorescein is water-soluble and can usually be removed with normal cleaning, this testing method may leave stains on fabric, carpets or wallpaper and **owners must be warned of this.**

Diagnosis

It is very important to properly identify the culprit(s) for the indoor house-soiling. Clients frequently blame a particular animal, usually because they have seen it eliminating in the house. However, other cats may also be involved. It is possible to use fluorescein dye to identify the urine of each cat in the household so that the identity of the soiling cat can be confirmed (Box 15.8). Recent research has shown that the fluorescence of urine spots from fluorescein-treated cats may vary with urine pH. The fluorescence of fluorescein varies with pH, such that it only strongly emits light under UV illumination when it is in a neutral or alkaline solution. In acidic solution, it may hardly glow green at all. Spots should therefore be sprayed with a buffer solution of sodium bicarbonate (baking soda), which will produce a pH of around 8, before testing with a UV lamp. If faecal soiling is involved, then a small amount of indigestible material is added to each cat's food for several days and the faeces are inspected. Crushed sweet corn works very well because it is easy to identify in the faeces and does not upset digestion.

A behavioural diagnosis should only be attempted after medical underlying and contributory factors have been investigated. A diagnosis is then reached after collecting a detailed history and making diagrams of the soiling locations. Causes of house-training breakdown are many and varied and detailed history-taking and in-depth consultations are essential to get an accurate picture. Post-trauma breakdown is relatively common and examples of trauma can include a period of enforced confinement, fear of the litter tray owing to administration of medication, or negative associations with the tray as a result of medical problems. Inappropriate facilities may be at the root of inappropriate toileting problems and so it is important to consider the type of litter used in the tray, the sort of tray that is being offered and also the location of that tray. The cleaning regime may also be relevant since most cats are reluctant to use trays that are dirty, while some others will fail to bond successfully to their latrine if it is cleaned too frequently. Other potential causes of a breakdown in house-training include challenges to security in nervous individuals, overcrowding within a small-sized territory where there is competition over the resource of the latrines or where access to the trays is controlled and manipulated by one individual within the household. There is also the issue of old age and debilitation (Box 15.9).

Recent research has demonstrated a direct connection between psychosocial stress and FLUTD. Feline idiopathic cystitis (FIC) is a complex condition that involves neurological changes in spinal pain fibres and biochemical changes in the bladder wall. The precise aetiology is not fully understood but cats with an anxious personality are predisposed to FIC and it is proposed that the condition arises from a combination of physical and psychological factors. Black and white cats and Persian cats are commonly affected and FIC may account for a significant proportion of FLUTD in cats. Urine samples of FIC cats may be sterile or may contain crystals, plugs or traces of blood. Diagnosis is confirmed by double-contrast radiography or ultrasound imaging of the bladder to reveal mural thickening.

Box 15.9   Typical causes for inappropriate elimination

- **Lack of privacy in latrine locations:** Litter trays that are placed too close to feeding areas or cat doors, or sited in busy places where the cat does not feel safe to go to the toilet. A previously satisfactory location may become unacceptable if the presence of new pets or children constantly disturbs the cat. New cats in the neighbourhood may overlook the litter tray from outside, again reducing privacy.
- **Inappropriate substrate:** Certain scented, pine or wood-pulp based litters are aversive to cats. When urinated on they may release odours that the cat finds repellent, especially if the litter tray is hooded or enclosed. Substrate depth is also important with cats preferring a depth of around 3 cm.
- **Competition and excessive latrine use:** If several cats are using the same litter tray then it quickly becomes soiled and cats may be forced to find somewhere else. Cats may be forced to displace each other in order to gain access to the solitary household latrine. Cats prefer to use separate toilets for urine and faeces wherever possible.
- **Despotic control of entry/exit points:** Feline despots may perch close to cat doors and threaten other cats as they come and go. Nervous cats may not have the confidence to go in and out so they cannot use outdoor latrines. Threatening of cats leaving or entering the litter tray may also occur from cats within the same household.
- **Specific fears:** Cats that are moved to a noisy or stressful location may be unwilling to go outside to use latrines. They may stay inside and soil the house if not provided with a litter tray.
- **Negative litter box associations:** If the cat has been attacked or disturbed while using a particular latrine, or if it has experienced pain on micturition, then it is likely to choose a different toilet location the next time it needs to eliminate.
- **Inability to use or find litter trays:** Elderly or debilitated cats may be less willing to travel to find a latrine so they may resort to soiling in the house. They may be unable to make use of high-sided or covered trays.
- **Medical illness:** Cats with PU/PD, incontinence, FLUTD or recurrent or chronic diarrhoea are unlikely to maintain a normal or acceptable pattern of elimination.
- **Punishment:** Cats that have been punished for eliminating in the wrong place may refuse to go to the toilet in the presence of the owner. Litter trays tend to be placed in public areas like the kitchen or utility area which means that the fearful cat ceases to use them for fear of being punished further.

Treatment

Medical aspects of elimination problems must be resolved. There is a close relationship between stress and FIC so dealing with social and environmental stress is an important component in resolving this condition (Box 15.10).

Typically, it is possible to identify one or two environmental changes that have initiated the house-soiling problem. This may be something as simple as a change of cat litter. However, it is very important not to treat the problem at this superficial level. If a single inconsequential change has caused the cat to house-soil then it is very likely that there are other underlying problems that also need to be addressed. Not to do so may mean consigning the cat to a life of stress and impaired welfare.

Treatment of house-soiling, therefore, involves dealing with general environmental and social issues that cause stress, as well as the specific aspects of latrine location and type. Aggression between cats sharing a household is often overlooked because actual fights may be uncommon and most of the threatening behaviours between them are subtle.

Overall resource levels should be increased and resources should be distributed so that individual cats and cat-factions can make use of them without coming into conflict with each other. This also helps to undermine the activities of feline despots who try to monopolise specific

---

Box 15.10   Prevention: inappropriate elimination

- Latrine preferences are learned early in life as kittens explore their environment to find suitable latrine sites.
- Specific preferences are conditioned according to the kinds of substrate and location that are available to the kittens.
- Confinement to newspaper-covered areas without proper latrines can lead to inappropriate preferences that can be very difficult to overcome.
- It is essential to provide kittens with latrines that resemble the kind of litter tray and substrate that the kitten can use when it is homed.
- Litter trays should be large and have low sides, so that kittens can use them, otherwise they may learn a preference for eliminating on the newspaper around it. This also enables the kittens to discover a suitable toilet location when they are following their mother.
- Several similar trays should be provided so that kittens have choice and easy access to them.
- Adult cats should be provided with litter trays that are located in quiet locations and deep-filled with a mineral-based or clumping type litter.
- Outdoor latrines may also be constructed (Advice sheet 1).
- New cats should be introduced in an appropriate manner and with an accompanying increase in resources.

resources. Additional cat flaps may be needed if aggression between cats is preventing certain cats from using outdoor latrines.

The cats should be provided with a range of suitable latrines, inside and outside the house. Cats do not share latrine facilities so, in multi-cat households, the optimum number of latrines should be one per cat plus one extra. This number of cat litter trays is obviously a horrific prospect for the owner of a lot of cats. The answer is to provide cats with outdoor latrines in the owner's garden. With the current fashion for hard landscaping, cats may have few opportunities to use good outdoor latrines and may have to travel across several gardens to find somewhere suitable. In winter, these toilets may become sodden or frozen, making them unusable. For this reason, many house-soiling problems are worse during the winter.

Outdoor latrines are actually very easy to construct. To create an outdoor latrine, dig a hole about 45 to 60 cm deep and 60 cm square, fill the bottom two-thirds with pea-sized gravel and then top up with soft white sand of the type used for children's playgrounds. (Hard yellow builder's sand is not suitable.) These outdoor toilets should be hidden in flowerbeds behind shrubs and tall plants to give the cat privacy. These latrines are essentially self-cleaning but it is sensible to regularly use a litter scoop to remove faeces in the same way as with a conventional litter tray. The sandy part of the latrine should be dug out and replaced every 6 months. One outdoor latrine is unlikely to be enough and different cats will have different preferences for location. At least two latrines should be provided.

There are often concerns that other cats will come into the territory to use the outdoor latrines. This is a possibility but rarely causes a problem. In fact, the presence of nearby latrines tends to strengthen the boundary of the resident cat's own territory. Information about improving indoor and outdoor environments for cats is included in Advice sheets 1 and 2, Appendix 3.

Indoor latrines should be made as appealing as possible. They should be positioned in quiet locations and deep-filled with a scent-free mineral-based litter. In some cases, soft sand or a mixture of soft sand and litter is attractive to cats and the sand content can be reduced gradually once the cat has shifted its location preference to the designated litter tray. F3 diffusers (Feliway®, CEVA Animal Health) are traditionally used to treat spraying problems, but can be used to make a latrine location more attractive. The diffuser is placed very close to the litter tray in a confined area. This can be effective for cats that choose to eliminate on piles of the owner's clothing or on the owner's bed because these locations are associated with increased security. F3 diffusers may also be used to reduce general social stress in the household. In this situation, the diffuser should be allowed to warm up for at least a couple of hours before allowing cats to have access to the room where the diffuser is installed.

Conversely, inappropriate latrine sites should be made less appealing (Box 15.11). There are a number of ways to do this including changing the floor substrate to make it less pleasant to stand on or placing small bowls of food close to the location so that it becomes designated as a feeding station instead of a latrine. The best guide for how to modify a particular latrine site is the cat's reason for choosing it in the first place. For example, a dark and secluded corner can be made a lot less discrete by moving furniture, putting in a loud radio close by or illuminating the corner with a bright spot lamp. A battery-powered lamp, activated by infrared, can be bought very cheaply from a hardware store and installed in a small corner where it will switch on every time the cat approaches. This can act as an effective deterrent.

Cats that are inhibited and fearful, and therefore unable to utilise improved resources because of their apprehension, may benefit from psychoactive drug therapy. Selegiline (Selgian®, CEVA Animal Sante) is not licensed for use in the cat but it can be used at a rate of 1 mg/kg, once daily, for the treatment of specific fears, a condition for which it is licensed in the dog (UK). This drug increases confidence and exploratory behaviour but takes 4 to 6 weeks to show efficacy. It should be continued until the cat is fully utilising resources and has not eliminated in the house for 8 weeks.

Where signs of chronic anxiety are apparent despite the use of F3 diffusers, then an SRI or SSRI type drug, such as clomipramine or fluoxetine, may be appropriate.

Box 15.11   Altering inappropriate latrine sites to make them less appealing to the cat

(This must only be done when a potential alternative has been made available)

- Cover the location with thick polythene: urine will then drain towards the cat's feet when it is standing on the sheet.
- Cover the location with a large sheet of silver foil: some cats do not like to stand on this.
- Apply strips of double-sided sticky tape to either of the above to make them even more repellent.
- Place small bowls of food on top of the latrine sites, so that they become feeding stations. Cats are usually reluctant to urinate near sources of food.
- Illuminate dark corners with a bright spot lamp so that any privacy is taken away.
- The same effect can be achieved using a small, battery-powered lamp activated by infrared, which will turn on each time the cat approaches (these are very inexpensive).

Trial treatments for FIC have included polysulphated glycosaminoglycans and amitriptyline. Response to glycosaminoglycans was variable, with some individuals responding extremely well and others less so. Treatment with amitriptyline has produced good results, with the effects being attributed to the noradrenergic effects of the drug. Amitriptyline is 5:1 selective in favour of noradrenaline (norepinephrine) over serotonin re-uptake inhibition, whereas clomipramine is 5:1 selective in favour of serotonin re-uptake. However, both drugs do have significant effects on noradrenaline re-uptake and clomipramine may be a suitable alternative if there are concerns over adverse effects with amitriptyline.

In all cases, psychoactive drug therapy should only be considered after reaching a specific diagnosis and taking into account the risks of disinhibition of aggression. Obstructive urinary tract disease should be ruled out before initiating therapy with SRI or SSRI drugs which have a risk of increasing outflow obstructions through their effects on acetylcholine transmission (Box 15.12).

Prognosis

Cats with a history of inadequate house-training, or inappropriate substrate or location preference are likely to relapse on occasion during periods of stress, or if the owner makes changes to existing toilets. These cats may always be a short step from reverting to using their own preferred toilet sites so it is important to stick to environmental modifications that work.

The prognosis for cats with house-soiling problems is good as long as owners can accept that there may be brief relapses in the future. Even if the domestic indoor and outdoor environment is optimised and relationships between cats in the household have been improved, there is always the possibility that new cats to the neighbourhood may upset the situation.

INDOOR MARKING

Indoor marking and house-soiling often occur together in the same household and in a multi-cat household several

---

Box 15.12   Treatment: inappropriate elimination

General environmental and social issues:

- Increase resources available to the cat and strategically locate them for easy access by the various cats and factions within the household.
- Give the cats indoor–outdoor access with an electronic coded cat door.
- Switch feeding to activity feeding.
- Provide more choice of resting and hiding locations.
- Install F3 diffusers (Feliway®, CEVA Animal Health) to reduce anxiety and improve inter-cat relationships in the house.
- Use scent swapping to improve group odour.
- Consider temporarily isolating and then reintroducing cats if there are problems of aggression.

Latrine number, location and substrate:

- Latrines should be relocated to quiet areas.
- Litter trays should be deep-filled (3 cm) with a mineral-based or clumping litter (not pine or wood-pulp based or scented).
- In some cases, using pure sand or a 50% mixture of litter and sand as a substrate in trays is attractive to cats.
- A mixture of covered and open litter trays may be tested to see which the cat prefers.
- Additional outdoor toilets should be provided.
- Total latrine number may need to be as many as one per cat plus one extra.
- A specific latrine location may be made to feel more secure by locating an F3 diffuser next to it.

Owner behaviour:

- Stop punishment of inappropriate elimination.

Psychoactive drug therapy:

- Selegiline: specific fear with behavioural inhibition that limits normal behaviour.
- Clomipramine/fluoxetine: chronic anxiety (concomitant signs of stress such as over-grooming).
- Clomipramine/amitriptyline: FIC

Box 15.13   Immediate action: indoor marking

- Introduce an appropriate cleaning routine (see box titled 'Removing urine contamination' and client handout in appendix).
- Protect property from further damage (see Box 15.3 and Advice sheet 4 in Appendix 3).
- Stop punishment of cats when they are caught spraying.
- Install F3 diffusers (Feliway®, CEVA Animal Health).

cats may be involved. An important part of reaching a behavioural diagnosis must be to identify the culprits. Fluorescein dye or sweet corn may be administered in the same way as for house-soiling problems, starting with the cats that are least likely to be involved in the problem (see Box 15.8 on the use of fluorescein for identifying the origin of urine deposits). More than one cat may be involved and it should be remembered that, in some cases, the culprit for indoor marking may not be a resident cat at all. Intact male cats and despots may enter the homes of other cats to take food and then leave urine marks within the home. In these cases, treating the resident cats will have no effect on the marking behaviour and, in fact, increasing the level of resources available within the home may raise its value and therefore encourage the despot to try to take it over. In such circumstances, an electronic coded cat-door would need to be fitted (Boxes 15.13, 15.14).

Diagnosis

Diagnosis involves several steps:

- Identify the culprits.
- Assess the health status of all group members.
- Map the location of resources and the progression of urine and faecal marks within the home.
- Assess the structure of the social group within the home in order to identify potential conflict.
- Identify specific situations in which marking occurs.
- Detail the cat's behaviour before, during and after the incidents.

The function of marking behaviour is to identify the significance of certain locations to the 'sender' and 'receiver' of the mark. Scent marks, therefore, act both as a memento of previous experience in a location as well as a signal to others. When a cat encounters the facial and flank marks on inanimate objects in the core part of the territory, they signify that this location has been safe in the past and when a cat leaves another face or flank mark, it is relabelling that place as safe based upon its current experience. The odours that cats share when allogrooming and allorubbing help to identify the group so that these and the core territory odours are a memento of previous interactions. Other odour marks are intended to enable cats to maintain distance from

one another. Both claw marks and urine spray marks contain pheromone chemical signals that are intended to signal to cats outside the social group that they are entering an area that is also occupied by other cats. The home range that surrounds the core territory is quite large and is intensely defended. Beyond this home range, the wider territory controlled by the cat or cat group may be very large. Feral and wild cats may hold territories that are more than 1 to 2 square miles. However, it is clear that cats may need to pass through areas of each other's territory and the boundaries are not absolute. Claw and urine marks are therefore intended to warn other cats to avoid certain locations at certain times so that they do not come into conflict with each other. This works well when there is a large enough territory for the different types of odour marks to be deposited in a meaningful way that allows the cats to avoid potential enemies and remain close to their affiliates. Natural social groups are made of related female cats and juveniles, with adult males and surplus females being displaced from the group at maturity. Intact males will range over much larger territories, visiting different groups of females to mate.

Box 15.14   Prevention: Indoor marking

- Introduce new cats carefully and with an accompanying *increase* in resources for the group.
- When redecorating, building or making changes to house layout, install an F3 diffuser (Feliway®, CEVA Animal Health) to maintain core territory odour signals. Allow paint to dry and the room to air thoroughly before allowing the cat(s) back into it. Harvest facial and flank odours from the cat(s) and apply these to doorways and furnishings in the newly decorated area. If the cat is particularly sensitive to change, it may be better to arrange a cattery stay during major projects of redecoration or renovation, especially if they involve core territory areas for the particular cat.
- Provide adequate resources for the group.
- When cats are temporarily removed from the group (such as when going to the veterinary clinic) they should be reintroduced carefully after trying to relabel them with the group odour.

Contrast this with the situation in the domestic environment. Pet cat groups are made up of unrelated and neutered males and females with widely differing rearing backgrounds. Some may come from a genetic and rearing background that does not favour sociable living in a group. From the owner's perspective, the expectation is that the cat's core territory will match the internal living space of the home so that facial and flank marking are seen indoors and spraying or claw marking is only performed outdoors. However, instead of being one large contiguous area, each domestic cat's territory may consist of several small patches that are distant from each other. Each cat is forced to travel across several other cat's territories in order to get to a latrine or hunting site. This increases the amount of feline traffic through gardens and increases the likelihood that each cat's core territory will be overlooked by cats outside. If underfed, despotic or intact male cats enter the homes of resident cats, then this further undermines the perception of the owner's home as 'core' territory.

So several scenarios emerge. If the core territory is threatened by being overlooked or invaded by cats that are not part of the group, then the boundary of the core territory can retreat into the house and the resident cat(s) will use spray or claw marks to delineate a boundary at the edge of the core territory, which happens to be within the home. These cats may end up inhabiting the upper rooms of a house as core territory and then spray marking or middening on the ground floor, but the situation often starts when urine marks appear at windows or external doors, or around the cat flap.

If the relationship between cats within the home is flawed then, rather than one group, there may be two or more factions co-existing within the home. They may have little tolerance for each other. Most domestic cat groups are of mixed gender and are not actively engaged in mutual kitten rearing, so there is no positive reason for the cats to co-exist other than their own individual social preferences and affiliations. The continued function of the group is highly dependent on whether present resources are plentiful enough to maintain the whole group without competition. Within domestic cat groups sharing a home, it is possible to identify patterns of interaction by analysing greeting, affiliative and aggressive behaviour between cats (see Fig. 15.3).

Groups can contain several types of individual and subgroup:

Cliques or factions: Groups of three or more cats that show greeting and other affiliative behaviour toward each other but may be aggressive to other members of the domestic group.

Pairs: Pairs of cats, often littermates, that greet and show affiliative behaviour toward each other.

Social facilitators: These cats will often offer and receive greetings and show affiliative behaviour with cats from several factions or cliques. They may also associate with other cats outside the group and serve to maintain group odour between individuals and subgroups that rarely interact directly with each other.

Satellite individuals: These offer and receive little or no greeting or affiliative behaviour with the other cats in the home. They may be involved in minor or passive aggressive incidents with other cats in the group, often as the recipient of threat.

Despots: These individuals may deliberately monopolise resources and create opportunities to intimidate other cats inside and outside the home.

Identifying the social structure of the group may give insights into why the relationship between resident cats has broken down. For example, the loss of a social facilitator cat may cause aggression to begin between factions because no other individual is maintaining the group odour. The same situation can occur when the owner goes away on holiday or when a social facilitator becomes ill or infirm. The role of a particular individual may change according to its health status. A pair or faction may break up if one cat suffers from pain, hyperaesthesia or some other condition that changes its acceptance of grooming or affiliative behaviour. It may change to become a satellite individual. A polyphagic hyperthyroid or diabetic cat may consume more food or despotically control access to it, leaving the rest of the group resource deficient. Investigating and treating marking problems that relate to social difficulties between cats can be demanding (Box 15.15).

Box 15.15   Typical causes of indoor marking

- **Loss of core territory facial or flank marks:** Usually due to redecoration or change of house.
- **Loss of maintenance of group odour:** Temporary or permanent loss of a social facilitator cat, absence of the owner or housing of group members apart (at a cattery) so that odour is not mixed between individuals and factions.
- **Failure of odour recognition of a specific individual:** Individual odour may be altered or lost if a cat is taken away for grooming or veterinary treatment such as dental work. The cat may also return home with the odour of an unfamiliar cat on it. The returning cat may be regarded as an intruder. This can cause aggression or the cat may never regain its previous role in the social group.
- **Introduction of a new cat:** This may exceed the population that can be supported by existing resources or the new cat may upset existing social relationships (through despotism, competition or by increasing stress in the group). The same effect is apparent when a recently introduced kitten reaches maturity.
- **Illness:** Conditions that alter the cat's emotional state or interaction with other cats (hyperthyroidism, senility, pain, hyperaesthesia, debilitation) or need for resources (conditions causing polydipsia or polyphagia).
- **Excessive population density outside the home:** Existing overpopulation, new cats introduced to an area or when a cat owner moves a group of cats into a new home in an area where many cats already live.
- **Unfamiliar odours brought into the house:** Non-resident cats may spray close to a front or garage door so that this odour seeps into the house. Owner's shoes, clothing or bags may pick up odours from outside.

Treatment

Underlying medical conditions should be investigated and treated. Regardless of the cause for the marking behaviour, it is useful to increase available resources so that cats have easy access to them and perceive their core territory to provide a surfeit of the things that they need. F3 diffusers help to create a sense of core territory and can considerably reduce tension in cat groups. Soiled areas should be protected according to the guidelines in Box 15.4 and in Advice sheet 4, Appendix 3. This prevents soiling from becoming ingrained and harder to remove (Box 15.16).

In the case of spraying caused by an external threat from cats, the perceived threat must be reduced and the boundary of the core territory strengthened. Basic changes might include installing an electronic coded cat flap so that outside cats cannot gain access to the home and the use of glass etch spray on windows. Glass etch spray is applied in several coats until the window is effectively opaque. Light will still enter, but it will be diffuse. This has several functions:

- It removes the opportunity for non-resident cats to use visual threats (posture, eye contact) to intimidate resident cats in their own home.
- It also prevents the resident cats from using internal vantage points to threaten cats outside and encourages them to go outside instead.
- This, in turn, helps to prevent reactionary spraying on areas around the window, which are intended to be a deterrent to the outside cat.

Glass etch is not needed on all windows, only on those that are known to be used as vantage points by indoor cats, are associated with areas of spraying or which provide outdoor cats with a view indoors. It may be removed after marking has stopped for a period of 8 or more weeks and can be shaved off the window in strips using a razor blade or scraper. This makes the change back to normal transparency more gradual.

The intensity of core territory facial and flank marks can be enhanced using F3 diffusers. These should be positioned in each of the rooms in which the cats spend a lot of time and used at a rate of 1 per 50 to 70 m². F3 may have no effect if used at less than this rate.

Having made the core territory safer, the aim is to enable the cats to re-establish a pattern of territorial defence outside. The cats should be given several vantage points that face into the garden but have no view back to the house. This prevents non-resident cats from using these perches to threaten the owner's cats. Non-resident cats may have favourite places from which they use long-distance visual threats to intimidate the client's cats. These should be removed or altered so that they are unusable. Flat-headed nails (8 to 10 cm long and 6 to 8 cm apart) knocked into the top of a fence will allow cats to walk along the fence but will prevent them from sitting comfortably on it. Pieces of sharp plastic doormat or plastic anti-burglar strip can be put onto the top of concrete posts or roofs so that perching is uncomfortable. If a particular perch cannot be made unusable, then the view from it can be blocked using fencing or plants. Glass and other hazardous deterrents should not be used because these may cause injury to the cats.

Softwood posts make good clawing places and they should be installed at the edge of the territory so that the resident cats are able to leave appropriate territorial scent marks. Rub them against existing scratch places and then break up the surface with a wire brush to make them appear attractive to claw. It is also sensible to place claw posts or pads near to the cat door inside the home so that the cat can leave a territorial scent mark without spraying. The cats should be provided with outdoor latrines around the edge of the garden as these also help to strengthen territorial boundary and reduce the need for resident cats to cross other territories to find a latrine. Information about these ideas is included in Appendix 3 Advice sheets.

If indoor marking has been caused by conflict between cats in the home, then comprehensive environmental enrichment should be provided. The aim is to provide separate factions with their own resources so that they can effectively live separately from each other while sharing the same domestic space. This ability to co-exist without competition actually increases the likelihood that the cats will begin to associate with each other.

Box 15.16 Proper use of pheromone products

- F3 diffusers (Feliway®, CEVA Animal Health) must be used at a rate of 1 per 50 to 70 m², in accordance with the manufacturer's instructions.
- Diffusers should be left switched on at all times and must not be moved from room to room.
- Diffusers should be installed strategically, one in each of the locations where individual cats or factions of cats spend time. Installing a single diffuser in a hallway between rooms will not generally produce an effect in the rooms.
- When F3 diffusers are first installed the cats should be kept away from the diffuser for the first 1 to 2 hours to prevent them from spraying onto the diffuser. Being plastic, the diffusers will initially release a combination of smells that some cats may find objectionable.
- If a diffuser becomes contaminated with urine it should be thoroughly cleaned; otherwise it will release urine odours along with the F3. Some diffusers may need to be thrown away.
- F3 spray can be used to spot mark new objects that are brought into the house (clothing, bags, new furniture).
- F3 spray can also be used as a deterrent for scratch marking in the home: one squirt is applied daily to the claw marking location. An alternative claw-marking location should be provided nearby.

The mixture of facial and urine marking odours impairs the sense of core territory for the cats. Urine marks are also self-perpetuating because the marker feels compelled to refresh them periodically. For these reasons, it is very important to remove urine odours thoroughly using the cleaning methods detailed in Box 15.3 and Advice sheet 4. Scented products and those containing ammonia should not be used to clean up spray marks because they may intensify urine odours and leave an objectionable smell that encourages over-marking. F3 diffusers may be used to intensify the core territory facial and flank odours and these scents may be harvested from the cats and then spread around the house.

Group odour is crucial to maintaining a multi-cat household free of conflict and it is often apparent that relationship breakdown occurs when cats are unable to maintain this for themselves. In the same way as for treatment of inter-cat aggression in the household, it is possible to classically condition an association between the odour of a specific cat or cat-faction and the presentation of food or play. The scent is harvested from the facial and flank regions of the individual cats (or factions) onto separate cloths. The cloth from one individual or faction is then regularly presented to one of the other cats before giving food or play, until that cat shows a positive response to that odour. That cat's cloth is presented in the same way to the group or individual represented by the cloth. Initially the presentation of the odour may cause some alarm. However, after repeated presentation, each cat should begin to rub against the cloth when it is presented which indicates that the odour has been fully accepted. The body odour of the factions or individuals may then be merged, by exchanging odours between them (Fig. 15.4). In situations where there is overt aggression between cats, it is best to isolate them for a period of 1 to 2 weeks and reintroduce them as if bringing in a new cat for the first time.

Marking sites can be made less attractive for cats in a number of ways, but it has to be remembered that, if the motivation is strong, this will merely displace the activity elsewhere. Deterrent methods must therefore be used in combination with other environmental modifications. Cats are generally reluctant to spray or midden close to feeding sites, so small bowls of food may be put close to spraying locations. This also increases the number of feeding places. Odour deterrents should be avoided because these may actually draw attention to spray sites or produce odours that the cat will deliberately over-mark. Sheets of aluminium foil or plastic can serve to protect the floor around a spray site and may deter cats from going there. These methods are best used for isolated locations where it is imperative that the cat does not spray, such as around electrical equipment (Box 15.17).

Claw marking often exists as a sub-problem in indoor marking cats. Claw marks have a similar territorial function to urine spraying and the rate of claw marking may increase along with other forms of indoor marking. Providing cats with good claw-marking sites that fit with their need to defend territory can be an effective way to displace the

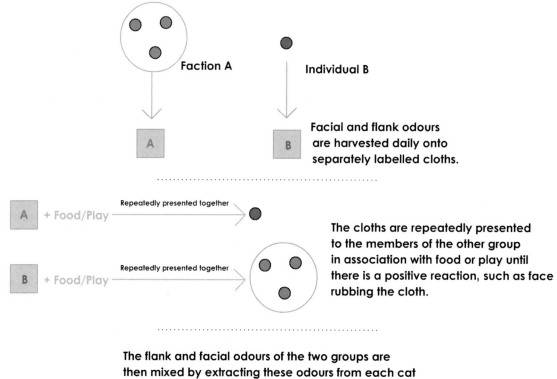

Faction A

Individual B

A   B   Facial and flank odours are harvested daily onto separately labelled cloths.

A + Food/Play   Repeatedly presented together

B + Food/Play   Repeatedly presented together

The cloths are repeatedly presented to the members of the other group in association with food or play until there is a positive reaction, such as face rubbing the cloth.

The flank and facial odours of the two groups are then mixed by extracting these odours from each cat onto one cloth and then rubbing all the cats with it.

Figure 15.4   Protocol for transferring odours between cats.

are made more attractive by rubbing them against existing clawing sites and then raking them with a wire brush to simulate real claw marks. Bold vertical stripes made with a permanent marker pen will draw attention to the object as a suitable clawing place. Undesirable claw marking can be deterred by daily application of F3 spray, combined with the provision of a nearby alternative scratching place. Client information on the provision of clawing places is provided in Advice sheet 5, Appendix 3.

Psychoactive drug therapy is often prescribed for cats with indoor marking problems but this will not offer a solution. The underlying reasons for the indoor marking must be addressed. Medication does have a role in long-standing cases where the number of marked sites is large, where marking has become habitual or where there is an emotional problem that may benefit from temporary drug

---

Box 15.17   Altering spraying sites to make them unattractive to the cat

- Place small bowls of food close to the marking location and combine this with an increase in the overall number of feeding stations throughout the house.
- Use plastic or aluminium foil sheets to cover flooring around the spray site, as some cats will not tread on this.
- Position a scratching post in front of the site to provide an alternative method of marking.

---

pattern of marking from spraying to clawing. Most owners find this desirable. Claw marking posts or pads may be positioned close to windows, doorways and cat doors. They

---

Box 15.18   Treatment: Indoor marking

General changes:

- Provide additional resources around the home, including extra resting, feeding, drinking and latrine sites. These should be located so that each faction or individual cat has easy access to its own set of resources close to a location where it spends time.
- Soiled sites should be cleaned properly (see Box 15.3, and Advice sheet 4 in Appendix 3).
- The cats should not be punished or threatened and chased when spraying as this may increase stress or encourage the development of spraying to gain attention.
- Strategically instal F3 diffusers (Feliway®, CEVA Animal Health).

External threat:

- Install one or more coded electronic cat flap to prevent entry by non-resident cats. Transparent cat doors should be sprayed with a solid-coloured paint so that they are completely opaque, otherwise non-resident cats may threaten residents through it.
- Use glass etch spray to prevent outside cats from seeing into the home through windows close to where the resident cats have sprayed, or which overlook resources.
- Install scratching posts, vantage points and latrines in the garden so that territorial control is shifted from inside to outside.
- If a stray entire male cat has moved into the area it should be trapped, neutered and homed away from the area.

Internal conflict:

- Follow general advice on resource distribution, giving each faction its own feeding stations and other resources. Consider providing an additional cat-door if one cat is guarding it.
- Introduce activity feeding.
- Use scent reintroduction and scent swapping to re-establish a group odour.
- Consider isolating and reintroducing cats in accordance with guidelines on dealing with inter-cat aggression.
- If cats have spent time away from the group, reintroduce them appropriately.

Unfamiliar odours coming in from outside the home:

- Regularly clean doorways, paths and walls where non-resident cats are spray marking (scrub with a solution of biological washing powder and hose clean).
- Fit draft excluder around doors and frames to prevent odours from coming in and install a weatherboard to the bottom of external doors so that urine marks do not run down the door and into the house.
- Take off outdoor shoes and put them on a high shelf when entering the house.
- Apply a squirt of F3 to bags when they are brought into the house.
- Allow new furniture to air for several hours before allowing the cats access to it. This allows plastic and other odours, that may trigger spraying, to disperse. Apply F3 spray to the furniture regularly until cats are voluntarily face and flank marking it.

Box 15.19   Withdrawing treatment

- Environmental modifications that are made outside should be permanently maintained, but glass-etch on windows, food bowls that have been used as spraying deterrents and other minor environmental modifications should be gradually removed after 6 to 8 weeks without spraying.
- Psychoactive drug or F3 diffuser therapy should be gradually withdrawn after 6 to 8 weeks without spraying or after the temporary environmental modifications have been removed. Drugs are withdrawn over a 4 to 8 week period, depending on the duration of therapy. At least two dose decrements are required, first halving the daily dose and then doubling the dose interval.
- Feliway® diffusers are allowed to run out completely, one at a time, after drugs and temporary environmental modifications have been removed.
- If inter-cat hostility exists in the household then F3 diffusers should be continued until the cats have fully re-established their previous allogrooming and allorubbing affiliative behaviour.

Box 15.20   The decision to use psychoactive drugs for indoor marking

Psychoactive drugs may be of value when:

- Individual cats are showing signs of chronic anxiety (SRI/SSRI) or inhibition of normal behaviour (selegiline).
- The case is longer than 6 months' duration.
- Response to environmental change has been incomplete.
- Spraying is a reaction to specific fear (selegiline).
- A rapid resolution is demanded and the client can be relied upon to complete environmental modification.

Risks of using psychoactive drugs include:

- Disinhibition of aggression: SRI/SSRI/benzodiazepine drugs.
- Clients may assume that changes in behaviour are solely due to medication, so they do not comply with behavioural therapy or environmental modification.
- There may be a relapse if drugs are withdrawn before environmental and social factors have been remedied.
- Potential adverse effects of drugs: fatal hepatic disease after oral benzodiazepine administration, cardiovascular effects of SSRI/SRI drugs.
- Interactions with concurrent medication or disease: drugs that affect the function of cytochrome P450 can interfere with the metabolism of SRI/SSRI drugs (e.g., cimetidine). SRI drugs should be used with care in cats with thyroid disturbance, or with bladder disease (risk of outflow obstruction).

---

support. Analysis of the general emotional state of the animal is important. SRI/SSRI drugs such as fluoxetine and clomipramine are beneficial for cats that are habitual indoor markers, or show a pattern of anxious, reactionary spraying. Selegiline benefits behaviourally inhibited cats that will not explore their environment, or that display fearful reactions followed closely by reactionary spraying when they see certain cats lurking outside the home. These drugs will not help confident cats that show no signs of anxiety or fear and are merely using spray marks, albeit inappropriately, as part of a calmly considered strategy to control territory in the house. Hormonal preparations have no role in the treatment of indoor marking (Boxes 15.18–15.20).

Prognosis

Cats with a history of indoor marking are likely to relapse at some point in the future because this behaviour is normal and situations outside the owner's influence may create the conditions for a new bout of marking. Typical times when marking may re-emerge are after redecoration, a house move or the introduction of a new stressor (new baby, new pet). Spring and summer bring a social turmoil for cats as these are times when they are most active and territorial space is hotly disputed. The presence of young entire females may lure intact males into a neighbourhood where they may settle and despotically wreak havoc on the local cat population (Box 15.21).

It is possible to minimise the risk of recidivism by continuing to offer an excess of resources and maintaining a suitable core and garden territory for the cats. If a new bout of marking is anticipated, then the environmental changes and F3 diffusers may be temporarily reinstated.

Box 15.21   Cooperation between cat owners

- Cat ownership is increasing which means that local feline population density may be very high, and rising.
- The problems of house-soiling and indoor marking that affect one cat owner may also be affecting others.
- Indoor and outdoor environmental modification can have a much more dramatic effect on the welfare and behaviour of cats if all cat owners in a neighbourhood make the same changes.
- Veterinary practices should encourage neighbours to work together to solve problems that arise from overpopulation and inter-cat conflict.
- Distribution of advice leaflets and running educational evenings can help and will gain good publicity for the practice.
- It can be beneficial for clients to be educated in feline behaviour, social structure and resource requirements.

ADVICE SHEETS THAT MAY BE RELEVANT TO THIS CHAPTER

In Appendix 3

1. Improving the outdoor environment for cats
2. Improving the indoor environment for cats
3. Multi-cat households
4. Cleaning routine for house-soiling and indoor marking
5. Claw marking
6. Introducing a new cat to the household

Chapter **16**

Feline aggression problems

INTRODUCTION

Within the general population, house-soiling and spraying are considered to be amongst the most common major problems, with aggression featuring far less than it does in the dog. However, recent figures from the annual report (2003) of the Association of Pet Behaviour Counsellors (APBC) showed that 23% of referred feline cases involved aggression toward other cats, making it the second most commonly referred problem after indoor marking (25% of cases). A further 13% of the reported feline cases involved aggression toward people. Aggression is therefore a significant concern for many cat owners. Data on referral rates of feline aggression cases to individual behavioural clinics varies widely, with some clinics experiencing referral rates of 13% of their total caseload and others 25%.

Other work, carried out by a research team at Southampton University, has shown that 13% of owners reported aggression to people and 48% aggression to other cats. These figures were obtained directly from a sample of the general cat-owning population, rather than from those seeking professional help, and they indicate that aggression problems may be even more prevalent in the general feline population than in the referral population.

There may be many reasons for this difference. First, many cat owners may be unaware of the welfare and safety risks associated with aggression problems. Secondly, the owners of aggressive cats have the option to exclude these animals from the domestic home so they become 'outdoor' cats. Thirdly, and most importantly, many cat owners may not be aware that anything can be done to help the situation and therefore do not seek help. Such obstacles to seeking advice place an additional demand on the veterinary practice to ask questions about feline behavioural problems during routine consultations, rather than to expect clients to raise the subject themselves.

Feline aggression is also often regarded as less serious than canine aggression and, as a consequence, cases may not be referred until they have become serious. Unfortunately, such an approach is not only detrimental to prognosis but also increases the risk of injury, so it is important for owners to understand how serious the consequences of feline aggression can be. Physical injury to people or animals and zoonotic infections are a very real danger since the cat is equipped with weapons in the form of claws and teeth. When feline aggression is targeted toward people, the danger it poses should never be underestimated. When the victims are children or elderly people with frail skin, it is important to emphasise to owners that the potential injuries from cats are serious. The rate of bacterial contamination in cat bites is several times that in the dog because bite punctures tend to be deep and a majority of cats harbour *Pasteurella multocida* and other pathogens in their mouths. The victims of cat bite or scratch injuries may therefore be subject to what is commonly called 'cat scratch disease' and should seek medical attention (Box 16.1).

The nature of aggressive responses in cats is strongly related to their natural behavioural responses and to their social and communication systems in the wild. The cat has a range of subtle body postures and facial expressions which can be used to diffuse tension and avoid physical conflict and, for a solitary hunter, this is important in order to prevent injury and consequent threat to the individual's survival. In addition, cats use a range of vocalisations to further increase the success of communication so that fighting is usually the defence strategy of last resort (Box 16.2).

Immediate intervention

In the UK cats are generally not regarded as property, and therefore the implications of aggression by cats is very complex. Fights between cats belonging to neighbours can cause a great deal of ill-will but are unlikely to lead to successful litigation. However, injuries caused to a person or an animal while in the home of the cat might be deemed the responsibility of the cat owner. Such injuries can, in some circumstances, be horrific (Box 16.3).

It is therefore the owner's duty to protect people and other animals from harm. Muzzling is not generally a viable option for cats but the same basic safety provisions, such as exclusion from the room and provision of physical barriers between cat and victim, may be made as for aggressive dogs (see Chapter 11).

The cat's primary response to threat is to avoid it or escape from it. The most critical aspect of managing aggressive cats is, therefore, to enable the cat to manage its fear in a non-aggressive way. Giving the cat escape routes and reliable places to hide will reduce its need to display aggression.

Box 16.1　Dealing with cat bites

Only 25% of dog bites will contain *Pasteurella multocida*, compared to 50 to 74% of cat bites. Other bacteria may also be present, including *Staphylococcus aureus*.

This means that all cat bites that cause skin penetration or bleeding should be treated medically without delay. A course of antibiotics and anti-tetanus may be required.

Immediate cleaning of the bite is also important, whether or not there is penetration:

- Wash for at least 5 minutes with a soapy solution under a free-flowing tap.
- Clean gently around the wound with a brush or cloth but do not scrub as this will cause bruising.
- Cover the wound with a loose dressing to prevent further contamination.
- Once the wound has been cleaned, apply pressure to stop the bleeding.

Even if the skin is apparently unbroken but the victim experiences fever or headaches, together with localised swelling, redness, and pain soon after the bite, then medical intervention should be sought urgently.

Box 16.2　Warning signs of aggression

Clients must be made aware of warning signs that indicate that the cat is likely to behave aggressively. This will enable them to avoid getting hurt, as well as to reduce unintentional intimidation and provocation of the cat. Important warning signs include:

- tail twitching
- flattening of the ears
- stiffening of the shoulders and legs
- dilatation of pupils
- hissing and spitting.

It is very important that clients do not attempt to soothe or calm the cat when it is showing this behaviour. Cats that are frozen in a self-defensive crouch are very close to launching an attack when provoked. Clients should look away from the cat and slowly move away.

Box 16.3　Immediate action in cases of feline aggression

- Do not use punishment to control aggression.
- Prevent cat from coming into contact with the target of the aggression. This is especially important where the target is vulnerable (children, the elderly or infirm).
- At times when this is impossible, the cat should be supervised. Consider the use of a harness and leash in these situations.
- The cat should have easy access to an escape route whenever placed in contact with the object of aggression. DO NOT ATTEMPT TO HANDLE A CAT WHEN IT IS IN A FRIGHTENED OR AN AGGRESSIVE STATE. IF FOR SOME REASON THE CAT *MUST* BE HANDLED THEN KEEP THIS AS BRIEF AS POSSIBLE AND KEEP THE CAT AT ARM'S LENGTH, AWAY FROM YOUR NECK AND FACE.

Risk assessment and prognosis in aggression cases

As with dogs, there is little scientific data to provide a reliable means of prognostication but the same basic issues remain when considering safety during the treatment of feline aggression problems:

- Will the cat bite (again)?
- What harm may it do if it does?
- Can the cause for the aggression be treated?
- What ongoing risk will the cat present after treatment?
- Whilst treatment proceeds, can people and animals be kept safe from the cat?
- Are the owners willing and capable of accepting and safely managing the immediate and long-term risks?

There is also a need to consider the amount of warning that precedes an attack and how often such attacks may occur. Infrequent but severe attacks that occur without much warning represent a genuine threat to safety and carry a poor prognosis.

As with dogs, there is an absolute necessity to follow up and manage these cases and to make sure that clients do not place themselves or others at risk. Predictability of aggressive behaviour is critical, as is preparing the owner with a plan of action should aggression be seen (Box 16.4).

Box 16.4   Follow-up for risk assessment

- Treatment of aggression cases is absolutely conditional on owners following the advice they are given in the treatment plan.
- At the first consultation the owner must be given a simple set of safety measures to lower risk of further incidents (supervision, isolation of the cat from contact with at-risk individuals, etc.)
- Dates should be set for the completion of environmental modifications that make up part of the safety and management strategy.
- With high-risk cases, follow up should be soon after the initial consult (within 2–3 weeks).
- Reassessment must concentrate on compliance with the safety measures, the owner's ability to complete the tasks set and their ability to maintain records and make accurate interpretations of the cat's behaviour.
- If the owner has been unable or unwilling to carry out safety measures, this indicates that future risk for this case will be high. This is particularly true if the owner is allowing at-risk individuals, such as children, to be in unsupervised contact with the aggressive cat against safety instructions.
- Treatment should proceed only if the owner can be persuaded to follow advice.

In many cases, cats show inhibited behaviour and subtle initial signs of fear or anxiety. Clients must be able to identify these in order to fully understand the cat's behaviour.

Prognosis depends upon the owner's commitment to carry out what may be a lengthy course of behavioural therapy, along with making potentially permanent changes in the cat's husbandry and environment.

In cases where cats are being asked to live in large feline groups with several unrelated individuals, it is important to consider the welfare implications for the cats concerned and, in cases of inter-cat aggression within the household, re-homing should be considered as a viable treatment option rather then a sign of therapeutic failure. Despotic cats that terrorise the neighbourhood carry a poor prognosis unless there is considerable cooperation between owners with regard to confinement, either permanent or on a rota basis.

The nature of the aggressive behaviour is important. Defensive behaviour has a better prognosis because it is possible to reduce the perception of threat and to provide the cat with alternative opportunities for dealing with fear (such as through escape or avoidance behaviour). Offensive aggression carries a more guarded prognosis unless full recovery from some medical underlying pathology can be achieved. Hyperthyroid cats, for example, carry a good prognosis for reform once the underlying pathology has been treated.

Other indicators of a good prognosis include selection of alternative coping strategies, such as retreating and hiding in cats that are fearful or anxious, and improvements in effective feline communication between warring cats in the same household. Decrease in both the intensity and the frequency of the aggressive incidents should be seen as favourable prognostic signs. Owners often find it difficult to be objective regarding progress in cases of feline aggression and there can be a considerable differential between actual change and the owner's perception of alterations in the cat's behaviour. It is therefore essential to persuade owners to keep a daily diary and to record all aggressive incidents, together with notes about the context or trigger for the behaviour. Likewise, a record should be kept of affiliative behaviour because a shift in the balance between these types of behaviour is a strong indicator of change.

Treatment versus referral

As with canine aggression, success depends upon the owner's ability to manage and alleviate risk while therapy proceeds. The general practitioner's immediate responsibility is to provide good safety advice while arrangements are made for an appointment or referral is arranged.

If, after an initial discussion with the owner, the problem does not have some obvious cause or means of management, then referral may be the best option. Depending on the level of behavioural experience within the practice, cases that are complex or involve significant immediate risk are going to be best referred, rather than dealt with in-house.

Specific indicators for the need to refer would include:

- an unreliable or unmotivated owner
- lack of specific behavioural knowledge and expertise within the practice
- owners who are unable to grasp the seriousness of a particular problem
- situations where serious injury is a risk (especially where the target of aggression is a particularly vulnerable: a child, elderly or infirm person)
- the risk the animal presents is not easily reduced by obvious changes in management
- the owner anticipates prosecution resulting from the cat's behaviour.

As with dogs, the apparent predictability of attacks is of crucial importance in managing and treating aggressive cats. Very rarely is aggression truly unpredictable unless the stimulus that triggers it is an internal one that is not obvious to the observer; for example, certain kinds of pain or medical disorders. Once the pattern of the cat's behaviour has been established, then management is much easier and it is also possible to identify any departures from this pattern which might indicate that the problem is expanding or getting more dangerous (Box 16.5).

Box 16.5   Predictability of aggression

Aggression is often labelled as 'unpredictable' when this is rarely the case. Usually there is a discernible pattern to the cat's behaviour:

- Any warnings the cat has given (eye contact, posture, growling, hissing).
- Any avoidant behaviour the cat has carried out, including freezing.
- Timing (certain times of day).
- Relationship to events or activities (territorial trigger, arrival of a visitor, play, grooming, feeding, owner departure from the house, etc.)
- Presence of certain stimuli (a noise, another cat, unfamiliar people, etc.)
- Relationship to the actions of a person (raised hand, shouting or shrieking, sudden movements, cornering the cat, picking the cat up).

To safely treat aggressive cats, the motivation for every aggressive incident must be thoroughly understood and a pattern of behaviour identified if possible. The owner should be asked to describe what happened at each event and not to interpret what happened. The first priority is to use this information to prevent injury. If attacks were *truly* unpredictable then this would constitute a serious and unavoidable risk that would not be acceptable.

The sequence of aggressive behaviour

The cat's primary defence strategy is to escape or avoid conflict. Cats do not possess a repertoire of appeasement behaviours to halt or modulate intraspecific aggression so physical confrontation may result in serious injury to both parties. As solitary hunters, survival depends on individual fitness so cats tend to avoid conflict in order to protect themselves.

If escape is impossible, then cats will frequently freeze and deliver a range of threatening behaviours, including postural and vocal signals that are designed to repel or hold the threat at bay. Meanwhile, the cat is re-evaluating its opportunities for an escape. Attacks may be sudden and brief, and again aimed at repelling the threat so as to reopen an opportunity for escape.

Cats will most often become aggressive when conflict is over a survival resource (including territory) or when escape from conflict is impossible; such as when the animal is debilitated or confined.

The feline aggressive sequence shares some similarities with other species; non-specific increases in body tension and threatening eye contact, for example. In addition, there is a range of feline aggressive displays which involve whole body and facial components. The cat may attempt to present itself as an active threat by increasing its apparent stature (piloerection, sideways body arched posture), or it may attempt to reduce the threat it poses by flattening onto the ground and adopting a self-defensive posture. These whole-body postures are a reliable indicator of the cat's attitude to a situation but they are relatively static and do not indicate the moment-by-moment shift in the cat's reaction. For this, it is better to look at facial signals such as head and ear position and other expressions involving the mouth and eyes.

One very important point is that the transition from a static defensive posture to an attack may be very sudden in cats. It is therefore very important to be able to read and appropriately respond to changes in facial signalling that indicate the cat's increasing sense of vulnerability and which may precede an aggressive outburst.

Classification of aggression

As with dogs, the term 'aggression' can be used to refer to a number of different behavioural responses, ranging from hissing and spitting to infliction of physical injury. Aggression should be considered to be a perfectly normal feature of the feline behavioural repertoire and the term 'aggressive' should not be used to define a cat's personality. The natural feline predatory sequence contains aggressive elements and these are learnt and perfected through play. Social conflict may also be manifested in normal and appropriate aggressive displays which are designed to diffuse tension and avoid physical confrontation. Within the context of problem behaviour, it is therefore essential to determine the motivation for aggressive behaviour and to identify elements of normal feline behaviour, such as predation, play or socially related aggression.

There have been various schemes suggested for categorising feline aggression. The first question to consider is whether the aggression is normally motivated or not. Normal aggression is contextually appropriate and usually relatively well-controlled and predictable, so it carries a good prognosis as long as the cat's behavioural needs can be met within the domestic environment. Abnormal aggression can result from physical illness or inappropriate learning.

The approach to categorisation used here will be to define aggression in terms of its immediate target, its motivation, its offensive or defensive or frustration-related nature and then to attach labels according to the circumstance or context of the aggression. It is always important to remember that every cat is an individual and every behavioural problem must be treated on that basis.

History–taking

Inter-cat aggression presents a particular problem because many of the aggressive incidents are not directly observed by the owner or may be misinterpreted when they are. Observation of the cat during the consultation is important but house visits may be preferable and, when they are not possible, consultation observation is best augmented with video footage of the cat's normal behaviour in its own surroundings. It is not acceptable to stage aggressive events for the purpose of making a diagnosis since this involves a serious risk of injury (Box 16.6).

Box 16.6   Important aspects of history–taking

- Historical description of aggressive incidents (starting with the first that the owner can remember). Details of each incident should include location, persons or animals present, context, time and target of the aggression.
- The cat's body posture and facial expression before, during and after each incident give strong indications of its emotional state and intent.
- The victim's response before, during and after each event should be recorded.
- Relationship between cat and other animals in the household (allorubbing, allogrooming, play, aggression, fear-avoidance).
- List of all situations in which low-level aggression behaviour is seen (hissing, spitting, growling, eye contact, body posture).
- List of stimuli or events that elicit fear or anxiety.

How intense are the aggressive displays?

Many owners find it hard to accurately describe their pet's posture and, therefore, visual images of cats, such as

Leyhausen's table of feline postures, can provide easily recognisable illustrations when asking owners to describe their cat's body language (see Chapter 4). This makes it easier for owners to identify behaviour before and after an aggressive event.

In addition to obtaining details about the behaviour of the aggressor, it is also important to establish the response of the victim (human or animal). Aggression may be reinforced by an unexpected or seemingly inappropriate reaction and even the retreat and escape behaviour of the victim may have a reinforcing or provocative effect. A fleeing victim is likely to be chased. High-pitched screams, rapid movement and confrontational or punitive measures can all lead to an escalation in tension and a more overtly aggressive response. This is especially true in aggression that is motivated by fear or is seen in association with predatory drives.

In cat-to-human aggression, it is common for the person to counter aggression with aggression in the mistaken belief that physical size is likely to win the day and some form of 'domination' of the cat will enable the person to prevail. However, this is more likely to be provocative and to lead to an increase in conflict and in the intensity of the aggressive response.

During the history-taking process, it is important to ask questions about the circumstances surrounding the aggressive incident, in terms of both the physical and social context in which the behaviour occurred. For example, if the cat was in a restricted environment, such as a narrow passageway, it is more likely that the behaviour was defensively motivated than if it were in the middle of an open space. If the cat showed aggression to its housemate when it was aroused by the sight of another cat outside the window, it is likely that the aggression was not primarily intended for the housemate but was being redirected. Questions about the people and animals that were present at the time of the incident, together with their responses, will form an important part of the history-taking process. Information about the physical environment, in terms of space available, routes of access and potential for escape, will also be relevant. Physical restriction is not the only important factor in terms of the environment and it is also necessary to consider restrictions in terms of behavioural choice. Cats use physical conflict as a last resort in the wild and, when aggression occurs readily within the domestic environment, it is advisable to examine the environment in which the conflict occurs from a feline perspective. Cats live in a three-dimensional world and make extensive use of vertical space in their environment. It is therefore important to consider this when investigating cases of aggression within the household, since lack of available vertical space may lead to a decrease in the cat's ability to regulate stress and a consequent increase in incidents of aggression, either toward owners or other cats within the social group. Availability of suitable retreats where cats can hide is also an issue in multi-cat households since hiding is an important coping strategy in response to challenge or change in the environment. Space is only one of the important resources within the home and availability of food, water and litter facilities should also be considered. Lack of access to these resources, or competition over them, may be a source of stress for feline inhabitants and lead to aggressive interactions.

AGGRESSION TOWARD PEOPLE

The most common motivational causes of aggression from cats to people include:

- fear
- anxiety
- frustration
- misdirection of predatory instinct.

These produce offensive and defensive patterns of aggression. In some cases, the human victim may not be the primary target for the aggressive behaviour and a diagnosis of redirected aggression may be made but, from a therapeutic point of view, the motivational diagnosis, which is appropriate to the cat's response to the primary target, will be all-important in formulating a successful treatment plan.

FEAR-RELATED AGGRESSION TOWARD PEOPLE

Tolerance or appreciation of human contact is learned as a result of early experience during the sensitive period. In many cases, aggressive cats are the product of an unsatisfactory start in life and problems start to arise. For example, a lack of appropriate handling between 2 and 7 weeks of age will cause a cat to grow up to be wary of people and to have

a predisposition toward defensively aggressive behaviour if it is placed in a situation where it feels threatened. Experience teaches these individuals that their aggressive behaviour is very effective at maintaining distance between themselves and any person of whom they are suspicious. Before long, the aggressive display is used as a pre-emptive rather than a reactionary behaviour. This results in a noticeable change in the cat's strategy for dealing with fear. Early in the course of the problem, the cat will show noticeable signs of fear, attempting to use defence strategies such as running away or hiding. However, over time it will begin to select aggressive responses more readily so that a more offensive pattern of behaviour is seen. By the time some of these cases are brought to the attention of the veterinary practice or referred for specific professional advice, the initial fearful motivation for the behaviour may be obscured by the cat's overt hostility and offensive behaviour.

It is important to question the owner about any previous traumatic experience involving people, the use of inappropriate punishment for behaviour in the past or the presence of inappropriate and unintentional reward of the present behaviour (Boxes 16.7, 16.8).

Cats that are exhibiting fear-related aggression toward people will often adopt characteristic postures and use defensive vocalisation prior to a defensive paw swipe, which is intended to drive the threat to a greater distance. The response of the person may be significant in the progression of the problem behaviour and it should be remembered that the owner's attempts at reassurance often reinforce fear and aggression by increasing social pressure on the cat and thereby increasing the perception of threat. In situations where owners try to deal with the aggressive behaviour by punishing the cat, an anticipation of the owner's apparent aggression may increase the cat's fear further and lead to an escalation of the problem.

Diagnosis

Fear-related aggression is a motivational diagnosis and it can be associated with a variety of contexts. In some cases,

---

Box 16.7   Immediate action: fear-related aggression toward people

- Identify all fear-eliciting events and stimuli.
- Take measures to avoid exposure to these events and stimuli (where possible), other than during therapy.
- Keep the cat supervised or under control whenever encountering any fear-eliciting events or stimuli.
- Avoid the use of threat or punishment to stop aggression.
- Avoid handling or interacting with the cat directly when it is fearful or aggressive (even when it is showing fear and aggression toward a cat outside the home).
- Where it will not create additional risk, provide the cat with an opportunity to escape from the situation in which it is fearful.
  DO NOT ATTEMPT TO HANDLE A CAT WHEN IT IS IN A FRIGHTENED OR AGGRESSIVE STATE. IF FOR SOME REASON THE CAT *MUST* BE HANDLED, THEN KEEP THIS AS BRIEF AS POSSIBLE, AND THE CAT SHOULD BE KEPT AT ARM'S LENGTH AWAY FROM THE HANDLER'S NECK AND FACE.

Box 16.8   Prevention of fear-related aggression toward people

- Kittens should be reared in complex and stimulating environments that include contact with many different people and other animals.
- They should experience a wide range of domestic noises and events so that these do not produce fear, anxiety or stress in the future.
- Immature animals should not be exposed to fearful or threatening situations or events.
- Physical punishment should NEVER be used in the training of cats or kittens.

it may therefore be beneficial to add a contextual label as part of the diagnosis. For example, a cat that is aggressive when handled by the owner may be diagnosed as displaying 'aggression associated with handling' that is fear-motivated and a cat that is fearful of strangers and shows aggression to the owners when visitors are present may be diagnosed as a case of 'redirected aggression' which is motivated by frustration of the fear response. In both cases 'fear-related aggression' is the underlying motivational diagnosis and treatment of the cat's underlying fear is crucial to the success of treatment; the contextual labels help the owner to understand when the behaviour may occur and to take steps to avoid it.

Treatment

It is unusual for cats to show fear-related aggression toward people outside the home environment unless cornered or handled (such as when at the veterinary clinic). Fear-related aggression toward people in the home is treated using desensitisation and counterconditioning procedures, often supported by pheromonotherapy.

The general method employed is:

- Identify the general class of target.
- Grade the response to the target according to appearance or behaviour. Some cats are more aggressive toward men or children and may react differently according to their clothing, what the person is carrying or how they are moving. List all those features which affect the cat's response so that they can be introduced during training.
- Find a group of willing volunteers who will be able to act as stooges for training.
- Prepare the home environment with suitable escape places for the cat to use.
- Begin training with the least fear- and aggression-evoking examples of the target class, at a distance which does not trigger aggression.
- The cat may be kept on a harness and line for added safety.
- Provide the cat with food rewards as a lure to leave the escape place and explore the environment with the target present.
- Over a number of sessions, bring the person closer making sure that, at no point, is fear or aggressive arousal elicited. The person may also walk or run around faster, make noises, move about or carry items in a way that would previously have evoked more fear and aggression. These changes are introduced gradually, systematically and with sufficient distance to avoid aggression or fear.
- Introduce progressively more fear-eliciting persons only as the cat ceases to respond to the less-evocative ones.

By identifying the elements of a person's appearance to which the cat responds, it is possible to do a lot of training

with a limited number of volunteers who can be dressed or disguised. Above all, in this example, it is important to note that 'unfamiliarity' is an element of the fear so the volunteers must not try to befriend the cat at any stage during training. Familiar individuals may only be used during training if they can be disguised or kept at a distance so that the cat cannot recognise them.

In some instances, clicker-training may be an effective way of training cats to respond appropriately to the presence of people. The cat is first trained to associate the sound of a click with the delivery of a small food reward. This is achieved by clicking and then dropping a piece of food approximately 20 to 30 times until there is some sign of positive anticipation on the part of the cat.

Clicks are then only delivered when the cat carries out a specific behaviour, such as sitting. Once the cat is reliably sitting to get a click this behaviour can be 'named'. Just as the cat is about to sit, the trainer says the command word that is intended to cue the behaviour: for example, saying 'sit'. After doing this a further 20 to 30 times, most cats will have been trained to sit, on cue, reliably.

Cats that have already begun to associate the presence of visitors with the availability of food treats may be asked to sit and then repeatedly clicked and treated while they stay calm. Alternatively, the cat may simply be clicked and rewarded repeatedly throughout the period that it remains calm, despite the person's presence. The limitation to this kind of training is that the sound of the click may produce a startle response that increases fear and anxiety and cats can sometimes appear to be more difficult to motivate through the provision of food than their canine counterparts (Box 16.9).

Pheromonotherapy may be used to assist behavioural therapy. The pheromone F3 (Feliway®, CEVA Animal Health) can be used to reduce general anxiety so that the home or training environment is less threatening and it has been particularly beneficial in cases of cat-to-cat aggression within the same household. F4 (Felifriend®, CEVA Animal Health) is a social pheromone used by cats to identify familiar individuals and, when applied to unfamiliar individuals, this can increase the cat's tendency to approach and show affiliative behaviour. This can also be useful because it reduces escape responses. Combinations of pheromone therapies are especially helpful when the target of aggression is a member of the family or regular visitor to the household of a cat that has been recently re-homed. F4 may produce dissonant emotional states (which can induce a panic reaction) when the person or animal to whom F4 has been applied is already familiar to the cat from some aversive encounter and therefore invokes visual triggering of hostile responses. Further work in this area is essential but, at the moment, F4 should be used with care, applying it only to unfamiliar individuals, preferably from species with which the cat was socialised as a kitten.

In some cases of fear-aggression, the use of psychoactive medication may be useful to support behavioural therapy. In the case of fear-related aggression selegiline (Selgian®,

CEVA Animal Health), used at a dose rate of 1.0 mg/kg, once daily, may be used to reduce apprehension. The effect of this drug is to increase exploratory behaviour and confidence in fearful situations. It can also enhance the perception of reward and thereby improve responses to counterconditioning procedures. However, by encouraging the animal to approach closer to the target of the fear-related aggression, there is an increased risk of injury if the person startles the cat by making a sudden noise or movement. This appears worst during the initiation of treatment (the first 4 to 6 weeks of medication).

Serotonergic drugs such as fluoxetine and clomipramine (Clomicalm®, Novartis) may be used to reduce aggression where anxiety is a causative factor. However, in many cases of fear-related aggression, anxiety over the consequences of launching an attack may be the only thing that prevents it. Reduction of anxiety in these cases can cause disinhibition of this anxiety, producing greater risk of attacks and injuries. Great care must therefore be taken when considering the use of any psychoactive drug; they can only be used safely and effectively after a thorough assessment of the case and in combination with a well-organised behavioural therapy plan and management to reduce risk of injury. **No drug is currently licensed for the treatment of feline fear-related aggression, so informed consent must be obtained at the time of prescribing** (Box 16.9).

Box 16.9   Treatment of fear-related aggression toward people

- Explain to the owner the signs of fearful arousal and other behaviours that will enable them to understand and predict the cat's behaviour more effectively.
- Avoid uncontrolled exposure to fear-eliciting situations and events.
- Identify and grade the stimuli and events that evoke fear.
- Desensitise and countercondition the cat to these stimuli and events, starting with stimuli that evoke the least response.
- Identify contexts and other stimuli that contribute to raised fearful arousal.
- Desensitise and countercondition the cat to these contexts and stimuli.

Prognosis

Prognosis strongly relates to the owner's expectation of therapy; however, clients who expect that a cat will become overtly friendly and tactile with all family members and visitors to the house may be disappointed.

Part of creating a good prognosis is therefore to teach clients about normal feline social behaviour and the kinds of activity from which cats derive pleasure. A balanced relationship involving appropriate levels of contact, greeting behaviour and play is likely to succeed. Cats that wish to avoid contact with certain visitors should be allowed to do so because this represents a safe and normal response to fear which is far more desirable than an aggressive attack.

If clients can be satisfied with this kind of situation, then the prognosis is generally good. However, cats that have already inflicted injuries without any deliberate provocation are potentially an ongoing danger. For example, cats that rush out from hiding places and attack without warning cannot be safely managed. This is why it is very important to differentiate motivations such as misdirected predatory play from genuine fear-related aggression, because the two often have different treatments and outcomes.

FRUSTRATION-RELATED AGGRESSION TOWARD PEOPLE

Frustration results when a situation fails to produce an outcome that is in line with the individual's expectations. Frustration is believed to have the same emotional basis as fear with the difference that, in humans, there is an ability to label the emotional experience differently according to the kinds of event that precede the emotional state. In other words, we are able to label frustration differently from fear only because we are able to rationalise the circumstances leading up to the frustration. Frustration is also able to evoke the same kinds of behavioural response as fear, including escape and aggression.

Expectations are conditioned by previous experience, with the heaviest emphasis on experience gained during the sensitive period. Anecdotally, there is an association between hand-rearing and frustration-related aggression. This presumably results from inappropriate expectations about human contact and some deficiency during the weaning process in terms of teaching kittens to cope with the withholding of potential reward. The process of transferring from a liquid to a solid diet is successfully accomplished during hand-rearing but the behavioural component of the weaning process, which is designed to teach the kitten to be an independent adult, is often lacking (Boxes 16.10, 16.11).

Box 16.10   Immediate action: frustration-related aggression toward people

- Cease punishment and confrontation as these intensify frustration and fear.
- Switch to some form of ad-lib feeding.
- Give the cat free access to all areas of the house and garden, unless there are places where the cat may be an increased threat to the owner (such as sleeping on the bed).
- Avoid picking the cat up as this can trigger aggression, especially when the cat is put back down again.

The weaning process is an important part of the kitten's behavioural development and changes in the queen's behaviour toward the kittens at this time will have a significant effect on their behaviour as adults. For the first 3 weeks of life, the queen spends up to 70% of her time caring for the kittens and, at this stage of development, they receive reward for their suckling behaviour on a continuous schedule. From the 3rd week onward, this behaviour begins to change and the kittens begin to show more demanding behaviour toward the queen, who in turn becomes less tolerant of them and begins to spend increasing amounts of time away from the nest. At this stage, the queen may discourage the kittens from suckling by adopting certain body postures and, even when she allows them to commence suckling, she may move away before the feeding routine is complete, leaving the kittens to drop from her nipples one by one as she exits the kittening box. In effect, the kittens have now been placed on an intermittent schedule of reinforcement and the reward of a full feed is not always available to them. This results in a sense of frustration but the kittens learn to deal with that emotional response and return to a steady state of emotion without recourse to aggression. As the kittens develop further and become more mobile and independent, the mother begins to take a back seat in the feeding process and the emphasis moves from the provision of milk by the queen to the supply of nutrition from prey items which are brought back to the kittens. In the early stages, prey will be killed by the queen; later, the kittens will need to learn how to dispatch their own prey so disabled and then active live prey will be supplied by the queen. The killing of prey also contains elements of delayed reward and frustration so kittens learn to tolerate what is essentially a normal emotional state. In this situation, frustration is also focused on the natural process of killing prey, rather than at the parent or other conspecifics. By the end of this stage of the weaning process, the kittens are far more independent and look away from their mother in order to find food. She is no longer the provider of their nutrition and, as their relationship in the context of feeding alters, so does the level of social dependency. The kitten is now ready to act as a solitary hunter and to start to practise the adult behaviours that will ensure its ultimate survival. During the hand-rearing process, the first stage of continuous nutritional reinforcement is adequately fulfilled, but the process of feeding on demand is often continued past the 3rd week of life because people are concerned about ensuring the kittens receive enough food. This means that early tolerance to frustration is not conditioned. When the time comes to introduce solid food, they often find that the kittens are reluctant to sample the new food and, in order to encourage them to eat, hand rearers will often put food onto their fingers. One reason for the lack of interest in solid food may be that, in mammals, some chemicals and flavours derived from the mother's diet will find their way into her milk and provide the first step in conditioning food preference. Replacement milk

does not contain any such flavours so hand-reared kittens fail to recognise the solid food with which they are presented. There is also a lack of maternal feeding behaviours for the kittens to model. One of the consequences of this is that the person remains the focus of the feeding experience and, instead of the kitten being encouraged to function independently, it is encouraged to remain in close contact with its rearer. This can lead to problems later when the owner is unable to deliver rewards when they are expected. The kitten also fails to develop a tolerance to frustration because the feeding process does not involve any delayed reinforcement or predatory behaviour.

Obviously, hand-rearing is not the only risk factor for developing aggression associated with frustration, and cats that have been weaned normally by their mothers can go on to develop aggression of this sort if they are continually rewarded for demanding behaviour during kittenhood.

Diagnosis

Frustration occurs when an anticipated event does not happen or fails to meet the individual's expectations.

Box 16.11   Preventing frustration–related aggression toward people

Hand-rearing of kittens should mirror natural weaning as seen in domestic cats:

- Very small amounts of liquidised solid food should be mixed into replacement milk so that the flavour of solid food is familiar before weaning begins.
- By 3 weeks of age, some feeds should end before the kitten is fully satiated and some meals should be replaced with solid food.
- The first few solid meals may be composed of a dish of replacement milk with small amounts of solid food placed in it. Gradually, the milk is withdrawn for these meals.
- Dried food is also made available.
- From week 4 to 5 onwards, feeding should also begin to involve some aspects of play. Games that involve food finding are a good way to train some simulated predatory behaviour: a fishing toy can be used to playfully lead the kitten to some food treats or a small bowl of food.
- Direct human involvement in feeding is phased out over this period, in favour of play.
- If possible, the kitten should be shifted towards activity or automatic feeding. Activity feeders can be made out of old plastic drinks bottles with holes cut in (so that dried food rolls out). Electronic feeding bowls that automatically uncover a portion of food, or which dispense a small activity ball containing food every hour, are another good way to reduce human involvement in feeding.

For example, when the owner does not open a door or a can of food quickly enough, or when a person tries to walk away from a cat when it expects interaction to continue. Often the aggression is not an isolated behaviour and the cat also displays other frustration-related behaviours, such as excessive vocalisation or indoor marking, in situations where it appears to be thwarted by circumstance. Frustration-related aggression may be made worse if motivation is abnormally increased by illness. For example, in cats that are suffering from polyphagia due to hyperthyroidism or diabetes mellitus.

There is also usually a history of hand-rearing or a pattern of regular reinforcement of demanding behaviour throughout the cat's life.

Box 16.12   Treatment of frustration–related aggression

- Give the cat control over access to resources and activities (food, outdoor access, etc.)
- Provide automatic and activity feeders.
- Stop all games that involve the cat interacting directly with hands and feet.
- Substitute play for cuddles and tactile interactions.
- Use fishing toys and other toys that focus play away from the owner.
- End games with the cat getting a small amount of food.
- Provide a wide range of environmental enrichment, including a regularly changed collection of lightweight toys for object play.
- Avoid picking the cat up as this removes control and can trigger aggression, especially when the cat is put back down again.

Treatment

A fundamental problem for these cats is that access to important resources is controlled by the owner who is often inconsistent. Most cats will not willingly tolerate having to wait for access to food or access to different areas of their territory but they are able to cope with this frustration. Cats with a low tolerance for frustration may lash out.

The first step in treating these cats is to reduce human involvement in the provision of the resources and activities the cat requires. The cat should be given back control.

For example, giving the cat ad-lib food access, perhaps using activity or automatic feeders, together with independent indoor–outdoor access. Food may be topped up but should always be available.

Play should be substituted for cuddling and other tactile interactions which may place the cat close to the owner at times when frustration could trigger a dangerous attack. Some cats become frustrated when play ceases abruptly, so all play should involve fishing toys, laser pointers and other devices that distance the owner from the play. Hand and foot movements should be minimised so that play does not become directed onto the owner. If possible, play should end with some kind of consummatory act, such as the toy leading the cat to a pile of favourite food treats. This simulates a normal end to predatory behaviour. The owner can then leave the context and put away the toy whilst the cat consumes the food (Box 16.12).

Prognosis

Prognosis depends on the severity of the attacks and whether at-risk individuals are present. It is absolutely essential to make a detailed list of individual attacks so that their pattern and severity may be accurately appraised. Cats with frustration-related aggression require ongoing management and, unless handled appropriately, there will be a risk of biting and clawing in the future. The severity of attacks varies hugely, with some cats inflicting multiple deeply penetrating bite and scratch wounds and others only inflicting minor injuries. The severe attacks can sometimes occur even when the victim is resting or sleeping so that avoidance is impossible. In some instances, the bites may be directed at the face and neck, which increases the risk considerably. However, the character of the attacks is usually quite consistent in each individual case so a prognosis may be provided. If the character of the attacks is predictable and preventable and they are of low intensity, then the prognosis is good. If the attacks are severe and at-risk individuals (children, elderly, infirm) are involved, then the prognosis is poor.

MISDIRECTED PREDATORY BEHAVIOUR TOWARD PEOPLE

Although often classified with other forms of aggression, predatory behaviour is functionally and mechanistically different to aggression. Cats are highly adapted to carry out a specific pattern of hunting behaviour. They have a small stomach and pared-down biochemical processes which are designed to cope with a large number of small fresh meals each day, rather than a single large one. One very common misconception among cat owners is that hunting is a behaviour which is performed in order to satisfy hunger. In fact, these two aspects of feline behaviour are independent of one another. A hungry cat will engage larger prey and deliver a kill bite more rapidly but a well-fed cat will still continue to hunt. Innate hunting responses are triggered by stimuli such as sudden movements or shrill noises.

As a result, a cat that is denied the opportunity to engage in hunting real prey or appropriate toys, will often display predatory behaviour toward other rapidly moving objects, such as human ankles and hands (Fig. 16.1). Human shrieks and protests simply drive the behaviour on. The behavioural sequences involved in predation are practised and perfected through object play so that, in some texts, the terms 'misdirected play' or 'play-related aggression' are used to describe a predatory form of behaviour that occurs in the absence of any genuine prey.

It is, however, important to remember that there is an underlying functional motivation for the behaviour, which is predation (Boxes 16.13, 16.14).

Diagnosis

When taking the history, it is important to fully characterise every incident:

- The cat's posture before, during and after an 'attack'.
- The contexts in which the attacks typically occur.
- The triggers that appeared to initiate the predatory sequence (first sign of stalking the target).
- The stimuli or events that prompted the final attack.

The behavioural history usually indicates that the problem began with inappropriate play, directed at hands and feet or involving chasing games. This has been actively encouraged by the owner; for example, games that involve running fingers over the backs of sofas or encouraging attacks on feet or hands under the duvet. The games become less enjoyable as the cat becomes larger and able to

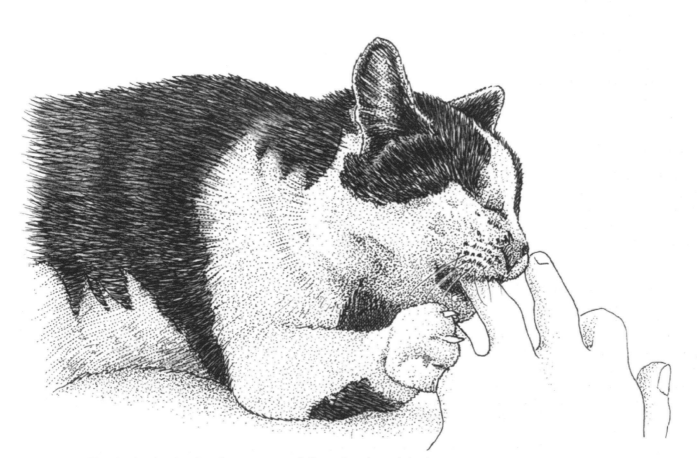

Figure 16.1   Play that involves hands or feet can cause misdirected predatory behaviour.

inflict injuries. There is a progression to more serious ambushes in which the cat waits for the owner and then lunges at or attacks them. There may be an element of frustration that the owner no longer playfully reciprocates the behaviour.

In many cases of misdirected predatory behaviour, the attack, or the preparatory stalking behaviour that preceded it, is being inadvertently rewarded by the human response. The cat gains attention, further play or simply revels in the victim's reaction to being pounced on.

One feature of predatory behaviour that differentiates it from play, is that the claws are usually extended and the bite is not inhibited. Bite intensity is under control of reflexes fed with information from local mechanoreceptors around the mouth so that the victim's movements will drive the bite to intensify. Elderly people and children are particularly at risk from this sort of behaviour and injuries are likely to be serious.

Treatment

All encouragement for misdirected predatory behaviour should cease; no more games with hands or feet as a target. When pounced on, the victim should stop moving and make no sound. This removes any reinforcement for the behaviour and reduces the risk that struggling will trigger deeper biting or raking with claws. The attacks may be startling and painful so the client may need to wear heavy trousers and long-sleeved clothes as a protection. Reinforced trousers may sometimes be needed. These are easily available from motorcycling shops and may be made from ballistic nylon or Kevlar reinforced fabric. These resist bite and claw penetration very well. The need for protective clothing is not permanent, and can be phased out as

the cat starts to use the environmental enrichment and alternative predatory targets.

Environmental enrichment should be provided, including activity feeders, timed feeders and a wide range of small lightweight toys to encourage object play. Simple items such as ping-pong balls covered in glitter or painted with marker pens and large feathers are perfectly suitable. The selection available to the cat should be changed regularly during the day so that there is always something new to attract the cat's attention.

Play with these toys may be further reinforced with attention (not touch), further stimulation using a fishing type toy or the provision of food treats.

Certain times of day are often peak periods for misdirected predatory behaviour. The cat is a crepuscular hunter so that its peak periods of activity will be early morning and evening. The owner should try to provide several short periods of play during the times when the cat is anticipated to be at its most active. Fishing toys and laser pointer games are appropriate since they distance the owner's hand movements from the play. However, caution should be exercised with the laser pointers since an element of frustration can develop if the cat is never able to actually catch the 'prey' and physically handle it. For this reason it is advised that laser pointers should never be the sole source of predatory activity but should be integrated into a play programme with other toys that the cat can actually catch and 'kill'.

Cats will often have favourite places from which to launch their predatory attacks, or stalking. Access to these should be blocked off.

> **Box 16.15   Treatment: misdirected predatory behaviour toward people**
>
> - Cease play directed at hands and feet.
> - Reduce reinforcement during stalking and attack behaviour (stop moving, do not make any noises).
> - Wear protective garments, or at least keep hands, legs and feet covered.
> - Provide an enriched play environment.
> - Provide suitable play at times when the cat is expected to be active.
> - Block access to the locations from which the cat launches its attacks.

> **Box 16.14   Preventing misdirected predatory behaviour toward people**
>
> - Provide kittens with a range of toys for object play: small, lightweight toys and larger objects. Real fur toys are available.
> - Change the selection of toys that are available several times each day to maintain a stimulating environment.
> - Encourage play that involves fishing toys, laser pointers and other devices that focus play on a toy rather than on hands or feet.
> - Provide activity feeders such as perforated plastic drinks bottles filled with dried food.
> - Do not play games where the cat is encouraged to regard hands or feet as suitable targets for play.
> - If the young cat does pounce on a person, they should remain still and provide minimal feedback for the behaviour (no struggling, no sudden movements or noises).

Prognosis

Prognosis is guarded if the cat's targets are children or vulnerable individuals or if serious injury has already been caused by the predatory attacks. If behavioural methods are working, then some improvement ought to be seen within 4–6 weeks.

Sustained improvements are seen only if environmental enrichment and proper play continue to be provided, and often this strengthens the positive aspects of the cat–owner relationship.

AGGRESSION ASSOCIATED WITH HUMAN INTERACTION

It is not uncommon for owners to report that their cat is perfectly friendly at a distance but is prone to showing aggressive behaviour in association with close physical contact or restraint.

There is a significant crossover between this form of aggression and others owing to the mixture of emotional motivations that may be present:

- Fear: resulting from experience of punishment or mishandling.
- Play: especially where play continues to a point at which it becomes frustrating for the cat. Usually claws remain sheathed and biting is inhibited, but it may still be painful.
- Resentment of contact: when owners pick the cat up or force contact with it.

Some cats will initiate interaction with their owners and then suddenly bite and attack after the person reciprocates contact. Immediately prior to the incident, the cat appears to be enjoying physical interaction. There has been some debate as to the possible motivation for these sudden assaults. It has been suggested that the cat's threshold for tolerance of handling is reduced either due to a lack of habituation as a kitten or as the result of an internal conflict between adult feline behavioural responses and the perpetuated juvenile responses of a domestic cat. Certainly, the greeting behaviour of cats is at odds with that of their owners. Greetings between cats are often restricted to a 'tail up' approach accompanied with a trill or chirrup and blinking eye contact. Only in a minority of these encounters do cats actually make physical contact; in most cases they will simply sit close to each other for a period. Owners often misinterpret the initial feline greeting behaviour as an invitation for physical contact and it is possible that this is offensive or irritating to the cat, especially if it is picked up and carried by the owner against its will. Many owners will also attempt to sustain contact beyond the tolerance of the cat, holding onto it as it tries to get away. The effect of this inappropriate owner behaviour is that the cat may become wary of getting close to the owner, or allowing physical contact (Boxes 16.16, 16.17).

Diagnosis

Aggression is often seen when the person reciprocates the cat's initial greeting or when the cat is approached. Until this point, the cat may be showing affiliative behaviour such as slow blinking or 'tail up' and will often show a relaxed body posture. The cat appears to enjoy a brief amount of physical contact but then suddenly turns aggressive without warning, often grabbing the owner's arm with its front legs and raking with the back ones. After the incident the cat will often move away and begin to exhibit displacement behaviour, such as grooming, which indicates that the cat is experiencing an amount of unresolved emotional conflict. The owner describes the cat's behaviour as unpredictable and suggests that the cat suddenly enters a state of confusion or panic as the interaction proceeds. The lack of predictability often relates to inadequate ability to correctly interpret changes in the cat's body language as it is approached or handled, combined with the owner's expectation that the cat ought to understand that the approach is intended to be friendly.

Box 16.17   Prevention of aggression associated with human interaction

Owners need to understand how to interpret basic feline modes of communication:

- Normal greeting behaviour between cats.
- The lack of importance of physical contact during greetings.
- Facial and body postures that indicate the cat's mood and intention.

This knowledge should be applied so that greetings between owners and their cats are sensitive to normal feline ethology and expectations.

They also need to understand the effect of certain kinds of handling:

- Fear or alarm caused when a cat is picked up and thereby loses its ability to engage an escape response.
- Holding and preventing the cat from getting away from contact is frustrating and alarming to it.

Box 16.16   Immediate action: aggression associated with human interaction

- Cats that become aggressive when handled must not be punished or restrained.

Temporary safety advice to owners might include:

- Stop picking the cat up or restricting its escape from social contact.
- Allow the cat to initiate contact but do not reciprocate by stroking or handling the cat.
- Do not approach the cat to handle it. Instead talk to the cat from a distance and allow it to come to you if it wants.

A complication of this form of aggression is that a substantial proportion of the cats with this problem may be suffering from undiagnosed feline hyperaesthesia syndrome; displaying the classic signs of rippling skin and hypersensitivity to touch. Feline hyperaesthesia syndrome is therefore an important differential in cases where cats are showing unpredictable aggression in association with owner interaction and a multidisciplinary approach involving dermatology and behavioural medicine is to be encouraged. Other causes of pain should also be ruled out.

Treatment

Underlying medical problems should be investigated and treated.

The pattern of interaction between owner and cat must be altered:

- Train the owner to give eye contact and vocal greetings instead of physical contact or handling. The owner must resist the temptation to pick the cat up.
- The owner must also be able to identify early signs of aggression and irritation, such as growling vocalisation, tail swishing and ears folded back.
- Identify the maximum amount (duration) and type of contact that the cat will tolerate before becoming aggressive. Owners should restrict physical contact to a maximum duration that is less than half of this value in order to minimise aggressive responses.
- Introduction of physical contact should be planned, systematic and increased in response to the cat's improved behaviour.
- The owner should substitute appropriate play for times when they might otherwise try to handle or cuddle the cat.

Owners may be reluctant to comply with these demands but this is made easier if the ethological basis is explained and an analogy is drawn with acceptable human greetings in different cultures. Hugging and kissing are the norm in many societies, even when introduced to strangers; whereas, in parts of Northern Europe, especially the UK, this would be considered socially uncomfortable. Following the social conventions enables the individual to fit into a social group without causing offence or stress. So it is with cats; forcing excessive physical contact is against normal feline social norms.

Cats need to learn about social interaction with humans and be conditioned to tolerate it. The situation is compounded once the cat has been forced to put up with interaction that it does not like and this creates negative associations with the approach of a person that must be overcome before touch contact can be reintroduced.

Fortunately, clients who change the character of their interactions with their cats will often be rewarded with increased trust and a greater amount of affiliative behaviour so that future compliance is usually high. However, it is important that they do not attempt to re-establish a tactile relationship with the cat as soon as it begins to become more approachable as this will undermine trust and the cat will regress rapidly.

Interactions should be limited to very short, planned sessions and always terminated before agitation begins. The owner needs to learn how to read body language and predict when tension is increasing. Tail twitching, flattening of the ears, stiffening of the shoulders and legs and dilatation of pupils are all signs of increasing arousal and risk of aggression. If the cat begins to show aggression during handling, it is important to avoid touching the cat's abdomen, even if it rolls onto its back or side. Severe lacerations are possible if a hand or foot is rapidly pulled away whilst the cat is latched onto it. Struggling and sudden movements of the hand also drive the cat to hold on tighter or to bite more deeply.

Whilst it may be painful, the most appropriate response is to remain still and make no noise. It is therefore advisable for owners to wear protective gloves and thick sleeves during treatment sessions. The primary aim of treatment should be to gradually work towards the situation where the cat is on the owner's lap, unrestrained. Once this has been achieved, it should be possible to gradually condition the cat to accept increasing levels of restraint and handling and eventually to accept being lifted from the ground, but this may take some considerable time.

Food rewards may be used during training but cats are rarely motivated to work for their daily food ration and the treats that are used will need to be of sufficient value that they genuinely represent a reward. Owners may need to experiment with a wide range of food rewards in order to discover what the cat really likes. Access to the chosen reward is restricted to training sessions alone as this helps to increase their perceived value.

The first step is to condition a positive association with the presence of a person by offering a food reward without any request for physical interaction. As treatment progresses, the cat should be rewarded for permitting increasingly direct contact from the person. It may help for the owner to be given a listed sequence of behaviours which should be rewarded. The handler must not progress to the next step unless the cat shows no signs of arousal or distress.

A typical sequence of actions might include:

- approaching person
- sitting on furniture close to person
- sitting unrestrained on person's lap
- tolerating brief stroking along the back
- tolerating brief restraint
- tolerating, and ultimately accepting, increasing amounts of stroking and restraint
- tolerating being lifted briefly off the floor
- tolerating, and ultimately accepting, being picked up.

This is another condition in which a permanent change in owner behaviour is important to continued success.

Clients should be taught to notice and appropriately respond to normal feline greetings such as:

- eye contact with slow blinking
- trills
- sitting close to the person without touching
- tactile contact.

Owners should be taught to reciprocate these kinds of greetings in a similar manner, for example, calling the cat's name in a high-pitched voice, or making slow-blinking eye contact. They must realise that the cat that sits in close proximity has already made its greeting and may not, on this occasion, have any desire to be touched. Physical contact should generally be restricted to times when the cat initiates it (Box 16.18).

Box 16.18   Treatment: aggression related to human interaction

- Identify maximum duration of contact that the cat will tolerate. Contact duration must not exceed this amount during training, and should generally be restricted to less than half the maximum duration.
- List the tactile interactions that the cat will and will not tolerate (see text).
- Condition the cat to associate the already well-tolerated interactions with the delivery of a food reward.
- Once the cat shows positive signs of anticipation during these sessions, then the client may proceed down the list towards the less well-tolerated types of contact.
- The owner should be taught how to recognise signs of rising aggression and irritation so that training does not provoke an attack.
- Play and other interactions should be substituted for touch until the cat is genuinely confident to be handled.

Prognosis

The prognosis for these cats is usually good as long as owners do not allow themselves to relapse into inappropriate behaviour as the cat becomes more affiliative. Owners must regard the changes in their own behaviour towards the cat as permanent and not merely a temporary means of winning over or convincing the cat. The prognosis is guarded to poor if the cat's attacks have been serious and unanticipated, such as when a person is attacked whilst walking past the cat without any intention to touch it.

AGGRESSION TOWARD OTHER CATS

It is now widely accepted that, in situations of aggression between cats in the same household, aggression can be manifested not only in active aggressive behaviour but also in a more passive manner through strategic use of marking behaviours such as indoor urine spraying. Passive aggression is therefore a differential diagnosis in cases of indoor marking.

Although people enjoy keeping more than one cat in a household, the population density in the home and in the urban area around it is not necessarily compatible with natural feline behaviour. In order to understand and accurately diagnose cases of aggression between cats, it is therefore important to appreciate the natural social behaviour of the cat and the potentially unnatural demands that life in a domestic environment puts on our feline companions.

The motivation for aggression in any particular case should be determined through a combination of observation and history-taking. The list of possible differentials is similar to that relating to aggression toward people and includes fear-related aggression and misdirected predatory behaviour. In addition, cats are more likely to show territorially motivated aggression toward other cats and, in these cases, consideration of natural feline social systems is crucial to understanding the behaviour and offering realistic means of controlling it.

Other common types of aggression between cats sharing a household include:

- despotic behaviour
- inter-male aggression
- maternal aggression.

Aggression between cats in the same household

Aggression between cats in the household is motivated by the underlying emotional responses as aggression towards people. These include fear, frustration, predatory behaviour or play. Often aggression problems in multi-cat households will relate to a combination of these causes, so accurate and comprehensive history-taking is an essential part of reaching a diagnosis (Boxes 16.19, 16.21).

Box 16.19   Immediate action: aggression between cats in the same household

- Where fighting has caused injury to one or other of the cats, they should be kept separate to prevent further fights and injuries.
- Each cat should be provided with a complete set of resources (food, water, a selection of toys and resting places and a latrine).
- If aggression has started immediately after the introduction of a new cat, then the cats should be separated, as above; likewise, if aggression has started after reintroduction of a cat that has been out of the household for a period.
- Fights must be broken up before they result in injury, but owners must be careful not to get injured. Picking cats up while they are in the middle of a fight can result in very damaging redirected aggression towards the person. Instead, try to distract the cats away from the conflict by using remote distractions such as noise.

Redirected aggression is also common, especially when aggressive display toward cats outside the house is thwarted and the cat turns its attention to an easier target within the house, such as another nearby cat.

Feline play often involves rehearsal of predatory behaviour, which is fine when it is directed at inanimate objects. However, other cats in the household are just as likely to become mock-predatory targets as their human counterparts.

Inter-cat aggression within the household is most likely to occur at certain key times such as when a new cat is being introduced to the household. This may be due to fear of the new cat or to more general effects on the availability of resources such as resting places, owner attention or food. Another important high-risk event is when a cat that has been temporarily hospitalised or housed in a cattery returns home. Poor socialisation of one or more of the cats in the home and the presence of social stress within the household are also factors that need to be considered (Box 16.20).

> **Box 16.20 Common causes for aggression between cats in the household**
>
> - Illness or debilitation.
> - Social pressure due to excessive population density.
> - Inappropriate introduction procedure with a new cat.
> - Temporary isolation of individual cats leading to failed recognition when they return, or loss of group odour.
> - Fear-related aggression.
> - Predatory or play-related behaviour.
> - Redirected aggression (frustration).

Diagnosis

As with house-soiling and spraying problems, it is important to fully understand the nature of the cats' relationships with each other and the way they make use of their domestic territory.

Some basic information is vital:

- A plan drawing of the home and garden indicating the location of feeding places, latrines, resting places and any other resources the cats might need.
- This drawing should also include information about places that each cat prefers to use (resting places, etc.) and any locations of spray marks or inappropriate elimination.
- The relationship between the cats can be determined by looking at the pattern of allorubbing, allogrooming and other affiliative behaviours, such as tail-up greetings, between individual cats. It is often found that small factions or cliques exist within the whole group with some cats remaining peripheral to the social group. There may also be 'super-social' individuals who show affiliative behaviour toward, and are accepted by, members of all of the factions. These cats

may be instrumental in preventing outbreaks of aggression between factions.

- Observation of passive-aggressive behaviours between the cats; chasing, resource guarding and other similar behaviours that indicate social conflict between factions or group members.

> **Box 16.21 Prevention of aggression toward other cats in the household**
>
> - Provide adequate resources so that competition does not develop.
> - Several feeding, drinking and latrine sites distributed around the home to enable cats to have a real choice of location for these activities. Latrines may also be created in the garden (see Chapter 15).
> - Consider the local cat population density and whether it can cope with the addition of another cat before attempting to introduce one.
> - Choose cats that come from successful multi-cat households or that have sociable parents.
> - Introduce new cats correctly (see Box 16.22).
> - Provide plenty of opportunities for appropriate play.

Treatment

The ultimate aim of treatment is to produce a fully functioning cat group in which there is maximal affiliative behaviour and minimal aggression. Treatment of aggression within cat groups should only proceed where there is a genuine likelihood that the environment can be permanently modified to meet the cats' needs. This may mean giving the cats access to more space, a larger number and diversity of resources and, possibly, indoor–outdoor access if the cats are currently kept inside. Part of the solution to some inter-cat aggression problems may be to identify and re-home despotic cats or to sensitively reduce the overall cat population in a household by re-homing certain factions en masse. In the latter case, the resolution is to produce several functioning cat groups that live separately. Some owners are fortunate enough to be able to provide two or more separate 'homes' for their cats within their property, by using outbuildings. Making this kind of decision requires an in-depth analysis and understanding of the social dynamics of the group and how it accesses resources. A good solution that improves the welfare of all the cats should never be regarded as a failure, even if the cats are unable to continue living with the owner. One significant problem in cat ownership is 'animal hoarding', especially in the case of inter-cat aggression within the household. Suspected animal hoarders should be carefully and sensitively counselled and, if unwilling to sensibly re-home and depopulate, then they should be reported to local authorities. Animal hoarders or collectors should not be supported in their attempts to keep excessively large populations of cats (Box 16.23).

Box 16.22   Introducing new cats to the household

Before introducing a new cat, it is important to assess the likelihood that resident cats will accept it. An already stressed group of cats, including a despot, will not readily accept a new cat. Their existing problems take priority. Ethologically insensitive direct introduction of cats carries a strong risk of fighting and long-term intolerance between cats. Future stressors, such as the addition of further cats to the neighbourhood, will unmask this brooding problem, potentially to instigate spraying and inter-cat aggression. Proper introduction of a new cat is therefore very important.

- Provide the new cat with its own room containing a latrine, food, water and a variety of resting and hiding places. Installing an F3 diffuser (Feliway®, CEVA Animal Health) will increase the sense of familiarity and security in this location.
- The resident cats should be provided with several feeding stations, places to drink and additional places to rest and hide. An F3 diffuser is also useful to increase their sense of security.
- Allow the new cat to become fully confident in this new location and with all members of the family. This may take a few days, after which the cat should be eating, resting and approaching visitors to this environment normally.

Stage 1: Scent introduction:
- Prepare several disposable cloths, each labelled with a cat's name.
- Use the labelled cloth daily to collect odours from the face and flank of the cat with whose name it has been labelled. The cloths must not be mixed up or stored together.
- Whenever going to greet, feed or play with either cat, it should be briefly presented with the opposing cat's cloth to smell and investigate. The cloth can be wrapped around the person's hand or, alternatively, a more passive introduction can be achieved by placing the cloth on the owner's knee while interacting with the other cats in the household. Initially, this may trigger a degree of alarm (the cat may back away, hiss or freeze). At this stage it is important not to force contact as the cat may become aggressive.
- If there are multiple cats in the household, then the resident cats should be presented with the new cat's smell and the new cat with odours from different cats in the group.
- With repeated presentation of the cloth, the cat should ultimately ignore the odour or may react positively to it. When both cats are reacting in this way it is time to move on to stage 2.

Stage 2: Scent swapping:
- After harvesting the odour from the cats, the cloths should be put together in a bag so that odours mix.
- This combined odour is then used in the same way as above.
- Once there is a positive reaction to this combined odour, then the client should mark themselves with the mixed odour so that, when the cats greet, they are unintentionally self-marking with this new odour. The cloth should be rubbed on objects that the cat regularly rubs against, including the owner's legs.
- Odour swapping may then switch to using a single cloth as long as each cat accepts being rubbed with the scent from the others.
- Once all cats are accepting this new odour and are actively rubbing against the clothed hand and other objects that have been marked with the cloth, then it is time to move to stage 3.

Stage 3: Allowing the new cat to explore:
- The new cat should be allowed to explore and utilise the rest of the house while the other cats are excluded or shut in an inaccessible room. This allows the new cat to learn all the hiding and escape places so that, as the cats meet, it does not feel vulnerable.
- Once the new cat is using the resources in the home confidently, then it is time to move on to the next stage.

Stage 4: Limited face-to-face introduction:
- The cats need to begin to see each other but without any risk of carrying out an attack. This can be managed using a glass door or mesh screen. Some child gates are made from a mesh that provides a partial barrier. Mesh barriers are best as they allow some diffusion of body odours that are involved in identification. If neither is possible, then a part-open door may be used (open so that cats can see each other but not get through).
- The cats are given food on either side of the screen at normal feeding times, or are distracted with a game.
- It is also useful to rub the door or screen with the odour from the cats so that there is maximum chance of recognition of scent.
- The cats are encouraged to play and feed progressively closer to the screen as long as there is no aggression.

Continued

Box 16.22 Introducing new cats to the household—cont'd

- Once the cats are showing no aggressive or fearful behaviour, they can be allowed to meet face-to-face after an initial meeting through the door or screen. If owners are particularly concerned then houselines can be used to give some sense of control, but it is important for the cats not to feel unduly restricted.

It is important to continue mixing odours between the cats and applying their 'group odour' to the owner and common marking places in the house until the cats have begun to rub against each other or groom each other. At this point, F3 diffusers and other environmental changes may be taken away gradually.

The total time for the introduction process may vary from a couple of weeks to a couple of months but there is no shortcut if harmony is to be achieved.

When treating aggression between cats sharing a household, it is important to address the basic factors that encourage cats to spontaneously form groups in feral or wild situations:

- An excess of resources (food, resting places, latrines, water).
- Instant access to available survival resources.
- Sufficient space (including 3-dimensional space).

Box 16.23 Identifying animal hoarding

'Animal hoarders' may present themselves as having 'rescued' animals, when often they have trapped or imprisoned them. These people are often well-known to genuine local representatives of re-homing charities who will have nothing to do with them. Indeed, animal hoarders may already be the subject of local authority prosecutions for welfare or nuisance violations. The definition of Animal Hoarding provided by HARC (Hoarding of Animals Research Consortium) and incorporated into Illinois Law is:

- More than the typical number of companion animals.
- Inability to provide even minimal standards of nutrition, sanitation, shelter and veterinary care, with this neglect often resulting in starvation, illness and death.
- Denial of the inability to provide this minimum care and the impact of that failure on the animals, the household and human occupants of the dwelling.

It might be expected that animal hoarders would not seek veterinary intervention for their animals. However, animal hoarders may exhibit a fundamental lack of insight into the conditions in which the animals are kept so that they will regularly ask for medical or behavioural help. In some cases, this may also be an attempt to maintain a degree of respectability as a defence against future prosecution. It is essential that veterinary surgeons and behaviourists do not fall into unwittingly supporting or defending the actions of clients who are animal hoarders. This behaviour is easily passed off as eccentric but it impacts on the health and welfare of the animals, the owner and neighbours. HARC is seeking recognition of animal hoarding as a form of mental illness.

This is in addition to any innate (genetic or acquired) tendency toward sociability in the individuals making up the group.

The first step to treating inter-cat aggression is therefore to reduce apparent competition. Providing each cat faction within a household with its own collection of resources will immediately reduce stress. The cats no longer have to queue for access to resources in close proximity to cats from opposing factions. Reduced contact in competitive situations will allow the cats to live in greater isolation from each other but this, in fact, also enables them to associate with each other without the complication of competition for food or space.

In order to maximise available space for the cats, it is also important to make the best use of the outdoor environment. Provision of extra resting places, perches and latrines outside will reduce competition for indoor resources. Access to outbuildings increases indoor space available to the cats, as does providing sheltered perches. Some owners are reluctant to give cats access to outdoors and in some countries cats are not permitted to roam free. In these cases, constructing a secure outdoor run may be a viable method of increasing available space.

Part of reducing competition is to reduce the value of the owner as a 'virtual resource'. The cats may regard the owner as a source of security or access to resources. They may be unable to gain access to food or go in and out of the house safely when the owner is not present to protect them and may come to depend upon controlling or communicating with the owner in order to carry out normal self-maintenance activities such as accessing a latrine. This is not appropriate, given the cat's ethology, and also means that cats tend to congregate around the owner, which places them in close proximity at a time when they are most desperate to get food or outdoor access. Free access to food in bowls, or activity feeders that always contain some food and are merely topped up by the owner at random, will enable the cats to maintain distance from one another. Likewise, cat doors (preferably more than one) are better than a 'human operated' back door.

Increasing access to space is also critical. The cat's primary means of controlling its interaction with other cats is to maintain distance from them. In the small rooms that are typical of most homes, it may be very difficult for a cat to feel safe because it is always forced into closer-than-desirable proximity to other cats. This tends to favour aggression because escape and avoidance are not possible. Fortunately, cats are able to make greater use of 3-dimen-sional space than humans and dogs, so giving them high perches in the form of shelves or cat furniture will enable the cats to re-engage avoidance and distance-maintaining behaviours. These should be provided indoors and out (see Fig. 16.2).

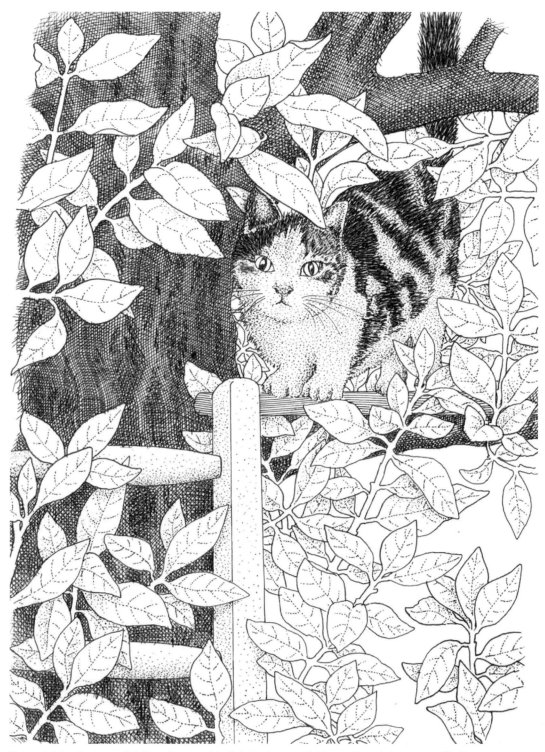

Figure 16.2   A range of hiding places and bolt–holes is essential to enable cats to use an effective escape strategy. Here, a platform is fitted into a tree so that the cat can observe the garden safely.

Cardboard boxes and other low-down bolt-holes provide an excellent escape route for cats that are regularly chased aggressively or during play. This enables the victim to take refuge without having to run too far and removes some of the reinforcement for chasing by the other cat. If the motivation for chasing is predatory play, then the owner should provide other play opportunities as an outlet for this motivation; such as play with a fishing toy and a changing supply of small, easily moved, brightly coloured toys.

The pheromone environment of functioning cat groups is quite special. Repeated face and flank marking of objects in the central section of the cats' territory, combined with allorubbing and allogrooming (rubbing and grooming of social partners) creates a strong sense of security and identity. This can be lost when factions of cats or individuals dissociate from one another. This is commonest when people are not present to transfer odours between cats or when a super-social individual within the group has gone. It can also occur when a house is redecorated, stripping odour marks from the environment, or when individuals are reunited after a period of separation (such as when hospitalised or having gone missing). The use of F3 diffusers can simulate the effect of dense facial and flank marking within an environment while the cats re-establish their own marks and exchange odours that identify them. The pheromone F4 ought to be very useful for treating inter-cat aggression within the household but, unfortunately, there have been problems with its practical use. F4 signals indicate familiarity but, with cats that have already had a number of aggressive encounters, there may be a dissonance between the memory of the visual appearance of the aggressor cat and the chemical 'familiarity' signal. This has been seen to trigger apparent panic and violent outbursts. F4 is not recommended for treating inter-cat aggression within the household but is very useful for reducing fear of unfamiliar people and other animals and for helping in the introduction of a new member of the household.

Individual acts of aggression between cats must be minimised. Vantage points used by despotic cats to observe access points and resources should be removed. Increasing the number of resource locations also makes despotism impossible.

A conditioned punisher such as a rattle can (see Advice sheet 14 in Appendix 3) may be used to disrupt aggressive behaviour at its outset; for example, to terminate threatening eye contact. When such an approach is used, it must not be readily connected to the owner and should not be used in such a way as to actually frighten either of the cats. The aim is merely to startle the cats in order to disrupt the behavioural sequence; but if used too late in the sequence when the cats show great body tension and are preparing to strike, it may actually trigger an aggressive attack. It has to be remembered that fear and anxiety are driving forces for aggressive behaviour and anything

---

Box 16.24   Treatment: aggression to other cats in the household

- Identify factions within the house.
- Identify the main aggressor(s).
- Consider fitting the aggressor(s) with a bell and collar so that other cats can evade them.
- Provide each faction with its own complete set of resources, located in an area where the cats already spend most of their time.
- Each faction should also be provided with an F3 diffuser (Feliway®, CEVA Animal Health) in the room where its resources are located.
- Provide additional hiding and resting places around the house.
- Increase access to 3-dimensional space by providing shelves and high cat furniture.
- Provide low-level bolt-holes, such as cardboard boxes, so that cats have easy access to an escape route when chased.
- Remove or block access to vantage points from which a despotic cat (or cats) have previously sought to intimidate other cats while they are accessing resources or moving from space to space (cat doors, doorways, corridors, close to latrines or feeding stations).
- Consider isolating factions or individuals if there is a significant risk of fighting or if previous attempts at reintroduction have failed.
- Proceed with an odour-introduction routine as detailed in the instructions on introducing a new cat (Box 16.22).
- F3 diffusers may be removed when the cats are freely associating without aggression and showing allogrooming and allorubbing between members of factions.
- Some deliberate odour swapping and the provision of additional resource locations may be needed to maintain permanent harmony.
- It may be possible to inhibit aggressive behaviours at the moment they start by using a conditioned punisher such as a rattle can. Care should be taken not to draw attention to the source of the punishment and to time it carefully so that it does not induce fear or trigger an aggressive attack when the cats are intent on each other.
- Increase play to reduce the incidence of predatory play directed at other cats.
- Additional drug or other therapies may be required.
- Consider re-homing if a feline despot is unwilling to share space and resources, if the welfare of the group is impaired or if social behaviour between the cats cannot be maintained. Do not introduce additional cats.
- Monitor frequency and intensity of aggressive behaviour.

---

that increases tension will probably favour fighting. Use of punishment is therefore not generally recommended. A better method of distracting the cats is to try to trigger a predatory behaviour that is directed at a toy. Most toys will not provide sufficient distraction but a laser pointer may be used carefully to break the cats' concentration and lure them away from each other into a game. The advantage of this particular toy is that several cats can be independently distracted by moving the dot to different locations.

Successful resolution of aggression is most likely if individuals recognise each other as part of the same group. This can be achieved by swapping odours between the cats and possibly by isolating factions or individuals so that a complete reintroduction is carried out, as if the cats were being brought into the house for the first time (see Advice sheet 6, Appendix 3). This may be the most appropriate course if the cats are likely to inflict serious injury on each other or where it is relatively easy for the owners to keep the cats apart in this way.

Prognosis

The prognosis for these cases depends upon several factors, including:

- owner compliance with environmental modifications
- the ability of the home environment to support the intended cat population
- sociability of individuals within the group
- the owner's expectation of the end result
- continued maintenance of the conditions that enable the group to co-exist (environmental enrichment, etc.)

Cats are able to co-exist successfully in groups but it is essential to prevent problems by choosing cats that are likely to be sociable and then introducing them in the right way. Re-homing some cats may be essential to provide the whole group with better welfare.

Aggression to other cats in the neighbourhood

The feline territory is divided into three zones:

1. The central core territory, which needs to be safe and secure.
2. The home range, which may be traversed by other cats as they go between different parts of their own territory.
3. The larger hunting range, which is also shared by larger numbers of cats in the local vicinity.

The sharing of access to territory means that time-share systems are important in avoiding conflict. Conflict is most likely in the home range when cat densities are high. Dawn and dusk are high risk times in terms of aggression and this may be due to the fact that prey is most active at these times and there is increased competition for this important resource, or simply a consequence of the increased chance of feline encounters because many cats are out and about at these times.

> **Box 16.25 Immediate action: aggression toward other cats in the neighbourhood**
>
> - Despotic cats may pursue others into their own homes and attack them there. The owners of such despotic cats should temporarily keep these cats indoors while preparations are made to limit the problem.
> - Neighbours should install electronic cat doors that do not permit entry by aggressor cats. This at least offers the cats a secure place to avoid fights.
> - In many cases it is possible to limit aggression by 'time-sharing' access to outdoors: allowing cats outside at times that prevent them coming into contact with each other.

Invasion of core territories and threat to resources within homes increases competition within the home and can increase the risk of conflict. When a feline despot is present within a neighbourhood, aggressive encounters between cats increase significantly. These despotic cats not only show intensely territorial behaviour but also make regular and repeated attempts to take over the territory of other cats, including their core territory or home range. They may enter the homes of other cats to attack or intimidate them, or to leave urine marks, leading to misdiagnosis of inter-cat aggression or indoor marking problems within the homes they are targeting. Entire male cats are more likely to be despotic, which is why stray males should be caught and neutered. However, there is no exclusive correlation between reproductive status and despotism, and other cats can behave in this way. Despotic cats are often most active at dawn and dusk, and their behaviour is often a source of tension between human and feline neighbours throughout the potentially very large area that the despot attempts to control (Boxes 16.25, 16.26).

Diagnosis

Aggression within a local cat population may be obvious to those who own cats that are the repeated victims of cat-bite injuries. Sometimes injuries are mistakenly attributed to foxes or other wildlife but this is actually very much less common. Inter-cat aggression in the neighbourhood is also an important underlying factor in house-soiling and spraying problems, as well as inter-cat aggression within the household. This is because the activities of local despots, or a very high feline population density, may cause cats to stay indoors where they then conflict with each other.

Aggression to other cats in the neighbourhood is more likely when the local population is destabilised by introduction of a newcomer, when there is one or more entire tomcat in the local population or when a feline despot is

---

Box 16.26 Prevention of aggression to other cats in the neighbourhood

- Neuter male and female cats.
- Do not introduce cats that have a history of despotism to already highly populated neighbourhoods.
- Be aware of local feline population density before introducing more cats to an area.
- Provide places in the garden for resident cats to claw mark so they can define the territory boundary.
- Provide outdoor latrines (sand pits) at the edge of the garden.
- Increase the cat's access to height in the garden by creating perches in trees and on walls/fences that look *away* from the house. This gives cats a chance to defend their own territory while preventing other cats from using the perches to spy on the cat's house.
- Encourage local cat owners to adopt activity feeding and other environmental enrichments that are known to encourage cats to live in harmony.
- Consider persuading cat owners to set up a local 'cat club' of people living in the neighbourhood so that they can swap ideas about improving gardens and homes to suit the cats better.

---

resident in the neighbourhood. Despotism is seen when a cat is actively displacing others from their territory or monopolising resources. Conflict is also at a peak when queens are beginning to call and territorial areas are disputed.

A territorial area closely corresponds to the survival resources it provides. The defence of territory is therefore linked to the defence of resources, so there is a reduction in territorial behaviour and aggression when there is a surfeit of resources within the neighbourhood.

Treatment

The majority of domestic cats are neutered and inter-cat aggression within neighbourhoods is consequently reduced but, in situations where two entire males live in close proximity, the risk of overt aggression is greatly increased. In such situations, the aggression can be very serious since reproductive, and hence genetic and evolutionary, success is at stake. Neutering before 12 months of age has been shown to decrease fighting by as much as 88%, which suggests that, in the case of male-to-male inter-cat aggression, hormonal influences are perhaps more significant than learning.

Intact male cats that are the cause of aggression should be neutered. If these cats are feral they will need to be trapped and relocated. Some make good pets once they have been castrated. If the intact male belongs to a local res-

ident, they must be contacted for permission to have the animal neutered. The surgery may be sponsored by a local charity or shelter organisation if the owner is unable to pay. In a minority of cases, the owner may be unwilling to have the cat neutered. This can be symptomatic of a general lack of care which may enable the cat to be removed on welfare grounds.

Aggression between entire males and females is rare, although it may occur if the female is not ready or willing to mate. The mating process is a very noisy event and it is not uncommon for inexperienced owners to misinterpret this as an episode of aggression. When owners report that entire cats are acting in a hostile manner toward one another, it is therefore important to consider the differential of normal mating behaviour.

Another hormonally related aggressive behaviour relates to the change in behaviour of lactating queens who can become increasingly aggressive toward other cats when they have a litter to protect. Such aggression may occur within the neighbourhood or inside the household and, while hostility toward other cats can be considered normal at this point, aggression toward owners in a domestic situation should not be accepted as part of normal 'maternal aggression'. Prospective owners should therefore resist the temptation to purchase kittens from a queen that is overtly hostile to them. Cats showing maternal aggression of this kind should be neutered so that further breeding cannot occur. If aggression is directed only at other cats, then the owner has a responsibility to house the cat securely to prevent this occurring.

In some cases, the general feline population is so large that resource density and individual territorial space are insufficient to prevent aggression. Neighbours may have to make a concerted attempt to improve the local environment so that cats may co-exist. The temptation to introduce more cats should be resisted. Time-sharing access to the garden may effectively reduce the population density that each cat experiences but this must be combined with

---

Box 16.27 Treatment: aggression to other cats in the neighbourhood

- Neuter male and female cats.
- Consider time-sharing outdoor access; stagger the times when cats are allowed outside using electronic cat flaps attached to a timer.
- Increase resources in the home and garden; indoor and outdoor latrines, more resting places, feeding and drinking sites.
- Introduce activity feeding.
- Schedule time for interactive play to coincide with peak periods when cats would otherwise be active outside.

improved resource access and environmental enrichment in the home (Box 16.27).

Prognosis

The prognosis is guarded because, in many cases, new residents will introduce new cats. Every change or increase in population brings further competition and instability. Successful management of a local overpopulation problem depends upon active participation by all cat owners.

ADVICE SHEETS THAT MAY BE RELEVANT TO THIS CHAPTER

In Appendix 3

1. Improving the outdoor environment for cats
2. Improving the indoor environment for cats
3. Multi-cat households
6. Introducing a new cat to the household

Further reading

Abrantes R 2001 Dog Language: an encyclopaedia of canine behaviour. Wakan Tanka, Naperville, Illinois

Abrantes R 2003 The evolution of canine social behaviour. Wakan Tanka, Naperville, Illinois

Bishop Y (ed) 2004 The veterinary formulary, 5th edn. Pharmaceutical Press, London

Bradshaw J 1992 The behaviour of the domestic cat. CABI, Oxford, UK

Burch M R, Bailey J S 1999 How dogs learn. Howell Books, New York

Chance P 1994 Leaning and behaviour, 3rd edn. Brooks/Cole, Pacific Grove, California

Dodman N H, Shuster L 1998 Psychopharmacology of animal behaviour disorders. Blackwell Science, Oxford, UK

Donaldson J 1996 The culture clash. James and Kenneth, Berkeley, California

Jevring C, Catanzaro T 1999 Healthcare of the well pet. WB Saunders, London

Kershaw E 1998 Go click. APBC

Lacey R The complete guide to psychiatric drugs: a layman's handbook. Ebury Press, London

Lieberman D A 1993 Learning, behaviour and cognition, 2nd edn. Brooks/Cole, Pacific Grove, California

Lindsay S R 2000 Handbook of applied dog behaviour and training volume 1: adaptation and learning. Iowa State University Press, Ames

Moore M (ed) 2000 BSAVA Manual of veterinary nursing. British Small Animal Veterinary Association, Cheltenham, UK

Neal M J 2002 Medical pharmacology at a glance. Blackwell Science, Oxford, UK

Pavlov I R 1924 Conditioned reflexes. Dover Publications, New York

Pryor K 1999 Don't Shoot the Dog. Bantam Books, New York

Reid P J 1996 Excel-erated Learning. James and Kenneth, Berkeley, California

Serpell J 1995 The domestic dog: its evolution, behaviour and interactions with people. Cambridge University Press, Cambridge, UK

Shiloh R, Nutt D, Weizman A 2001 An atlas of psychiatric pharmacology. Martin Dunitz, London

Silverstone T, Turner P Drug treatment in psychiatry. Routledge, London, UK

Stahl S M 2000 Essential psychopharmacology: neuroscientific basis and practical applications. Cambridge University Press, Cambridge, UK

Tennant B (ed) 2002 BSAVA small animal formulary, 4th edn. British Small Animal Veterinary Association, Cheltenham, UK

Thorne C (ed) 1992 The Waltham book of dog and cat behaviour. Pergamon, Oxford, UK

Turner D, Bateson P 2000 The domestic cat: the biology of its behaviour. Cambridge University Press, Cambridge, UK

Practice resources

Behaviour handouts. Lifelearn, Newmarket, UK

CABTSG Referral form. In this edition and available in electric form from www.cabtsg.org

Headstart for Kittens, The Blue Cross, Headstart Programme, Shilton Road, Burford, Oxon OX18 4PF

Headstart for puppies/kittens, The Blue Cross, Headstart Programme, Shilton Road, Burford, Oxon OX18 4PF

Mackinnon P Kind, fair, effective: the puppy class. Available from APBC, PO Box 46, Worcester, WR8 9YS, UK

Peachey E Running puppy classes. Available from APBC, PO Box 46, Worcester, WR8 9YS, UK

Seksel K 1997 Kitten Kindy. The proceedings of the first international conference on veterinary behavioural medicine. UFAW, Potters Bar, UK, pp 28–30

Recommended reading for clients

Appleby D Ain't misbehavin'. Broadcast Books, Bristol, UK

Appleby D How to have a contented cat. Available from APBC, PO Box 46, Worcester, WR8 9YS, UK

Appleby D How to have a happy puppy. Available from APBC, PO Box 46, Worcester, WR8 9YS, UK

Bailey G 1995 Perfect puppy. Hamlyn, London

Bessant C, Neville P 2000 Perfect kitten. Hamlyn, London

Heath S Cat and kitten behaviour: an owner's guide. Harper Collins, London

Patmore K So your children want a dog. Available from APBC, PO Box 46, Worcester, WR8 9YS, UK

Paws for thought. Wise Owl Productions (available from APBC, PO Box 46, Worcester, WR8 9YS, UK)

Appendices

Appendix 1

Case reference number_____

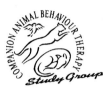

Referral Form for Animal Behaviour Case

This form is approved by The Companion Animal Behaviour Therapy Study Group and was produced after consultation with the Royal College of Veterinary Surgeons

Behaviour problems may arise both directly and indirectly as a result of concurrent or previous medical problems. Veterinary involvement is therefore essential in eliminating organic causes of the problem and prioritising the diagnostic and treatment strategy to be used in any given case. In order to safeguard the welfare of your patient and indicate your approval of referral, please complete the following form. Please note that until a case is released to another veterinary surgeon then you, as the client's normal veterinary surgeon, remain responsible for the treatment, advice and any prescriptions given.

Referring / Contact Veterinary Surgeon _____**MRCVS**

Practice Name_____

Address:_____   **Tel: (inc. STD code)**_____

_____

_____   **Fax:**_____

_____

Post Code_____

Client Name:_____   **Patient name**_____

Species/breed_____   **Age**_____**Sex (inc.neuter status)**_____

Address:_____   **Tel: (inc. STD code)**_____

_____

_____

_____

Post Code_____

Brief details of behavior problem   **Date first noticed**____/____/_____

_____

_____

_____

_____

Has euthanasia been considered?_____

I hereby acknowledge my approval for the client described overleaf to be referred for management of the current behaviour problem to:

Referral Practice Name:_____

Case reference number_____

Medical history:

Date of last health check___/___/___   Weight_____Kg

Please indicate if there are current or previous health problems concerning the following and attach appropriate details:

☐ Allergic reactions   ☐ Orolaryngeal region

☐ Cardiovascular system   ☐ Respiratory system

☐ Endocrinological system   ☐ Sensory systems

☐ Muscular skeletal system   ☐ Skin and adnexae

☐ Nervous system   ☐ Urogenital system

Please provide details of any blood screens performed including specific organ function tests and assays

_____

_____

Date and purpose of any general anaesthetics

_____

_____

Details of any ongoing medical conditions or treatments

_____

_____

_____

Summary medical history / medical records attached (delete as appropriate)

Further information attached Yes / No

Signed:_____MRCVS   Date____/____/_____

I ...., the owner of the above named animal, consent to the disclosure of clinical information regarding my pet by my veterinary surgeon for the purposes of referral.

Signed_____   Date____/____/_____

© CABTSG 2000

Appendix 2

CONTENTS

ADVICE SHEET 1

USING A HOUSELINE

The houseline is a way to exert control over your dog *safely* while you are training him to obey commands. You should use the houseline only under the instruction of your behavioural advisor. The houseline is used to help with training and is not a substitute for it. The typical times you may need to use the houseline would be to help you to:

- get a dog off a bed or the couch
- get a dog out of her basket
- take a dog out to the toilet
- move the dog out of the way or away from something.

Once you have a houseline, it is essential that you make full and proper use of it so that you can avoid any kind of conflict with your dog.

MAKING A HOUSELINE

The houseline is a 3-m long piece of fine rope or cord that is attached to the dog's collar using a standard leash clip. The cord must be of a type that will not get tangled up in furniture and which the dog cannot collect together, sit on and guard. A good choice is plastic coated steel washing line because it is also difficult to chew. The leash clip must be fixed on securely.

As an alternative, you can also buy ready-made houselines and certain leashes are also suitable.

The houseline is fixed to your dog's collar and left in place at all times when you are around to supervise your dog. Never leave the houseline on when nobody is at home to supervise the dog as there is a risk of entanglement.

USING THE HOUSELINE

The line is used in any situation where you want the dog to move and you would normally have to take hold of him or push him. This reduces the dog's fear of being grabbed or the tendency for some dogs to object to being moved.

The correct use of the houseline is as follows:

- Pick up the end of the houseline without looking your dog in the eye.
- Turn around and walk away from your dog.
- Call your dog and give the command you want him to obey (for example, the command, 'Freddy, off' to get him off the sofa). Use a calm and relaxed voice.
- When your dog obeys give him a reward (praise, food, etc.).
- Give your dog the command a second time if he does not obey at once, but keep your voice calm and relaxed.
- If your dog still does not obey and the line is now tense, then give him a couple of gentle tugs with the houseline so that you dislodge him from where he is. Then give your command again.
- Repeat this until he does what you want, and then give the reward.

It is absolutely essential that you keep your back to the dog until you are giving the reward.

Using the line is not meant to be a *challenge* to the dog; do not pull on it while facing or staring at him or else the dog will take the situation as a direct threat and may become aggressive.

Even if the dog becomes reluctant to move, it is better to pull with your back to the dog than to turn around and face up to him.

You should remain totally emotionless throughout this; show no irritatation if your dog does not respond perfectly every time and do not allow your voice to become loud or angry when using the line. Try to be gentle but persistent when you pull the line. You want the dog to assume that resistance is pointless but that the use of the line is neither painful nor upsetting.

RESULTS

To begin with, your dog will resist the houseline but you should see no aggression. If your dog does become aggressive, you must stop using the houseline and go back to your behavioural advisor for help. Dogs with arthritis or neck problems might find the use of the houseline painful so you must get your vet to check your dog over before using a houseline.

ADVICE SHEET 2

JUMPING UP

This training may be accomplished with or without a clicker. Please consult the handout about introducing a clicker before using one for training. If your dog shows signs of fear of the clicker noise, then contact your veterinary surgeon or behaviourist.

This is a method for teaching your dog to sit down and remain calm at times when he might want to jump up at you. Typically, dogs jump up when you come home or as you are walking around.

STAGE 1: BASIC PREPARATION

Start by training a 'sit' command, preferably using clicker-training.

Next, get a bum bag so that you can carry food around with you more conveniently and do the training of a basic 'sit' command in the places where your dog is inclined to jump up at you; the hallway, outside your bedroom door, in the back garden and any other typical places where your dog is used to seeing you and might get excited. These are the places where he misbehaves so you want to create a powerful memory of doing obedience training there.

It is important that, in each of these situations, you train your dog to sit and stay calm while getting a train of perhaps 10 to 20 consecutive clicks and food rewards. If he stands up or moves, ask him to sit and then start clicking and food rewarding again when he obeys. If he jumps up, then *look away* and say 'no' quite quietly. Do not look at your dog when you say 'no'. Once you have finished your little bit of training at one of these locations, then move on to the next one, giving your dog a signal that it is time to move.

Once you can see that your dog is responding well to this training, which may take a few days or a couple of weeks, then you can move on to the next stage.

STAGE 2: SPECIFIC TRAINING EXERCISES

When your dog jumps up, it is usually an expression of excitement and it is very hard for him to concentrate or think about doing anything other than expressing his pleasure at seeing you. That is why you started by doing lots of basic training so that deep inside your dog's memory there is an automatic 'sit' response. This makes it easier for him to understand what you are saying at times of stress and excitement.

Now you need to move on to training in situations that most closely resemble those in which your dog jumps up; for example, when you return and enter through the front door. This is a typical situation and the method can be adapted to others.

- Take your dog to the front door, with your bum bag and clicker.
- Step outside the door and wait a few seconds.
- Come back in and immediately ask your dog to sit.
- Give him 5 to 10 clicks and food rewards and then walk around the entrance area, giving a few clicks and dropping food onto the floor if your dog does not jump up. Then go back out again. Repeat this several times at each training session.
- Vary the amount of time you stay outside between a few seconds and a couple of minutes. Make sure that you walk away from the house so that your dog does not see you standing outside!

As you repeat this training several times each day, you will find that your dog starts to sit just as you come in through the door. You may not even have to ask. This is excellent, so click and reward your dog if he spontaneously does this.

To begin with, it is important that the 'click' is the only thing that tells your dog that he is doing the right thing. Avoid giving praise or touching your dog because this will make him get excited and he may stand up or run about.

Once you can see that he is responding well to training, then you can add in a little verbal praise and even stroking *if he remains sitting*. This must be in addition to the clicker training and you must stop it if your dog becomes unruly or excited in any way.

STAGE 3: WHEN YOU COME HOME

Now you should start to introduce exactly the same method as in Stage 2 to genuine situations when you come home.

- Always come in wearing your bum bag and clicker.
- Get your dog to sit and then give 10+ clicks and food rewards.
- Remember that your dog is very excited and may find it harder to stay under control, so you will need to give clicks and food rewards at high frequency if you are going to hold his attention.
- You need to keep giving them until he is calm and then keep giving clicks and rewards as you walk into the house while he stays calm and does not jump up.
- If he jumps up at any time, then look away and say 'no', as before. Stop and ask him to sit again.

You will find that your training transfers quite easily because your dog has already done so much of this kind of work before.

STAGE 4: STOPPING JUMPING UP AT OTHER PEOPLE

Precisely the same methods can be applied to stop your dog jumping up at other people, but only once you have trained your dog not to jump up at two or three family members who follow the routines above.

Then your dog will find it much easier and less frustrating to do training with visitors.

This method must only be used for dogs that do not show any kind of aggression towards people at the front door and that are always pleased to see everyone.

The difference with this stage of training is that *you* give the commands, clicks and rewards and the visitor just comes in and out.

Do not allow your dog to meet people at the front door when they first come to the house because this is a time when the dog is too excited.

Wait until the dog has calmed down and the person has been in the house for a while.

Then go through a similar routine to that in Stage 2:

- Get the person to go out for a short period and then come back.
- When you go to answer the door, ask your dog to sit and then start giving clicks and food rewards.
- Open the door.
- When the person comes in, keep your dog sitting for 20 to 30 seconds while the person stands still.
- Then get them to walk around while you give clicks and food if your dog stays calm and does not jump up.

- Then the person leaves and goes through the same routine again.

You will find that, just as in the other training sessions, your dog rapidly learns to stay sitting calmly while this person goes in and out.

Practise this with two or three different people until your dog stays calm throughout training. Then you can go through the same routine with a range of different people when they are genuinely coming into the house for the first time.

STAGE 5: FINISHING TRAINING

Obviously, nobody wants to have to keep doing training forever, and there has to be a point at which clicker-training is phased out. However, you must continue training until your dog is responding perfectly in real situations. If you stop too soon, you will find that your dog rapidly reverts to misbehaviour.

Instead, phase out training by giving fewer and fewer clicks and food rewards. There is more information about the best way to do this in Advice sheet 17.

ADVICE SHEET 3

REWARD AND PUNISHMENT

INTRODUCTION

All species of mammal use the same basic rules in order to learn about the world in which they live.

Through association, we learn about the connections between events and their consequences. This enables us to predict what is going to happen in the future and refine our response so that we make the best of what is to come.

Here are some of the basic rules that enable animals, and people, to learn:

- If two things happen at the same time then we assume there is a connection between them.
- If I do something and there is an immediate effect, then I will learn that there is a connection between what I did and what happened.
- The more often two things happen at the same time, the more strongly the association between them will become.
- The more important the events are, then the more likely we are to make the connection quickly because it matters to us.

We have all experienced the situation where we press a light switch and suddenly there is a loud bang as the light bulb blows. Our reaction is to freeze and think, 'What did I do wrong?'.

As rational individuals we know that the bulb was going to pop as soon as current passed though it again and all we did was to activate a switch to make this happen. However, we cannot stop ourselves flinching slightly in anticipation the next time we operate the light switch.

The important difference between animals and us is that we are able to think about and learn from what we have been doing in the distant past. Animals learn about what is going on *right now*, not what happened a year, a week, or even a few minutes ago.

Experiments have shown us that:

- dogs and cats learn associations most effectively if events are half a second apart.
- the ability to make associations begins to drop off after a gap of 2 seconds or more.
- if events are more than 2 minutes apart, little or no association will be made between them.

What is the importance of this for training?

- When you give a reward you are actually rewarding what is going on *right now*.
- Rewarding behaviour increases the chances of it happening again in the future.
- Rewards need to be given quite quickly; any longer than a couple of seconds will be too slow and you may not, in fact, be rewarding what you think. For example,

if you have asked your dog to sit but, as you go to give the reward, the dog stands up; then what are you rewarding?

The same kind of rules apply to punishment:

- The timing of punishment needs to be even more perfect because we do not want to punish the wrong behaviour or allow the dog to begin to get a reward from what it is doing.
- Punishment must be given as the dog *starts* to do something wrong; that way you will have a greater effect and the punishment you use need only be of the very mildest kind.
- If you wait until immediately *after* the dog has done wrong, there will be a problem; the dog may have enjoyed breaking the rules and may balance the punishment against the reward. Your dog will think 'That cake was fantastic so, given the chance, I happily trade getting the cake for getting told off again!'. The dog may also see the punishment as disconnected from what he has done; the cake was eaten a few seconds ago and you only caught your dog as it digested the last mouthful.
- If you punish long after an event has passed, the dog will have no recollection of what it did to be punished for and it will come to regard the person punishing as threatening and unpredictable. These dogs often look 'guilty' when in fact they are simply frightened, confused and submissive.

We also need to be aware of the importance of what is actually going on around the time of punishment. If we come into the house to find our dog chewing the sofa and the dog gets up and delightedly rushes towards us wagging its tail . . . should we punish or not? From our point of view, the dog's recent misbehaviour is the sole focus of our attention. For the dog it is completely different: our return home is the most important event in his whole day and that is all he is thinking about now. If we punish this dog, he is very unlikely to associate the punishment with the sofa chewing because the emotional impact of seeing us again has erased this event from his mind. If we punish now, we are risking making the dog very uncertain and anxious about what we will be like next time we come home and this may make him even more destructive.

Another good example is the dog that won't come back.

The dog has run up and down the field for 3 hours with you running behind shouting 'Come here!'. Finally he comes back wagging his tail. What do you do? If you shout and threaten him then, what are you punishing? Unfortunately, you are punishing the one thing that you do want, i.e., coming back! You might not want to heavily reward such a slow recall but punishing the dog will make him even more reluctant to come back next time.

Remembering that the dog's ability to make associations is limited to a relatively narrow time frame, we must also avoid 'delayed punishment'. If, for example, you come down in the morning to find cold faeces on the kitchen floor there is absolutely no point in using punishment. It is too late and your dog will have absolutely no idea why you are angry. Dogs are often submissive in these situations but this is not an indication that they are in any way guilty or aware that they have done anything wrong. Dogs are exceptionally good at reading body language so your dog knows you are angry and is trying to ingratiate himself so that you do not threaten or harm him. The fact that the dog defecates on the kitchen floor has nothing to do with wilfulness or dominance.

REWARD AND PUNISHMENT

These are two of the most misused words in the English language. When we say we punished an animal, what we are often saying is that we 'made them pay' for what they did wrong. But have we achieved the underlying aim of stopping him from misbehaving again in the future? If not, then the 'punishment' has done nothing more than give us an outlet for our anger.

When we punish, what we really want is for the dog's behaviour to change so that we see less of the problem behaviour in the future. So if we tell the dog off for doing the same thing every day for 5 months and at the end of that time the dog is still doing it exactly the same as before, then are we punishing the behaviour?

The answer is, unfortunately, no we are not!

Animals are very resilient to things that they do not like because, in the wild, they often face failure, defeat and injury. If a wild dog stopped hunting antelope because sometimes it got a painful kick in the face, then it would soon starve and die. The same effect is seen when punishment alone is used to stop misbehaviour. It will suppress the behaviour for a while but the animal will still occasionally retest whether the behaviour is worth trying again. Very quickly the problem behaviour comes back again.

The other risk with punishment is that it cause aggression: the animal feels threatened, frustrated and thwarted so it may react in the only way it can, by lashing out.

So, we must not use punishment as the only method of controlling behaviour and training animals because we won't get the results we want and we may cause other problems that are more dangerous.

Reward is also a slightly confusing term because what we see as a reward may not be very rewarding for the dog. Offering a food treat that the dog is not very keen on may be an offer of reward from our perspective but, to the dog, it is irrelevant.

Reward and punishment are inextricably linked. As anyone who has refused to give his or her child pocketmoney because of bad behaviour can tell us, withholding a reward is a form of punishment. So all the time that we are offering a reward for a good 'sit' behaviour we are also punishing the dog for continuing to stand up.

The actual definitions of reward and punishment are:

Punishment: A punishment is anything that causes a decrease in the likelihood of a behaviour happening in the future.

Reward: A reward is anything that causes an increase in the likelihood of the behaviour happening again in the future.

HOW CAN YOU USE PUNISHMENT AND REWARD EFFECTIVELY?

Punishment

Imagine the situation where you go out of your front door and a brick falls on your head. You look up and there is nothing going on that might explain why. The next time you go out of the front door the same thing happens and again you have no idea why. You get a builder to check the house and still you have no idea what is going on. After a week, you decide to go out through the back door from now on because you are fed up having a sore head. After a month of leaving via the back door, you decide to try the front one again . . . and a brick lands on your head. Having a permanently sore head is unpleasant and it is just as easy to use the back door so you choose never to go through the front door again.

Picture the same situation again but this time, when you look up, there is a crane looming over the house. You go back in and decide to avoid going through the front door again until the crane has gone.

What does this story tell us?

It shows that the best punishment is one where the exact mechanism for how it was delivered is unclear. You know that you did something that resulted in an outcome that you did not like but you cannot look more deeply into the situation to find a way of rationalising what happened, in order to carry on doing what you want without fear of punishment.

This can be translated to how we punish animals.

If every time your dog chews a book you sneak up and bop him on the head with a newspaper, the dog may learn not to chew books while you are around. He may also learn that you are a rather nasty person and begin to fear rolled-up newspapers or being stroked or crept up on while busy.

This has no effect on your dog's behaviour when you are out and simply makes him resent or fear you.

Perhaps one day he will turn and snap at you when you reach to stroke him while he is chewing a bone because he thinks you are going to hit him. Far from the ideal or intended result.

If, on the other hand, every time your dog goes to chew a book there is a cap underneath it that goes bang when the book is picked up, then the dog will soon discover that the only way to avoid the bang is to leave the books alone. Nothing predicts or signals to him what is going to happen so he has no other choice than to change his behaviour. The dog's owner may even appear to be something of a saviour as you reward your dog for coming away from the nasty book!

We call this 'remote punishment'; this is punishment that is very closely related to the behaviour that we do not want but is completely impersonal (nobody was seen to be involved in it).

This avoids all of the potential effects that the dog may associate his owner with punishment and threat.

However, like all forms of punishment, it still has to be used very carefully. We must not use any punishment that might frighten the dog too much. All we want to do is to interrupt the behaviour by very mildly startling the dog. So we must tailor the punishment to suit the situation and the individual; noise methods are not suitable for sound-sensitive dogs!

In any case we should always use the minimum intensity of punishment possible.

REWARD

We often worry that by offering dogs rewards for doing everything, we are bribing them but there is an immense difference between reward and bribe. Bribing is definitely wrong because it does not get us what we want and we enter a negotiation situation with the dog, which they may ultimately win!

Rewards are like a salary; we do the work and we get paid for doing it. Perhaps sometimes we get a bonus because we have worked particularly hard but it is obvious from the outset that 'no work' equals 'no pay'.

A bribe is an offer of money or favours that is used to motivate us to behave differently than we might otherwise wish to. We might expect to negotiate to get a bigger bribe because we know that we have to act against our better judgment in order to get it. Our price might go 'sky high', especially if we can see that the other person is desperate to get something out of us.

Bribes do not work unless they are really good because you have the chance to weigh up what you are willing to do.

It is exactly the same with training dogs.

If you hold out a food reward as a lure to get the dog in from the garden then he may come. But he may also hold out a bit longer to see if you go back to the cupboard to get something better to offer him. As you offer the food, you may see a familiar expression on your dog's face; 'Make me a better offer'. He knows he is negotiating a bribe!

If, however, you train the dog to work for food rewards in very simple easy situations and then gradually build up to more difficult ones, then the dog has not had a chance to negotiate. He learns that to get the food he must obey and, since he has little better to do, that is exactly what he does. After a while, he does what you say without even thinking about it.

Now, when he is called in from the garden he dashes in. No food is held out as a lure and he accepts whatever he gets as a reward when he gets in.

ADVICE SHEET 4

AGGRESSION AROUND FOOD

This is a simple method of training your dog to tolerate your presence and approach when he or she is eating.

Start using very bland dried food since dogs are distinctly less inclined to guard food that has an uninteresting texture or flavour. They also guard a smaller meal less ferociously than they do a large one; so small, frequent and dull meals are the best tool for this training.

STAGE 1:

- Get two food bowls and fill one with the amount of food that you are going to give the dog at this meal.
- Put this bowl in a place so that the dog cannot see what is in it but where you will easily be able to reach and take food from it.
- Sit down on a low chair and put the empty bowl a short distance from your feet.
- Take a handful of the food from the full bowl that is at your side.
- Hold it above the dog's head (far enough above him that there is no chance of his being able to reach or grab it).
- Ask the dog to sit.
- As soon as your dog sits, move your arm slowly down as if to put the food into the bowl.
- If your dog makes *any* move to take the food or growls, stop moving your hand. Wait until your dog stops growling, and ask him to sit again.
- When he sits, continue to move your hand to the bowl.
- Finally drop the food into the bowl, saying 'take it' as you do so.
- As soon as the dog finishes this food, hold another handful above him and repeat the same process.

Very rapidly, you should find that your dog sits spontaneously while you hold the food above him. Repeat this sequence until the food bowl you are dispensing from is empty but do not let your dog see that the food has run out. Just put the bowl out of reach and leave the room. Keep repeating this exercise until there is no sign of irritability at all.

Now follow a series of stages that increase in difficulty. You should repeat exercises at each stage until your dog is showing no signs of growling or aggression, before moving on to the next stage. If you are concerned about your dog's behaviour or the risk of being bitten, then stop training and seek further advice.

STAGE 2:

Carry out the same training method but add more food to the bowl while your dog is still eating. Add the food as your dog is just coming to the end of what is in the bowl. Gradually increase the amount of food you give the dog in each handful so that there is more food in the bowl each time you add extra.

STAGE 3:

Do the same training while standing up next to your dog, instead of sitting.

STAGE 4:

Take a step away from your dog after adding the food. Then step towards your dog again before adding the next handful of food.

STAGE 5:

Take several steps further away before approaching to add more food to the bowl while your dog is eating.

STAGE 6:

Give your dog a larger portion of the dull dried food in the bowl in one go and approach to add small amounts of extra-tasty food.

This training programme must be followed by all adults in the house but starting with the person the dog already shows least aggression to when they are present during feeding. Remember that the dog must get the extra food only if it does not growl or threaten the person adding it.

Once all people in the house have completed Stage 6, then you can do the last stage in training.

STAGE 7:

Put an initial amount of food into the bowl. Then several people take turns to walk up and add some treats to the bowl while the dog is eating, before walking away again.

As with all problems that involve aggression, you must not try to progress too quickly and you must stop if there is any chance of a threat or a hazard. Do not take unnecessary risks, and be prepared to spend as much time on a given stage as is necessary to complete it.

PREVENTING A RELAPSE

Once this process is complete, you should be able to approach the dog and add food with no complaint. However, it is important not to become too confident; to maintain this kind of learning it is essential to regularly put things into the dog's bowl throughout the rest of its life. This might be only every couple of weeks, but it helps to maintain the confidence that the dog has about you and avoids re-emergence of the problem.

ADVICE SHEET 5

REDUCING POSSESSIVENESS THROUGH PLAY

This training may be accomplished with or without a clicker. Please consult the handout about introducing a clicker before using one for training. If your dog shows signs of fear of the clicker noise then contact your veterinary surgeon or behaviourist.

Many dogs will steal toys during play, or find objects and refuse to give them up. This can be because they do not want play to end or because they want to retain possession of the object.

The more that we chase the dog around or try to barter with them for the object, the greater its value becomes and the more reluctant the dog is to give it up. The dog may also thoroughly enjoy being chased around, thinking this is as much of a game for us as it is for them.

There are many ways to deal with this but the best way is through play, using the rules of a game to train the dog not to steal things and to give them up when asked. Training through play avoids confrontation that can lead to aggression later on.

It is best to combine the strategy in this handout with those on Advice sheets 8 and 12 on 'click-touch training' and 'play and calm signals' because together these dramatically improve communication between the owner and dog.

Some general rules to follow are:

- Divide your dog's toys into those you play games with and those he likes to chew on his own.
- Any toys that he chews on his own he can keep but you must *never* play games with them.
- The toys you do play games with should be kept in a cupboard, somewhere out of your dog's reach, so that you have to go and get a toy to start a game.
- Now that you are in control of the play, you must make sure that you ask your dog for a game many times a day. It is best to ask for a game at a time when you would expect your dog to want to play, but also when he is quiet and not demanding one.

GAME 1:

At least two people are needed together with several identical toys to play with.

- Start a throw-fetch game in which the people throw the toy between them and also for the dog.
- You need to throw the toy between you a lot so that the dog can see that he is joining in with your game.
- If your dog runs away with a toy and won't give it back, ignore him and get out one of the other identical toys. Continue to play throw-fetch between you and run about so that your dog can see that you are having fun and he has excluded himself by running off with the other toy.
- If he comes back to join in, he must sit first.
- Once he is playing, you should craftily arrange to get close to the toy he has dropped so that you can quickly pick it up again.

Continue to play like this, making it clear to your dog that it is your game that he is joining in with and that selfish possessiveness gets him nowhere.

GAME 2:

One or more people are needed, together with food treats and several duplicate toys.

- Play a throw-fetch game with the dog.
- When he brings back the toy, hold up one hand with a second toy in it and the other with a food reward.
- Quietly say the dog's name followed by the command 'drop'.
- When he drops the toy, give the food reward and then throw the next toy without picking up the one the dog put down.
- While the dog is running to get the second toy, pick up the first.
- Continue this sequence.

WHAT IF THE DOG WILL NOT GIVE UP THE TOY?

Each time he does not drop, turn your head away and then quietly say 'no'. Wait for a few seconds and then try again. If after three requests your dog does not give up the toy, stop the game and ignore the dog for 2 minutes before trying again.

If two people are present, then play a variation on game 1 in which both of you play throw-fetch and deliberately exclude the dog if he will not give up the toy he has. As soon as he drops it, you can give the food reward and throw the next toy.

It will take a number of repetitions before your dog fully understands what is going on because there is a lot to learn in this game. It can be made easier if you use a clicker to pinpoint when your dog gets it right; give a click as he drops the toy and then give a food reward.

Do not get impatient or angry and try to keep your tone of voice happy and jolly. After playing this game several times a day for several weeks, your dog should have a good grasp of the fact that whatever he possesses has little value, and you will be able to start using your drop command to ask him to give you all sorts of things that he picks up. To begin with you must always give him some kind of treat as a reward for dropping what he has.

ADVICE SHEET 6

MUZZLE-TRAINING

There are some circumstances in which it is appropriate for dogs to be muzzled and, if the muzzle is to have the appropriate effect, it is important that your dog is happy to accept its use and does not regard it as a threat. Muzzle-training involves making positive associations with the muzzle and teaching your dog to anticipate reward when the muzzle is worn. There are different varieties of muzzles on the market but, in situations when a muzzle needs to be worn during the course of behavioural therapy, it is recommended that a 'Baskerville®' type is used. These muzzles allow your dog to breathe freely and also to pant should this be necessary in situations of stress or heat. Dogs can also drink while wearing the muzzle and the small holes in the basket allow you to post food rewards, enabling him to be rewarded while still wearing the muzzle.

In order to accustom your dog to the muzzle, you will need to take time to introduce it carefully and gradually and the following approach is recommended.

1. Put a piece of your dog's favourite food in the nose section of the muzzle and, holding the muzzle in your hand, bring it up to your dog's nose. He should respond to the food by sniffing and, provided that the muzzle is held very still and is in an open position with the neck strap out of the way, your dog will put his nose into the muzzle in order to remove the food. Repeat this exercise several times until your dog will happily place his head into the muzzle to retrieve the reward.

2. The next stage involves gently sliding the muzzle over your dog's nose as he eats the treat and removing it as soon as the treat has been consumed. On each occasion that you repeat this exercise, you should leave the muzzle in position for a little longer so that your dog gets used to the sensation of the muzzle around the face and eventually you should incorporate fastening the muzzle buckle into this routine.

3. Each time that you put the muzzle on your dog, you should use a command such as 'muzzle' so that your dog learns to associate this command with the action of being muzzled and can therefore predict the situation and not be startled.

4. When you are muzzle-training your dog, try to ensure that you go through the above process of putting the muzzle on, rewarding the dog and removing the muzzle in a variety of locations and at a variety of times. If you only ever use a muzzle in certain circumstances or in certain locations, your dog will learn to anticipate its use and this can lead to problems.

You should expect your dog to wear a muzzle only after he has been trained to accept it.

ADVICE SHEET 7

TERRITORIAL TRIGGERS

PREVENTING RISK

Territorial dogs are constantly making decisions about who should and who should not enter their territory. Unfortunately, the decisions they make are often incorrect and they continue to guard well after we have decided the person is a friend and not an intruder.

For this reason, no territorial dog should be left to make its own mind up about someone. Nobody should ever be left with a territorial dog or allowed to come and go from its territory unsupervised. The risk may be small, but it is a real one because many territorial dogs 'act first and ask questions later'.

A dog that is startled by someone may not have the time to go through the process of barking and guarding and may feel its only option is to attack.

BASIC PRECAUTIONS:

- Fit adequate gates and fencing; tall enough to stop jumping over and buried to prevent digging out.
- Lock all access points to the garden and house.
- Do not give keys to trades people or visitors.
- Never trust your dog to make the right choices.

THE REACTION TO PEOPLE AT THE BOUNDARY OF THE TERRITORY

We expect dogs to bark at people when they appear at the door; however, it really is not necessary. Rarely is anyone that comes to the front door likely to be a threat to the household; burglars tend to be a lot more discreet. So, almost everyone at the door is either a friend or someone who is doing a legitimate job.

The perfect guard dog is one that recognises that the front door is a normal entry for friends and that people passing by in the street are not a threat to security. It is therefore important that you minimise the number of things that focus your dog's territorial behaviour on the front door and the street outside your house.

What keeps dogs barking at the door?

In the context of territorial behaviour, barking has two main functions:

- It is a way to scare away a potential intruder.
- It is a call to arms. It alerts others in the household to come and deal with the intruder.

This behaviour is often rewarding. Every day that the postman comes to the door he gets barked at and the dog thinks that the barking has worked because the person left. Likewise the milkman, paper boy and refuse collector come and go. From the dog's perspective, its guarding behaviour is successful every time but these people insist on coming back every day for another try. This teaches the dog to be more territorial and, in fact, a lot of these dogs become fixated on following their daily territorial duties despite the fact that these people are absolutely no threat at all.

Barking is also rewarded in other ways. When the dog barks we rush to the door. The barking worked because it enabled the dog to call us so that we could help fend off the intruder.

Then, when we answer the door, we often hold the dog by his collar while the visitor stands on the step. This reinforces the dog's feeling that it has a role in deciding whether or not the person should come in.

What if we shout at the dog to tell it to shut up? In this case the dog may believe that we are joining in with the barking!

The way to get around all of these problems is to reduce the things that trigger territoriality and reduce the dog's responsibility for guarding the home.

REDUCING THE THINGS THAT TRIGGER TERRITORIALITY

- Move all deliveries to a box as far away from the house as possible and preferably out of the dog's sight. Lockable boxes are available at garden centres.
- Never take your dog to meet people at the door; not even friends that your dog knows.
- If it is possible (which is not always the case) restrict your dog to a part of the house that does not overlook a busy road or footpath.
- Alternatively, block your dog's view of areas where he sees things or people that he barks at.
- Do not go to the door when your dog is barking. Call the dog away from the door and then put him in another room until the visitor has come inside or gone away. Perhaps throw a few food treats down on the floor or give the dog an activity ball as a distraction while you deal with the door.

ADVICE SHEET 8

PLAY AND CALM SIGNALS

This training may be accomplished with or without a clicker. Please consult Advice sheet 19 about introducing a clicker before using one for training. If your dog shows signs of fear of the clicker noise, then contact your veterinary surgeon or behaviourist.

Many dogs become overexcited and then get frustrated when play comes to an end. They have not properly learned the signals we give when we want to start or stop play so when a game ends they try to demand more. These dogs also demand play at inappropriate times and do not take well to not getting their way. This is not because they are nasty or aggressive but partly because they want to play and think that we must too. They have not learned the signals that we use to say 'no, go away'.

This piece of training is designed to teach your dog to alter his mood and level of excitement according to your body language so that he understands when to play and when to stop. This training works best if you combine it with the exercises for reducing attention-seeking.

Like children, some dogs get over-excited during play and the games get rough and out of control. It is important to keep play under control and to cool things down before they get out of hand. This is particularly important when children are involved in play with the dog.

GENERAL RULES

- Divide toys into two types; those you join in play with and those your dog can enjoy on his own. The former are things like a ball or a tug toy and the latter are chews, bones and the like.
- Keep all toys that you play games with in a box out of your dog's reach.
- Your dog can still have full access to any chews and chewy toys but you must never play games with these under any circumstances.
- All play must be started and finished under your control; do not allow your dog to start play or continue it after you want play to end.

- After games, you must put away the toy you were playing with.

PLAY ROUTINE

- Take a bum bag full of your dog's favourite food treats and a clicker with you whenever you play.
- Then go and get a toy to play with.
- Take your dog calmly into the garden (or where you want to play).
- Ask your dog to sit and give 5 to 10 food rewards (or clicks and food rewards if you are using clicker training) for doing so.
- Start the game by giving your play signal: '(your-dog's-name), play'.
- Then begin to play and act really excited.
- After 30 to 60 seconds (before your dog has become over-excited) you must suddenly become calm and stop the game. Say 'no' and look away.
- Ask your dog to sit and give about 5 to 20 consecutive (clicks and) rewards while he sits and becomes calm. Do not start play again until he has calmed down.
- When you are ready to start play, give the play signal again and start another short game.
- For several minutes, keep alternating between play and sitting for treats.
- Finish the game by getting your dog to sit and stay calm for 10 to 20 rewards and then give a very small chew to occupy him for a few minutes.

In this way the game ends with your dog calm and anticipating a chew rather than over-excited and demanding more play.

You must use this routine every time you play a game with your dog, practising several times each day for short periods of 5–10 minutes at a time, always keeping excitement under control.

If you practise regularly, after three weeks or so you should see that your dog is responding very quickly to the signals you are giving and you can gradually phase out the clicks and food rewards. For further advice on how to phase out the use of rewards, see Advice sheet 17 entitled 'Using food rewards for training'.

ADVICE SHEET 9

THE 'COME AWAY' COMMAND

This training may be accomplished with or without a clicker. Please consult the handout about introducing a clicker before using one for training. If your dog shows signs of fear of the clicker noise, then contact your veterinary surgeon or behaviourist.

When puppies are young, they learn to control their fear by looking or turning away from things they find frightening and returning to their mother. This is a fundamental strategy for dealing with fear that some pet dogs do not learn. Instead they become more and more self-reliant and get into trouble by confronting the things they fear.

This training method aims to teach your dog to look or come away from things and return to you. Essentially, the dog learns to allow you to make decisions about what to do next.

PREPARATION

To do this training you must first introduce the clicker according to Advice sheet 19 and equip yourself with an extending leash and a bum bag full of treats or a toy. Start by doing training in the garden or a quiet park where your dog is relaxed and unlikely to encounter anything of which it might be fearful.

INITIAL TRAINING

- Allow your dog to walk around and explore while attached to the extending leash.
- Regularly stop and lock the leash. Take a few paces backwards and call '(your-dog's-name), come away' in a calm voice.
- When your dog turns to come to you, give a series of clicks until he is right next to you. Then give a food treat.
- Ask your dog to sit and continue giving clicks and food treats while he sits and watches you calmly.
- After 30 seconds or so, give your dog a release signal by saying 'walk on'. This tells your dog that he can go back to what he was doing before.

Once you can get your dog to come back to you in this way in a number of different places and situations, then you can try introducing it during some simulated situations involving the things he fears. In the following example the dog is fearful of a person, but your dog may be frightened of other things such as other dogs, or unfamiliar objects.

- Arrange for a person your dog might be fearful of to appear at a distance during a walk. The person should stay a long way away, perhaps 10 m or more, so that your dog's interest in them is minimal.
- Take a few paces backwards and lock the extending leash.
- Call '(your-dog's-name), come away' and begin to move away from the person.
- When your dog turns and comes toward you, start clicking.
- Give a food reward when your dog reaches you.
- Ask your dog to sit and give a series of clicks and rewards while he stays calm and gives you his attention.
- While you are doing this, the person should go away again.
- Then give the signal to 'walk on' before starting off on the walk again.

You should arrange that the person should reappear several times during your walk so that you can practise the exercise a few times. It is useful if the person appears a bit closer on some occasions so that you can check that your dog will turn away from them at a shorter distance.

Repeat this training until your dog will turn away from the person or thing that he fears immediately and reliably.

USING THE 'COME AWAY' COMMAND IN REAL SITUATIONS

Whenever you encounter real situations that your dog is afraid of, use the 'come away' command to call your dog and lead him away from whatever it is. Try to move your dog to a place where the frightening thing will stay at a distance sufficient to allow him to remain calm. Get your dog to sit down and then give a series of clicks and food rewards while the fearful thing goes away again.

ADVICE SHEET 10

THE INDOOR KENNEL

Your dog may need to be trained to spend time in an indoor kennel or crate in order to prevent him causing damage or soiling in the house. The indoor kennel must be introduced carefully and your dog must not be apprehensive of going into it. Using an indoor kennel is not cruel as long as your dog does not spend an excessive amount of time confined in this way and you provide lots of play and mental and physical stimulation when he is out of it.

Most dogs do very little when they are alone. They usually sleep and chew things while lying down. There is no reason why a comfortable and properly-sized indoor kennel cannot make an ideal sleeping and resting place for a dog. In fact, if a dog is correctly trained, he will see the crate as a safe place to be in; it will feel like a den.

HOUSE-TRAINING

Confinement in an indoor kennel is often an essential part of house-training dogs because most of them have a strong aversion to going to the toilet in their own bed area. You should follow a training method in conjunction with the use of an indoor kennel.

DESTRUCTIVENESS

Young dogs in particular have a tendency to chew things. An indoor kennel is an excellent place to leave a dog with his own things to chew so that he learns not to chew your property.

WHEN NOT TO USE AN INDOOR KENNEL

An indoor kennel should not be used for dogs that become distressed when they are left alone or for dogs that show reluctance to go into the cage. Dogs with phobia problems should not be shut into an indoor kennel when there are loud noises such as thunderstorms.

CHOICE OF INDOOR KENNEL

The most common type is a collapsible metal cage with a plastic base. These are ideal as they can be taken down and moved to other locations. The advantage of this is that, when the dog goes away from home for any period, the cage can go too, providing a safe and familiar place that the dog already knows.

The cage should not be bare; it must contain food, chews, water, toys and a comfortable place to sleep. Your dog should be able to stand up, turn around and lay down in whatever position he wishes without being cramped by the size of the cage. Many dogs like a den that is dark, so throwing a heavy blanket over the cage may help. Being a social animal, your dog will not like to be kept in a cage that is isolated from everything. It is best to position the indoor kennel close to where people usually spend most of their time so the dog does not feel left out.

TRAINING YOUR DOG TO USE THE INDOOR KENNEL

Your dog will come to like the indoor kennel if it is somewhere that he associates with the things that he likes. If he is fed there, has his chews there and gets attention whenever he is in the cage, then he will want to spend more time there.

- Make the indoor kennel as comfortable as possible for your dog to sleep in. Put his favourite bedding in there for him to sleep on. It may help to position the cage in exactly the same place where your dog normally sleeps.
- Allow your dog to use the indoor kennel as a bed at night but do not shut the door when he is in it.
- Feed all meals in the indoor kennel and leave food treats and chews there many times during the day for your dog to find.
- Regularly take your dog to the cage and put him into it before giving food treats or a chew.
- If you find your dog is in the crate, praise him.
- Leave a water bowl in the kennel for him to use.

During this initial period of acclimatisation to the cage, the door must always be left open. After a few days, you should see that your dog is happy to go in and out of the indoor kennel at will.

The next stage is to train your dog to go into the cage on command, using reward-based training. Once your dog is willing to spend longer periods in the cage on command and is choosing to go there to rest and sleep at night, then you can start to confine him in it for short periods during the day and over night.

- Put the dog into the indoor kennel to rest whenever he is tired, such as after a walk or vigorous game.
- Settle him into the cage at night and then shut the door.

The most important rules for the use of an indoor kennel are:

1. NEVER send your dog to the indoor kennel as a punishment because he may then resent going there.
2. STOP using the indoor cage if your dog shows signs of increased destructiveness, anxiety or violent attempts to break out of it.
3. Consult the behaviourist who is supervising your case if you have any problems.
4. Always provide an adequate supply of water for your dog when he is shut in the indoor kennel.

ADVICE SHEET 11

ATTENTION-SEEKING AND THE 'NO' SIGNAL

This training may be accomplished with or without a clicker. Please consult Advice sheet 19 about introducing a clicker before using one for training. If your dog shows signs of fear of the clicker noise, then contact your veterinary surgeon or behaviourist.

Dogs can turn almost any kind of behaviour into a method of attention-seeking. Frequently, they start out by seeking attention in a nice way, perhaps by nudging or licking, but they may go on to become more and more demanding. They can even end up biting, jumping on top of, or sexually mounting people. They will use anything that gets a response.

Attention-seeking can become a problem for the dog when he becomes over-dependent on reassurance from his owner. A dog that constantly seeks reassurance may not be able to cope very well without it and can become quite distressed when left alone or placed in a stressful situation. So stopping unwarranted attention-seeking behaviour is not a punishment; it is actually in the dog's best interests.

There are three main elements in stopping your dog seeking attention:

- Teaching your dog a 'stop' signal that tells him that asking you for attention will not work.
- Consistently actively ignoring all attention-seeking.
- Giving a lot of attention at other times when your dog is calm and relaxed or has done something you want him to do.

Please read this entire handout before starting any training.

THE 'NO' SIGNAL

What do dogs want when they seek attention? They want to be touched, or looked at or spoken to. Unfortunately, we often try to stop attention-seeking by looking sternly at the dog, pushing it with our hand and telling it to go away. This is little different from what the dog has been asking for and, for many dogs, it is better than being ignored. So their attention-seeking has been at least moderately successful. Being touched with a paw on the shoulder is a common 'let's play' signal that dogs use to start a game; so a young or playful dog may completely misunderstand the message we intend to give. We need to teach the dog a simple signal that shows him that his attention-seeking is going to get him nowhere, but without causing frustration and irritation.

You should repeat this routine for a few minutes several times each day. It works best if your dog is already trained with a clicker; the points at which you should use the clicker are indicated in the text.

- Two or more people sit or stand a few feet apart, each with a clicker and a bum bag or a food pot.
- One person starts by calling the dog and then asks him to sit or lie down in a calm voice '(your-dog's-name), sit'. Do not shout or get angry if your dog does not respond immediately, just wait for a moment and try again.
- While your dog remains sitting, give him a series of rewards (precede each with a click if you have a clicker). Remain very calm and relaxed, keeping your hands away from the food between rewards.
- If your dog stands up before you have finished your turn, then ask him to sit again in the same calm voice.
- After 5 to 20 consecutive rewards you can end your turn: look *away* from your dog and say 'no' calmly. There should be no anger or tension in your voice.
- When you have said 'no', the next person takes their turn by calling the dog over and going through the same procedure.

To begin with, your dog will be confused and will hang around the person who has just finished their turn, but quite quickly you will find that your dog immediately goes away from that person.

Continue to do this training every day until you can see that your 'no' signal is working effectively, both in practice and in real situations.

CONSISTENTLY IGNORING ATTENTION-SEEKING

To be effective you now need to use your 'no' signal whenever your dog seeks attention. To begin with, it helps if anyone else present then calls him away after you have said 'no'. They should ask the dog to sit and then give him some attention.

If you want to give your dog attention when he comes to ask, say 'no' and look away as before, but then ask him to sit or lie down. Continue to look away until your dog sits. Now you can turn to him and give your attention because he has done what you asked.

Key points:

- Use your 'no' signal with all forms of attention-seeking (even nudging and other friendly gestures).
- Never allow your voice to sound cross when using the 'no' signal.
- If there is anyone else present, get them to call the dog away after you have said 'no'.
- Once your dog is obeying your signal, you can cease the training sessions.

The most common times for dogs to seek attention are when you get up in the morning or come home. These are times when you must not give attention but you will also need to follow the specific training for these situations to avoid your dog getting frustrated and irritable.

GIVING ATTENTION FOR GOOD BEHAVIOUR

Your dog is used to getting plenty of attention and if you just ignore him all the time he will get frustrated and angry. Now that he is not getting attention for his misbehaviour, you must also start to give him attention for the behaviour that you to see more often. You need to make sure that you give your dog small amounts of attention very regularly throughout the time that you are with him. From now on, you need to make sure that you make a point of noticing and rewarding all of your dog's good, calm behaviour. The aim is that your dog gets at least as much attention as he was getting before, but for good behaviour instead of bad.

For example:

- Regularly say 'hello' to your dog as you walk past him while he is resting.
- Call him from his bed for a game several times each day.
- Stroke your dog gently while he is resting nearby.

You also need to get your dog to sit or lie down and wait calmly every time that you give him something. This includes:

- when allowing your dog in and out of the house
- when giving food (meals and treats)
- when giving attention
- when offering play.

ADVICE SHEET 12

CLICK-TOUCH TRAINING

This training may be accomplished with or without a clicker. Please consult Advice sheet 19 before using a clicker for training. If your dog shows signs of fear of the clicker noise, then contact your veterinary surgeon or behaviourist.

Dogs use certain kinds of pawing and touching to communicate with each other. One of the commonest is when one dog paws another on the shoulder as a sign that they are playing or want to play.

We also use touch to communicate with dogs but we have a completely different aim in mind. We want to restrain or to calm the dog. This means that when a dog gets over-excited or playful, we will reach out to try to hold them or calm them down but the dog gets completely the opposite impression and will begin to play even more vigorously, get more excited and may perhaps play-bite.

This piece of training is designed to teach dogs to associate hand contact with calmness and relaxation and is intended for dogs that show signs of one of the following:

- play-biting
- over-excitement when touched (including excitement urination)
- submissiveness when greeted or handled by a person of whom they are otherwise not frightened (including submissive urination).

This method should not be used with dogs that show any form of aggression when handled. **If your dog becomes aggressive at any time during this training, you must stop and discuss this with your behaviourist before continuing.**

GENERAL RULES

From now on your dog has to see that your hands are used for only one thing; calm and gentle stroking contact.

- You must not ruffle or tickle your dog's fur in a way that causes excitement.
- Do not grab or pull at your dog playfully or wave your hands around as an enticement to play games.
- You must not use your hands to smack or threaten your dog (holding up a raised hand and using scolding tone of voice).
- Never play rough games involving your hands; all play should be focused on toys such as those for throw-fetch and tugging games.
- Do not play wrestling games with your dog.

PREPARATIONS FOR TRAINING

- You will need a clicker and a pot or bum bag full of treats that you know your dog likes. The food treats must be very small so you can give a lot of them.

- Your dog must already be capable of responding consistently to 'sit' and 'lie down' commands.
- Your dog should be familiar with clicker-training and not frightened by the sound of the clicker.
- You should have taught your dog the meaning of the 'no' signal.

Consult the appropriate handouts if you are unsure about any of these.

TRAINING ROUTINE

- Get your food pot or bum bag and clicker.
- Ask your dog to sit or lie down (whichever is the easier for him). Give your dog 5 to 10 consecutive clicks and food rewards while he stays sitting.
- Now touch your dog with your free hand and, if he still remains sitting and calm, give a click *while your hand is still touching his body*. Then take your hand away.
- Keep your 'clicker hand' at your side and do not point the clicker at your dog during the training.
- It is absolutely vital that you do not touch or even reach towards the food until after you have given the click.
- If at any point your dog turns around to investigate your hand as you go to touch him, or if he wriggles around, shows submissive behaviour or stands up. Then take your hand away, say 'no' quite quietly and turn away for a few seconds. After this short pause, try again.
- If your dog stands up, calmly ask him to sit again before continuing.
- Repeat this sequence of touching, clicking while your hand is in contact and then rewarding until the session is over.
- Each training session should last for about 2 to 10 minutes, depending upon your dog's level of concentration.
- Repeat this training several times each day.
- Stop the training before your dog becomes bored or fractious.

Start by touching the front of your dog's chest area because this generally provokes less of a reaction. Once you can see that he is completely relaxed, then you can go on to touch the head, shoulders and the rest of the body including the legs. Do not touch any part of his body that causes growling or wariness.

Once your dog is accepting single firm touches, you can move on to single strokes. Touch your dog, make a calm stroke along his body and then stop moving the hand. Give a click at the end of the stroke while your hand is still touching.

You should then move on to stroking and clicking in this way all over the body and legs as before. Do this training in several different locations (in different parts of your home, at a friend's house, in the garden or park). It is also important to get several different people to carry out the same training. In this way your dog will behave well regardless of where he is or who is touching him.

THE END OF TRAINING

You will have completed training when you can touch your dog at any time without seeing any signs of the problem behaviour you are trying to treat. Then you need to phase out the training programme. There is advice about this in Advice sheet 17, but a summary is as follows:

- Stop clicking and rewarding every touch or stroke.
- Instead, click and reward after a randomly variable number of touches and strokes.
- Start by clicking and rewarding randomly after 1–5 strokes. Then after every 1–10, 1–20, etc.
- You must only go to a lower rate of rewarding when it is clear that your dog is still performing correctly and consistently.
- When your dog has learned to accept more strokes before he gets his click, the reward he finally gets must be a bit bigger so that it was worth waiting for.

The last step before phasing out training altogether is to keep one or two food rewards in your pocket and give your dog an occasional treat after you have been stroking him for a few seconds.

ADVICE SHEET 13

PREPARATIONS FOR PHOBIC EVENTS (FIREWORKS AND THUNDER)

Preparation is all-important if dogs are to get through fireworks or thunderstorms with the minimum of fear and stress. First you need to make a special place where your dog can go to get away from the sounds he fears. Most dogs will already have a favourite room to go to, in which case all you need to do is to modify this place to make it even more suitable as a bolt-hole.

Some dogs do not know where to go to escape and, for these individuals, you need to create somewhere for them to hide. It is best to choose a room that is naturally quiet and those that are located toward the centre of the house and have minimal numbers of windows are the most suitable.

It is best to prepare the refuge as far ahead of the firework event as you can. Your dog must always be able to get to this place whenever he is frightened.

ADVANCE PREPARATION: CREATING A REFUGE:

- Install a Dog Appeasing Pheromone (DAP®) diffuser in the home, preferably close to or inside the dog's hiding place. The DAP® diffuser is a device that looks like an air freshener that you plug into a wall socket. It produces a smell that is like a chemical that your dog's mother used to calm her puppies. DAP® diffusers are available from your vet and should be left operating 24 hours a day. If possible, install the diffuser a couple of weeks before a known event, like fireworks, as this will produce a more powerful effect. DAP® makes dogs feel much more relaxed and confident when they might otherwise be stressed.
- Put in lots of blankets for your dog to dig and burrow in, preferably placed in a corner where the dog has already tended to dig or hide. Include an old, unwashed piece of clothing, like a woolly jumper, so that your dog can smell your scent and feel comforted by your indirect presence.
- Try to minimise the amount of noise entering the bolthole room from outside. The dog must not see the flashes of fireworks or lightning, so close the windows and use heavy curtains to make the room dark.
- Bowls of food and water are essential and it is a good idea to make sure that your dog has emptied his bladder an hour or so before the storm or firework event starts.
- Leave a few special chews and things for your dog to eat in the hiding place in case he fancies something chewy to reduce his tension. However, do not be alarmed if he does not seem interested in them – some dogs are simply not interested in treats at a time like this.
- Moderately loud rhythmic music with a good beat is an effective way to mask the firework noises from out-side, so put a hi-fi system in the room and keep the volume at a loud but comfortable level. However, every dog is an individual and if yours is not very partial to music at other times you should respect his personal taste!
- The designated hiding place must be accessible to your dog at all times and it is vital that you make sure that doors are fixed so that they cannot accidentally shut and trap the pet inside or out of the room.
- Get your dog used to going to the hiding place 2 to 3 times each day during the run up to a firework display by taking him there and giving him some food or a favourite chew. This will help the dog to understand that this is a good place to go to.
- If you know that a firework display is due on a particular evening, then give your dog a large, stodgy, carbohydrate-rich meal in the late afternoon of that day. Pasta, mashed potato or overcooked rice are ideal and will help to make your dog feel calm and sleepy as the night draws in.
- Make sure your pet is kept in a safe and secure environment at all times so that he doesn't bolt and escape if a sudden noise occurs. Keep your dog on a leash in public places and make sure that gates, fences and doors are secure.

If your vet has given you medication to reduce your dog's fears, make sure you follow the prescription precisely.

WHEN THE NOISES START:

- As soon as the fireworks display starts, lead your dog to the hiding place and encourage him to stay there.
- Do not get cross with your dog when he is scared as it will only make him more frightened.
- It is tempting to try to soothe your dog to relieve his fears but this is the worst thing to do. It gives your dog the impression that there is something to be frightened of and may even reward him for being scared. Also, if your dog comes to think of you as the only person who can soothe his fears, he may panic if there are fireworks when you are not around to help.
- Ignore your dog when he is looking frightened and only show attention and affection when he has begun to relax. Then you can give your dog a game and some food treats as a reward.
- It is a good idea to try to keep your dog in a happy mood by playing lots of games and doing little bits of training using food rewards. This will stop him from falling into a state of anxious tension, but do not expect too much.
- Ignore the noises yourself and try to appear happy and relaxed. If your pet is only mildly fearful, you could try to engage him in some form of active game. Try to appear happy and unconcerned. It can help if you play a game with another pet in the household because the frightened one may be tempted to join in.

- If your pet is very frightened by the noises and cannot be encouraged to play, then lead him to the refuge you have created.

If your dog is really terrified of fireworks then you could give him some earplugs to block out some of the noise. Doggy earplugs are easy to get from pet stores and your vet, but you can also make them out of rolls of wrung-out damp cotton wool. However, it is important to take care and to make sure that you do not push them too far down into your dog's ear. You must also make sure that you remove them and throw them away afterwards. Care must be taken that the earplug is not so thin that it falls out, or so fat it hurts when you put it in.

Lastly, having got through fireworks this year, you need to start to do something about your dog's phobia problems. Many dogs can be treated using behavioural methods called desensitisation and counterconditioning. Specially made recordings of fireworks can be used to train dogs not to react to the noises they fear. CDs of fireworks, thunder and other noises are sold under the brand name 'Sounds Scary' and are available through your vet.

ADVICE SHEET 14

USING TRAINING DISCS OR A RATTLE CAN

Training discs or a rattle can are used to create what we call 'conditioned avoidance' behaviour.

The discs or can are in themselves not frightening; if you threw them across the room for your dog then there is a good chance that he would bring them back to you or try to play with them!

There is nothing special about the discs or can. They do not make a special sort of sound; they just make a noise that most dogs are not already familiar with. It is perfectly possible to create exactly the same response with a bunch of keys or a range of other objects but training discs or a rattle can are easy to use.

The way we use them is to create a connection in the dog's mind between the sound of the discs or can and failure to get an expected reward. We are all familiar with methods of punishment that involve taking things away; depriving children of pocket money, for example. The trouble is that we cannot tell a dog that he will be deprived of something because he cannot understand what we are telling him that well. The discs or can give us a way of achieving this, while also making the dog understand *failure*.

Training discs can be bought from most pet shops or you can make up a rattle can. The rattle can is just an old drinks can with a handful of small pebbles in it. The top is sealed with some tape. The sound is better if you scrunch the sides of the can a bit.

Introducing the discs or can is simple. It is possible to introduce the discs on your own but, if you find it hard to co-ordinate all the things you are supposed to do, then get someone to assist. If you need help, get the other person to control the food while you use the discs. Otherwise the procedure is just the same:

- Get some really lovely food treats that excite your dog and put them in a pot.
- Hold the fabric loop of the discs with the last three fingers of one hand so that the discs themselves fall comfortably between your thumb and forefinger. That way you can hold them silently but also use them to make a loud rattle if you relax your grip and shake your wrist. Alternatively, hold the rattle can by the top so that you can shake it easily.
- Take some small pieces of food in the other hand.
- Start by just putting some food down onto the floor, one piece at a time, for your dog to eat. Wave the food around as you bring it to the ground so that he shows real signs of anticipating something nice.
- Do not let go of the food as you put it onto the floor in front of your dog; let him take it from your fingers as they hold the food on the floor.

Do this 5 to 10 times so the dog is *expecting* food to be given.

Once your dog thinks he knows what is going to happen and is almost following your hand to the floor ready to get the food, then we are ready to go on to the next stage.

Now it is time for the discs or rattle can.

- Take a piece of food and go as if to put it on the floor as you have done before.
- As you put it down on the floor and your dog goes to take it, give the discs or can a loud shake behind your back.
- Snatch the food away before your dog can get it.
- Your dog will probably seem puzzled.
- Repeat this procedure several times.
- After a few repetitions your dog will probably back away a couple of paces when the discs or can rattle. You may see slight signs of anxiety, such as lip licking.

Repeat the procedure with the discs until your dog is startled by the sound of the discs (or can) and does not try to take the food. Usually this happens within four trials. It is very likely that the dog will seek refuge with another family member that is in the area. As soon as the dog runs to them after the sound of the discs they should be friendly and encouraging. This rewards the dog for showing the avoidance behaviour. That is all that is needed to introduce the discs and they can now be used in training.

The important thing about the discs is that the response to them is learned; the discs are not in themselves something to fear. The fear that is developed is a fear of *failure*; not getting a reward that was expected.

When used during training exercises, the discs must only be used to indicate some sort of failure; in other words, if you rattle the discs and the dog sometimes does manage to get the food, then the fear of the discs would disappear.

For example, when the discs or can are used to train a dog to stop barking at the front door, it is important that the person at the door does not go away until the dog *stops* barking. Remember that the reason why the dog may be barking is as a warning to the intruder to send them away. The dog will feel *rewarded* when they go and if, when the discs are used, the person does go while the dog is still barking, then the dog learns to ignore the discs.

From now on you should use the discs as a primary method of punishment wherever you want to stop your dog from doing something wrong. The situations in which you should use the discs are covered in the text.

Whenever you use the discs or can you should try to keep them slightly out of the dog's sight. Do not rattle them at the dog, otherwise he will realise what is going on and may come to ignore them. Occasionally, the power of the discs reduces with time and you need to 'recharge' them by repeating the introductory procedure.

ADVICE SHEET 15

HOUSE-TRAINING

For hygiene reasons, all dogs should be trained to urinate and defecate on command and in an appropriate place.

FIRST, SOME THINGS TO AVOID

Never use physical punishment (smacking) when a dog goes to the toilet in the wrong place as this will just make the dog more secretive and difficult to house-train. Rubbing a dog's nose in what it has done will teach the dog nothing, but it will make a horrible mess. If you find a mess that your dog has done earlier you must not punish him, even verbally.

DEALING WITH MISTAKES

Mistakes will happen, and your dog will occasionally soil in the house until he is fully house-trained.

- If you catch your dog making a mess somewhere, then say 'no' in a calm voice (not angrily) and quickly take him to the place where you want him to go to the toilet. Then reward him for finishing off there.
- If you find a mess your dog has done earlier, just clean it up. Do not get cross with him.

When you clean up, try to avoid strong-smelling cleaners like bleach or pine-scented disinfectant. These may mark the place with a strong smell that encourages the dog to use it as a latrine. Instead, use odourless cleaners after you have thoroughly cleaned the area with soapy water. After cleaning, apply a biologically-based scent-free deodoriser spray.

HOUSE-TRAINING METHOD

Dogs tend to need to go to the toilet within 20 minutes of a meal or a period of sleep. You should take your dog to the toilet area at these times and regularly every 90 minutes during the day (every 60 minutes for puppies) until you can see a pattern to when your dog needs to go to the toilet.

Designate a toilet place in the garden. It should be an obvious place, preferably somewhere that your dog has previously used. If you have to mop up urine in the house then wring the cloths out onto this toilet spot occasionally so that it is marked as a latrine.

- At the appropriate times, calmly put your dog on a leash and take him into the garden. Remain completely passive and do not interact with your dog in any way.
- Walk to the toilet spot and circle is a couple of times. Continue to stay calm and ignore your dog.
- Stand still and quietly mutter the command you want your dog to respond to.
- Wait for up to 5 minutes.
- If your dog goes to the toilet wait until he is almost finished. If you are using clicker-training, then give a click just as your dog is finishing going to the toilet. Give a reward, praise and attention. Let your dog off the leash to sniff around the garden. Play a game for a couple of minutes.
- If your dog does not go to the toilet, silently lead him back inside without even taking the leash off. Try taking your dog outside again a little later.

As you repeat this training, you should gradually raise the level of your voice to a normal level of speech when you give the command. You will find that your dog rapidly comes to understand that he should go to the toilet whenever let into the garden or given a command. You can test this by following the same house-training routine when you go to the park. In public places it may not be acceptable to allow your dog to run free, so you may have to use a strong extending leash to control your dog during play.

It is also important to restrict your dog's ability to make mistakes. Keep your dog supervised at all times when you are at home and take him to go to the toilet before you go out. Also consider using an indoor kennel to confine your dog while you are out. If you do use an indoor kennel, your dog must be acclimatised to it first (see Advice sheet 10). Talk to your behaviourist about this. Dogs will rarely soil their own bed area so this prevents accidents while you are not around. A normal dog may take 3 to 4 weeks to become reasonably well house-trained, but a dog that has grown up without any training, or that has been incorrectly trained using strong punishment, may take longer to learn.

ADVICE SHEET 16

ENVIRONMENTAL ENRICHMENT FOR DOGS

Wild dogs spend a lot of time finding and eating food. They wander in search of prey, hunt and catch it or scavenge for the remains of other animals' successful hunts. In the domestic situation, dogs eat all of their food in just a few seconds which means that they are left with an enormous amount of excess time. This results in under-stimulation, boredom and problem behaviour, such as destructiveness. To avoid this we need to make dogs work for their food in ways that simulate the sorts of things they would normally do in the wild.

If we do not provide suitable ways for dogs to use up their time and energy, then we run the risk that they will find things to amuse themselves, many of which we will not like. This is especially true for younger dogs that are, by their nature, more active and more inclined to find things to do.

Chewing behaviour is particularly important to dogs. They use it to soothe themselves when they are anxious and to occupy themselves when they are bored. It is impossible to suppress this behaviour but we can redirect it in a way that reduces damage to our own property.

SUGGESTED ACTIVITIES FOR DOGS

Activity feeding (food finding)

- Scatter part of the dog's food on the lawn for the dog to find (or in the park if there are no other dogs around)
- Use ready made activity feeders (Activity ball, Puzzle Ball®, Buster Cube®, Havaball®)
- Make home-made feeders from empty plastic bottles with the lid taken off (these can be suspended at dog height for the dog to knock food out of).
- Hide food in a number of locations around the garden (under pots, in buckets, etc.).
- Feed most of your dog's food through activity feeding in several short sessions each day.

Digging

Redirect this to a more suitable location, such as a country park.

Most dogs will mimic digging behaviour displayed by the owner: simply make an excited digging action on a patch of earth while saying 'dig, dig, dig'. The majority of dogs will learn to dig on command within a few minutes.

Submerge an empty bucket in the soil. Put a small dog chew in it and lightly sprinkle with earth. Show the dog so that it removes the chew. Repeat daily, each time increasing the depth of earth until the bucket is two-thirds full. You could also put a rock on the top or experiment with other ways of burying things.

Destructiveness

Some dogs (particularly young ones) need to have things to destroy. This desire to destroy things is part of growing up and declines as the dog matures. Likewise, anxious or unsettled dogs will show signs of increased destructiveness, which is also often temporary. Good targets for destructive behaviour include:

- empty cardboard boxes and cardboard tubes to tear up
- tightly-rolled-up newspapers to rip up (with food treats rolled inside).

Prey catching and handling behaviour

Play throw-fetch games to redirect chase behaviour.

Throw a ball, toy or Frisbee® back and forth between two people (let the dog get it occasionally and give a treat for success).

Provide toys for shaking and biting:

- squeaky
- with parts that flap when shaken.

Provide good safe targets for chewing:

- nylon bones
- edible chews as part of daily diet.

ADVICE SHEET 17

USING FOOD REWARDS FOR TRAINING

WHAT IS A SUITABLE FOOD REWARD?

Most dogs are willing to work for some kind of food reward; it is just a matter of discovering what it is they like. We tend to pick prepackaged dog treats because they are convenient and are marketed to look appealing but, in many cases, they are quite bland and flavourless so dogs are not that keen to work for them.

Dogs have very individual and sometimes surprising tastes so it is best to experiment with a wide range of highly flavoured foods.

Try *small* pieces of:

- fruit and vegetables
- sausages and cooked meats
- biscuits
- cheese.

It is easy to judge the value your dog places on the food treat by the level of anticipation he shows. A lot of wagging and enthusiasm means that your dog finds what you are giving him to be really delicious. It is a good idea to make a mental note of how much your dog likes various treats so that you can give better rewards for really good behaviour or when you need something that your dog will really work hard to get. Dogs that are a little frightened or anxious, or are simply very excited, may suffer from a dry mouth, so these dogs need moist rather than dry treats.

HOW TO USE FOOD

Food is an effective form of reward but the dog may become dependent on food treats and may not work without the lure of a food treat. This can be avoided by using clicker-training and by using food rewards properly. Some dogs do not respond at all to food rewards and prefer play or human contact as a reward. The following use food as a reward but, under guidance, you can use other rewards as an alternative.

The rules for using reward are:

Stage 1: Decide on the kind of behaviour you want to see and then reward the dog for doing it

Repeat the cycle of issuing commands, waiting for response and then giving a reward within two seconds of a response. In the case of clicker-training, the click is delivered as soon as the dog obeys the command and then the food reward can be given anything up to 5 seconds later.

The aim for this stage is to get your dog to respond consistently to every command but not to worry too much about how good each actual response is. It is also a good idea to give occasional extra-good bonus rewards at random so that your dog is always anticipating something really good.

Stage 2: Improving performance

For the first few performances, all you want is something *close* to what you want, then you can start to perfect it. During stage one a sloppy or slow sit is enough but during Stage 2 you want to give a better reward for a better performance. Decide what the *perfect* response is (for example, a really fast sit or greater concentration in a distracting environment). From now on, responses that are closer to the ideal get a better reward (nicer food or a bigger reward or both). Hone the response until the performance is *perfect*. You must continue to give your occasional bonus rewards but, instead of giving them randomly, you must give them for better behaviour.

Stage 3: Reduce the rate of rewarding, but leave performance intact

Once the behaviour is perfect, you need to reduce the dependence on reward and make the learning more permanent. The best way to do this is to make the dog work harder for each reward, but give bigger rewards. This is very simple: just ask the dog to perform several acts of obedience but only reward a few of them. Sometimes reward the first time your dog does what you want and sometimes the fifth, and so on. When you do give a reward it needs to be a bigger one, so your dog is anticipating something really good.

During Stage 3 your dog will have no idea whether his 1st, 5th or 10th performance is going to get a reward, but he knows that he will lose all that he has worked for if he fails to respond on the last occasion when the food is finally going to be given. This relies on the same piece of psychology that keeps people putting money into one-armed-bandits. After putting 20 coins into the machine, they cannot risk not putting in the 21st because that might be the time when the payoff comes. Instead, they use up every last coin in their pocket.

There has to be an upper limit to the size of the reward you give so, if you get down to rewarding every 50th performance, you cannot give 50 bits of food. But this is also exactly the same as the slot machine; the top prize pay-out is never as much as the money put into the machine. After a while, the dog is not working for an actual reward. It is working for the anticipation that one *might* come.

You can also alternate the reward. Sometimes give a pat on the head, sometimes food and sometimes a game; this also increases the addiction because the dog can never be sure what the reward will be. Concentrate on training one thing at each session of training and do not start giving random rewards until the dog is doing all of the things you want, exactly as you would like.

If you are using 'clicker-training', it is important to remember that the clicker must *always* indicate the delivery of a reward. To wean dogs off reward with a clicker you follow the same routine as above; start by clicking every behaviour you want, then click better behaviours and give a better reward after the click. Finally click and reward randomly and give extra good rewards, just as mentioned above.

Other general tips:

- Always precede *every* command with the dog's name said in a high-pitched musical voice (e.g., 'Freddy, come').
- When training at home, try to use a very quiet voice so that your dog gets used to concentrating on it.
- Do not shout or get cross because the dog will then be put off by the tone of your voice and will ignore what you are saying.

It is easy to understand why; if someone shouted angrily at you in a foreign language, what would you do? I would think about running away and that is exactly what a dog will often think about too.

By talking quietly, and always using the dog's name, you are teaching him to listen to what you are saying, which enables him to concentrate better.

ADVICE SHEET 18

FOOD FOR WORK

As the title suggests, this regime is designed to make your dog work to get his food so that he is less bored and his motivation to do training is improved. It can also be a good way to help combat obesity.

Wild and feral carnivores have to search for and catch their food. Food is essential for an animal's survival and the clearest measure of success they can have in any given situation is whether they get the food or not. Every step in the sequence of finding, capturing and killing the prey is essential to success, as failure at any stage results in the loss of a meal. So animals very rapidly learn to refine the way they hunt for food so that they maximise success.

Wild dogs learn to use their time and energy effectively, because, if they did not, they would starve to death. They have to spend a proportion of their time every day finding food and they are compelled to take advantage of easy opportunities. The food-for-work regime takes advantage of the dog's natural instinct.

It can seem cruel to alter the way that your dog is fed but remember that dogs are opportunists and scavengers; they were designed to live by their wits. The captive environment is unnatural to them and many dogs are very bored by a life in which everything is provided for them. That is why some of them develop bad habits; it is a way of using up their excess time and taking a degree of control over their environment. A food-for-work regime gives dogs something to think about and more to do.

The food-for-work regime is simply that; the dog only gets food through activity feeding or as a reward for performance during training.

The rules are simple:

- No complete meals out of a bowl. Only put a very small amount of food in the bowl at meal times.
- Gradually phase out 'bowl feeding' altogether.

- Give no indiscriminate titbits or treats. Your dog must work for every scrap of food.
- Follow the rules of how and when to reward (on other handouts).

It is important that, to begin with, your dog still gets some food out of a bowl at meal times, otherwise he will wonder what on earth is going on. After all, the aim is not to make your dog feel insecure about where his meals come from. After a couple of weeks you should gradually reduce the amount of food given from a bowl and, instead, give this food through activity feeding at meal times. You will probably find that your dog becomes more excited about feeding and really enjoys using the feeders.

The first step is to plan what you are going to feed:

- Measure out the total amount of food, including treats, that you are going to give each day.
- Divide this into portions that are to be given through activity feeding and portions for training.
- Save the best bits of food for use as rewards during training.

This makes every food reward into an opportunity. Perhaps getting food out of an activity feeder is hard work, whereas coming on command to get a food treat is so easy that the dog would be foolish to miss out. So command responses improve.

Next you need to plan your dog's feeding activities:

- For suggestions on activity feeding see Advice sheet 16.
- Plan some training exercises according to the training or behavioural plan you have been given.

Remember that your dog will be hungry and you need to provide several activity feeding and training opportunities each day. Training sessions may, on some occasions, be quite short but you need to do at least a couple every day.

Once your programme of behavioural therapy and training has finished, you can phase out the training part of the food-for-work regime and simply give your dog all his food through activity feeding.

ADVICE SHEET 19

INTRODUCING THE CLICKER

The clicker is a small plastic device which emits a loud clicking sound when the metal tongue inside it is pressed. It is used as part of the process of training dogs (or cats) and treating their behaviour problems.

Before using the clicker as part of training, it must be introduced so that the animal understands what the noise means. The animal is trained to associate the sound of the click with being given a reward (usually food). This uses the same principle of conditioning that Pavlov used to train dogs to salivate when they heard a bell.

Once this association has been made, the click can be used to indicate to the dog the *exact* bit of behaviour that we want him to do again.

HOW IS THIS DIFFERENT FROM TRADITIONAL METHODS?

Dogs and cats are best at understanding reward when it comes within just 2 *seconds* of their doing something. Beyond this time, learning is poor or non-existent. The clicker can be used to indicate precisely what is being rewarded, although the reward does not need to be given immediately after the click; there can be a delay of up to a few seconds.

This enables us to train at a distance and to choose a very precise moment to reward.

Clicker-training does not depend upon the animal learning a command word before it learns the action. Clicker-training can be used to teach quite complicated behaviour that would otherwise be very difficult to achieve.

HOW TO START

Some dogs or cats find the noise of the clicker too loud and alarming so the first step is to introduce it quietly.

- Get a pot containing some *small* pieces of your pet's favourite food treats and get the clicker.
- Muffle the clicker at first by sitting on the hand that is holding the clicker. Make a click and watch your pet's reaction. If he looks interested but relaxed, then give a food reward.
- **If your pet looks frightened or wants to get away, then you should contact the person who is supervising the treatment of your pet's problem to ask for extra help.**

If your pet was happy with the first click, then give several more clicks, each followed by a food reward. Try, if possible, not to reach for the food or hold any in your hand until after you have made the click.

Next, take your hand out from under your leg and give 20 or so more clicks, each followed by a food reward. **Again, if at any time your dog looks unsettled or fearful, then stop and contact your veterinary surgeon or behaviourist.** After this introduction, your dog or cat should look pleased or excited whenever he hears a click.

You are now ready to start training with the clicker, but remember the rules:

- Never give a click without giving a reward.
- Never use the sound of the clicker to get your pet's attention; you only give a click *after* he has responded to a command.
- Try to avoid handling food until you have given the click. Training works less well if you are fiddling with food all the time because your pet won't be concentrating on what he is doing when the next click happens.

The basic method for teaching commands using clicker-training is to lure the dog or cat into performing an action, or allow it to happen naturally, and then to selectively click and reward the behaviour that you want to train to a command. Once your pet is doing exactly what you want, you can then give that behaviour a 'name' so that your pet knows that this is what you want him to do when he hears that command.

Here is an example for training a 'sit' command:

- Sit down with a pot of your dog's favourite food treats on your lap, along with a clicker.
- Stay still and wait for your dog to sit down.
- Ignore or fend off all behaviour other than sitting.
- When your pet sits down, you should click as soon as his backside hits the floor and then give him a food treat.
- If your pet stays sitting then give another click and food treat, otherwise wait until he sits down again.

You should find that the amount of time your pet spends sitting down increases dramatically over the course of the first 10 minutes or so and that he stops doing all of the other things he was trying in order to get the food from you, such as jumping up or whimpering or running around.

When you know that your pet is sitting down again very reliably and quickly after collecting each treat, then you can start to introduce the word 'sit':

- As your pet begins to sit down spontaneously say '(your pet's name), sit' and then wait. As soon as he sits down give a click and food reward.
- Repeat this 20 to 30 times and your pet will have made the initial association between the command word 'sit' and what he should do to get the food.

You should now practise getting your pet to sit in a number of other situations, giving clicks and rewards for an obedient response.

ADVICE SHEET 20

THE 'LEAVE' COMMAND

You may already have trained your dog to leave things using another word, but it is important to start training this word again from scratch. It is very important to choose a command word that is easy for you to remember because you are likely to be using this command at times when an incident is about to happen and you need to regain control rapidly.

'Leave' or 'leave it' work very well because they are easy to remember but if you have already used these commands before, then you may want to use something else.

The purpose of this training is to teach your dog to look at you in preference to looking at other things. The 'other things' might include a stranger of whom the dog is fearful, a cyclist, another dog, some food on the pavement or almost anything else.

First you need to train your dog to look at you when there isn't much else to think about.

To do this training you will need a clicker, some food treats and a quiet place to train where there are no distractions. The function of the clicker must be introduced according to Advice sheet 19.

STAGE 1

- Take a food treat in each hand, holding them tightly.
- Hold one hand close to the dog so that he can investigate it but could also easily look into your face without moving his head very far.
- Keep the other hand out of the way.
- Say '(your dog's name)', leave' whilst the dog investigates your closed hand.
- As soon as he looks away from the treat, give a click and let him have the reward from the *free hand* (the one that the dog *was not allowed to investigate*).

It is important that the click is timed to the precise moment when the dog looks away from the hand being held out. Repeat this 20+ times, or until your dog is looking away from the hand each time you give the command.

STAGE 2

Repeat the same procedure as above, but this time only give the treat when the dog looks into your eyes (even if only for a moment).

Practise holding the hand with the food in different positions, on the floor, outstretched and even moving, so that your dog becomes used to looking away from the hand whatever it is doing.

Move on to the next stage when your dog will look into your eyes for a few seconds after being commanded to 'leave'.

STAGE 3

Choose a toy or other object in which your dog has moderate interest, and which will not prove so distracting that he will not be able to concentrate on the training. Put your dog on an extending leash so that you can exercise control.

- Place the toy on the ground and say '(your dog's name),' leave'.
- Give a click and then a food reward if your dog looks away from the toy and back at you.
- Pause for a few seconds and then say 'take it'.
- Play a short game, lasting less than 30 seconds, with the toy.
- Repeat this exercise, gradually allowing the toy to roll as you put it on the floor.
- The aim is to build up from putting the toy onto the floor, to rolling it gently, then rolling it faster and finally throwing it whilst still keeping your dog from chasing the toy by using the 'leave' command.

Progress will be slow and gradual and you must use the extending leash to prevent your dog from chasing the toy if he gets carried away.

STAGE 4

Now you can move on to applying the same basic training with a wider range of toys, objects or pieces of food that you have dropped.

You must only say 'take it' when your dog is allowed to interact with the object or eat the food that you have dropped *after* he has obeyed the 'leave' command.

Once your dog is able to 'leave' a wide range of test toys and objects, then you can use this command in real situations where you want your dog to leave something alone. In these situations, you may or may not have a clicker, but you should always reward your dog with food or play.

Appendix 3

CONTENTS

ADVICE SHEET 1

IMPROVING THE OUTDOOR ENVIRONMENT FOR CATS

Making alterations to the outdoor environment for your cat has the benefits of:

- increasing the space available to your cat(s)
- reducing competition for resources such as latrines and resting places within the home
- enabling the cat to successfully maintain the garden as territory.

Cats control access to their territory using scent marks and by watching and threatening their enemies form vantage points. The garden must therefore be filled with hiding and climbing places as well as posts for scratching. This will also tend to reduce undesirable scratching that is carried out indoors.

PROVIDING OUTDOOR TOILETS

House-soiling problems tend to be worse in the winter, which is probably because outdoor latrines become difficult or unappealing for the cat to use. Hard, frozen ground is difficult to dig and waterlogged, heavy soil is messy and unpleasant for the cat. Remember that cats are evolved from desert-living ancestors.

Outdoor toilets reduce your cat's need to have an indoor litter tray or can help to reduce the number of indoor litter trays needed in a multi-cat household. They can be constructed easily to make them low-maintenance and available for the cat to use all year round.

- Find a suitable location for the latrine at the edge of the garden, obscured by flowerbeds and bushes to give the cat some privacy.
- Dig a hole that is approximately 60–90 cm deep and 60–90 cm square.
- Fill the bottom two-thirds of the hole with pea-sized gravel for good drainage.

- Top up the hole with soft, white sand. Use playground quality sand and not the orange type used for building (known as sharp sand).
- Once your cat is using the latrine regularly, you can scatter a little earth over the top to disguise it.
- Use a litter scoop to remove any faeces, as you would with a conventional indoor tray.
- Dig out and replace the sand every few months to refresh the latrine.

Sand latrines get neither waterlogged nor frozen and they give the cat an easily accessible toilet close to the house. Some cats cannot find a proper latrine in their own garden and have to go several houses away to find a suitable location. Apart from increasing the probability of a house-soiling problem if that latrine ceases to be available, it also tends to annoy neighbours.

SCRATCHING PLACES

Outdoor scratching places should be provided at the edge of the garden so that the cat can control access to its territory. These are simply made from softwood posts which have been rubbed against existing scratching places to pick up claw marking odours. The surface is scratched with a wire brush to simulate scratch marks as this often attracts further scratching.

HIDING PLACES AND VANTAGE POINTS

Your cat needs some easily-defended vantage points in the garden where it can rest and observe other cats. There are many ways to do this:

- Fix shelves to fences and walls outside.
- Put wooden platforms into trees.
- Clear a shelf for the cat to sit on by a window in a garden shed.

The most important aspect of these places is that they must be set up to face *away* from the house and into the garden. In this way they do not allow other cats to use them to observe the house or cat flap. Block the view of the house using the natural arrangement of trees and shrubs in the garden, enhanced with planters and other features.

If your cat is hesitant to go out and hangs around the cat flap for long periods or often rushes in as if being pursued, then it is helpful to place a few hiding places close to the exit of the cat flap. For example, position a few planters outside so that, if chased, your cat may hide rather than run inside. This reduces the tendency to spray around the inside of the cat flap. It also means that your cat can sneak out into the garden without being watched by other cats. However, you may have to make other arrangements if you have a local feline despot or intact tomcat, as these cats may lurk right outside the cat door waiting to attack your cat.

If your garden is largely open space with no planted borders, this can prove difficult for cats. Unless the area is devoid of any form of threat, they find traversing large open spaces quite intimidating. If possible, try to provide plenty of shrubs, trees, and planters that break up open spaces and provide secluded walkways at the edge of the garden for the cat to use.

BLOCKING ACCESS BY OTHER CATS

Mostly, cats are not concerned when other cats traverse their territory because it is normal for this to happen. Problems arise when other cats lurk in the garden, using their own vantage points to observe and threaten your cat, either in its own home or when it tries to enter the garden.

Guidance on how to deal with this in the home is included in Advice sheet 2 about improving the indoor environment for cats, but it is also possible to modify the garden to deter other cats.

Steps to take:

- Identify all vantage points other cats use to observe your cat in the home and garden.
- Block the view from these places: plant shrubs or place planters and other obstacles to obstruct the view. For example, trellis fence can be erected at the top of a wall to stop cats from watching from a neighbour's garage or shed roof.
- Make vantage points uncomfortable for other cats to use: knock long (8–10 cm), flat-headed nails into the top of wooden fences or posts, spaced about 4 to 6 cm apart to stop cats sitting there. They will still be able to walk along and stand, but not be able to lurk and threaten. Alternatively, fix pieces of spiky plastic doormat or commercially available intruder-deterrent plastic spikes onto fences, posts, and other places where cats sit.

Do not use broken glass or other hazardous deterrents as they may injure cats very badly.

ADVICE SHEET 2

IMPROVING THE INDOOR ENVIRONMENT FOR CATS

Cats use and rely on their environment in a different way from other animals. The inside of the home should be considered the 'core' of the cat's territory. This is somewhere that the cat expects to feel safe and where it can eat, drink and rest in privacy away from potential enemies. Cats also make more use of three-dimensional space than people or dogs; they are keen to climb up high to vantage points where they feel safe.

It is important to provide cats with a home environment that meets their needs, especially in multi-cat households, residential areas that are overpopulated with cats or when cats do not have outdoor access. Otherwise, there is a significant risk of frustration, stress and behavioural problems, such as aggression, house-soiling or urine marking.

In almost all cases, it is preferable to give cats outdoor access but, when this is impossible some reason, it is even more important that the indoor environment provides all of the cat's needs.

RECOGNISING INDICATORS OF STRESS

Stressed cats are often hard to spot because, in most cases, they become quiet and introverted when they are unhappy.

Typical signs of stress include:

Excessive grooming: This may result in bald or sore patches.

Lack of activity: Cats that stop playing become reluctant to move about or eat. When in close proximity to each other, the cats may move very slowly as they are frightened of being chased or attacked.

Hiding: The cat spends most of its time hiding in the same place and will not come out to feed or interact.

Ease of startle: The cat is very jumpy and will startle at sudden movements or sounds.

Wariness or fighting around resources: The cat seems hesitant to approach cat-doors, food and latrines. When they are in these locations they may seem very nervous. Hissing and spitting may be seen when other cats approach.

A household full of very passive cats that seem to spend all their time sitting still and watching each other probably indicates a high degree of stress.

The cat's basic needs are for:

- space (including access to height)
- an abundance of resources (food, water, latrines, resting places)
- opportunities to perform normal behaviour (hunting, clawing, etc.)
- privacy.

Space

Cats should be provided with lots of opportunity to climb and explore. Provide shelves at different heights, cat furniture and clear the tops of cupboards and wardrobes so that the cats can gain access to them.

Resources

Cats need several places to eat, drink and rest. This gives them choice and means that, if two cats do not get along, then they need not compete for the same toilet or food bowl. Enabling the cats to live separate lives actually increases the chances that they will get along.

Choice over resting places is particularly important because cats move from one place to another regularly to avoid their own parasites (such as fleas).

A common formula for the number of separate latrines needed in a multi-cat household is 1 per cat +1. This means 9 cat toilets for 8 cats! This is because cats do not share latrines in the wild and they like to have separate ones for urine and faeces. Fortunately, it is possible to provide really good outdoor toilets for cats so that the number of litter trays needed is reduced.

Cats also have a different thirst response from dogs and people, which means that they may not consume enough water to maintain healthy kidneys and a healthy urinary system. Cats can be encouraged to drink more healthy amounts by providing them with a recirculating-type water fountain. These are available commercially and include a carbon filter to remove water impurities that cats dislike (such as chlorine). This makes the water taste more appealing, like rainwater. The water movement and provision of a running water slope make it much easier for the cat to drink.

Opportunities to perform normal behaviour

Clawing is often a problem because it is destructive and annoying for owners.

Further information about problem clawing is provided in Advice sheet 5 but it is even more important to give cats opportunities to claw so that it does not become a problem in the first place.

Cats typically claw:

- to stretch back muscles after waking
- to mark boundaries of territory
- to sharpen claws
- to gain attention.

Appropriate places to position clawing posts are therefore:

- close to resting places
- near to cat doors and in the garden
- in living rooms close to furniture (where the cat may claw for attention).

Cats have preferences for particular kinds of material to claw. Upholstered furniture is often used for claw sharpening and stretching. Soft wood is often used for marking boundaries. Experiment with providing the right surfaces to suit the cat's clawing needs. Encourage clawing by taking notice and praising when your cat claws on an object that you want to be used for clawing.

Hunting and play are important for cats, especially in the early morning and evening. These are times when it is important to encourage interactive games using fishing toys, laser pointers and lightweight toys rolled on the floor. Under no circumstances encourage play involving people's feet or hands because this can create problems of predatory aggression, especially for cats that are kept indoors.

At other times, the cat should be provided with a continually changing range of small lightweight toys to play with. Keep a selection of feathers, decorated table-tennis balls, furry mouse toys and similar small items in a box. Scatter a selection around the house daily. Real fur toys are particularly good because they act as a focus for predatory behaviour.

Variety is important:

- *Noise*: Toys that twitter or squeak when touched.
- *Movement*: Toys that move rapidly and unpredictably when they roll.
- *Texture, size and colour*: Bright colours, feathers, parts that sparkle or dangle or toys that mimic real prey.

Typically, cats get bored with play after about 10 minutes. This means that play sessions must be brief but frequent. If your cat appears to be getting bored with a particular toy part-way through a game, switch to something else or move the toy in a different way to attract your cat's attention.

In the wild, cats spend 6 or more hours every day hunting for, catching and eating their prey. They may make 100+ attempts to catch prey and only succeed in perhaps 10% of instances. In the domestic environment, all this activity may be absent, especially for indoor cats. It is also known that well-fed cats continue to hunt wildlife, but when they catch a bird or mouse they will take more time to kill it. This means that the wild animal's suffering is prolonged. Activity feeding provides a partial solution because the cat has to work to get food.

Activity feeders include:

Delidome® (available from online retailers): An electronic cat feeder that throws out small balls full of food every 1 to 2 hours for the cat to play with.

Empty plastic drinks bottles: perforated with food-pellet sized holes and part filled with dried cat food. The food falls out as the toy rolls along.

Food bowls: placed high on shelves for the cat to find.

Activity box: Fill a box with crumpled newspaper and small toys. Hide small dried food treats for the cat to rummage and find (freeze-dried prawns and smelly fish treats work well).

Indoor play and activity-feeding are obviously essential for indoor-only cats, but they also reduce the outdoor cat's interest in predatory behaviour, thus saving wildlife from predation.

Privacy

Privacy is, in part, provided by giving cats choice. A multitude of resting and feeding places helps to enable cats to vary the amount of contact they have with each other according to their mood. Covered litter trays provide added privacy, as do food bowls placed high on shelves.

Some cats, especially those which are elderly or infirm, also like to have ground-level hiding places to which they can run. Commercial options are available but empty cat baskets or cardboard boxes are suitable alternatives.

The indoor part of the cat's territory is somewhere where the cat should feel secure. In the wild this 'core' part of the cat's territory is never invaded or overlooked by other cats because it is surrounded by a space that the cat patrols and where it leaves scent marks to repel invading cats. Indoor-only cats are unable to do this and may feel very vulnerable if outside cats can look in at them through windows. Even cats that do have outdoor access may not be able to maintain a suitable buffer distance that keeps other cats away from their home.

It is important to block views from windows that are overlooked, perhaps close to places where your cat has urine marked or shown signs of aggression or fear in the past. This is easily achieved using 'glass etch spray' which is used to make bathroom windows opaque. Light still comes through but the cat cannot see clearly what is on the other side of the glass. Other cats tend to hang around less when there is no chance to threaten the indoor cat. Changes may also be made outdoors to deter other cats from lurking and menacing your cat (see Advice sheet 1).

The indoor territory should be available only to your own cat. To avoid problems of other cats entering the home, which can cause urine spraying or aggression between your own cats, it is best to fit an electronic cat flap with personalised coded collar keys that allow only your cats to enter.

GIVING INDOOR HOUSED CATS SOME FRESH AIR

Harness and lead

Some cats can learn to walk on a leash and harness if this is introduced while they are young. However, cats should not be taken on walks in the same way as dogs because this can be terrifying and distressing for them. Walks should be confined to a garden within easy access of the house so that the cat can build up familiarity with the landscape and odour marks that are there. If the cat shows signs of fear or anxiety, walks should be stopped.

Outdoor pen

Indoor cats should ideally be given access to an enclosed outdoor area. Free access is via a cat-flap so that the cat can choose when it goes in and out. A well-designed pen should mimic the outside world as closely as possible, providing a multitude of tree trunks, toys, scratching posts and high-up resting places. Introduction to the pen should be gradual, perhaps involving play or searches for food treats. The cat must always be able to return to the house voluntarily.

ADVICE SHEET 3

MULTI-CAT HOUSEHOLDS

DO CATS LIKE TO LIVE ALONE?

If you have a single, happy cat that has outdoor access and plenty of toys and resting places in the home, there is no reason to provide other cats as playmates. It is important to remember that cats are solitary hunters and they do not need to associate with other cats in order to survive. This means that cats can live alone perfectly happily. Provided that they have a sufficient supply of safe territory, food, shelter and affection from their owners, they will survive very well. Your cat is free to associate with cats outside and, if it is a sociable individual, it can find friends there. If, however, it is not of a sociable disposition then it can avoid other cats. Some cats definitely prefer to have their own home, without other cats in it, so it is important to think carefully before getting another cat.

WHEN IS IT BEST NOT TO HAVE SEVERAL CATS?

Some urban areas have a very high population density of cats and adding extra ones may cause tension and stress. Your own cats may not be able to carve out their own territory and could end up living indoors because they are too frightened to go outside.

If you intend to keep several cats indoors, without outside access, this can also cause problems. You will need to adapt the house to provide the cats with space and a whole host of resources and activities to save them from becoming bored or stressed by the absence of privacy from other cats.

IS IT BEST TO TAKE ON TWO CATS AT THE SAME TIME?

In the wild, cats do form their own communities which are made up of groups of related females. Cats are very intolerant of outsiders and are less likely to live happily with a cat to which they are not related. So if you want two cats to live together, it is best to get them as littermates. If you are unable to get two littermates, you can raise very young kittens as if they were from the same litter, provided that you take them on at a very early age; that is, before they are 7 weeks old.

INTRODUCING A NEW CAT INTO A HOUSEHOLD

If you do decide to take on an adult cat or older kitten as an additional cat in a multi-cat household, then you must introduce the new cat very carefully. Advice sheet 6 explains how to do this.

WHAT KIND OF CAT MAKES A GOOD SECOND OR ADDITIONAL CAT?

Research has shown that resident adult cats are more likely to accept the introduction of a new cat if it is significantly younger than them. They are far more intolerant of same-aged or older 'new' cats. Research also suggests that resident cats are more likely to tolerate a new cat of the opposite rather than the same sex and that, in cases of same sex pairs, two males are slightly more likely to be compatible than two females. Some older cats do feel intimidated by kittens as they may feel unable to stand up to physical play. Getting two young kittens reduces the pressure on the older cat because the kittens can play together.

REPLACING A HOUSEMATE AFTER AN ACCIDENT OR ILLNESS

Friendships between cats are unique and individual and they cannot be replaced by bringing in a new cat. If a pair of littermates has been raised together, their bond is particularly unlikely to be replaced. The remaining cat may experience genuine grief and may search for and call out to the missing sibling. Grieving can go on for a period of several months and is not a good time to introduce another cat. Hostility to a new cat may be very intense. If a new cat is introduced after grieving is over, then the bond is unlikely ever to be as strong as between the previous pair.

SUCCESSFUL INTEGRATION OF NEW CATS

Apart from introducing the new cat correctly, it is important to make sure that the cats have enough key resources so that they feel comfortable to co-exist without competition.

The provision of feeding sites for one or two cats will not be enough when a third or fourth cat is introduced, as each cat needs its own share of feeding, resting, drinking and latrine sites. Much like people, cats get along best when they have their own privacy and the amount of indoor space available may not satisfy this need. Greater access to height, with cat furniture, shelves and places to climb, will allow the cats a greater amount of usable space, even though the floor area of the house is unchanged. Please see Advice sheets 1 and 2 on adapting the indoor and outdoor environments for cats.

ADVICE SHEET 4

CLEANING URINE AND FAECES MARKS IN THE HOME

House-soiling and marking can begin for a number of reasons but, in some cases, it continues purely because the cat can detect the smell of locations where it has previously marked or gone to the toilet. Removing these odours is essential to stopping further soiling.

It is also important to protect the floor and furnishings to prevent urine or faeces from soaking in and leaving a permanent odour.

The best way to remove odours from existing sites is as follows:

Make up 3 sprayer bottles, labelled A, B and C. They should be filled in accordance with the following instructions:

A: A solution of *biological* clothes washing powder or liquid in water (approximately 1 part of powder/ liquid cleaner to 10 parts of water)
B: Plain water
C: Surgical spirit (clear surgical spirit, not coloured methylated spirit).

Each soiled site should be cleaned in the following way:

- Use paper towel to remove urine and faeces.
- Spray the area with bottle A.
- Wipe clean with paper towel.
- Spray with bottle B.
- Wipe clean and mop dry with paper towel.
- Spray with bottle C and allow to dry before allowing the cat into the area.

Do not use a reusable cloth for cleaning as this will spread urine odours from place to place as you clean.

It is advised that you test this cleaning method on a small and inconspicuous area of the carpet or fabric you are cleaning to ensure that it will not be damaged.

If you are cleaning curtains or furniture covers that can be removed and washed, then machine wash them according to the manufacturer's instructions.

PREVENTING FURTHER SOILING

Faecal odours are relatively easy to remove using the method above, but urine may seep into cracks in flooring and at the edges of furniture so that odours are hard to remove.

Particular problem areas are:

- wooden furniture
- joints between floorboards or panels of laminated flooring
- the junction between hard flooring and skirting boards, kitchen cupboards, etc.
- the top edge of skirting boards (baseboards)

- grouting between ceramic tiles (on floors or walls)
- electrical equipment and electrical outlets.

These, and any other potential traps for urine, must be cleaned and sealed so that urine odours do not penetrate.

Wooden furniture should be regularly waxed with a heavy-grade wax polish (not a spray) so that the surface is protected. The feet of wooden chairs and tables can sometimes absorb urine so these should be protected with a dab of varnish on the underside, if possible.

Joints between wooden floors should be sealed and painted over with at least two coats of a high-quality varnish. Gaps between floorboards are easily sealed with rubber or silicone bath sealant, which is available in many colours, before painting over with varnish.

The junction between a wooden or hard floor and the bottom of skirting board should be sealed with a rubber or silicone bathroom sealant.

The same method may be used to seal the top edge of skirting boards.

Porous grouting may be steam-cleaned or replaced with a waterproof equivalent, and then painted over with an appropriate sealant (sealant for terracotta tiles and grouting is available from most DIY shops).

Electrical equipment, such as toasters, kettles, televisions and audio equipment, may become targets for spraying as they heat up and release smells that cats find objectionable. Once they have been contaminated with urine, they will release urine odours every time they are switched on, which attracts further spray marking. Soiled cooking equipment should be discarded as it presents a health hazard unless it can be completely cleaned. Audio and TV equipment that has previously been soiled must be cleaned with great care. It may not be possible to remove all traces of urine. Audio equipment may need to be put into a glass-fronted rack or cupboard, away from access by the cat, and TV equipment could be covered with a polythene sheet when it is switched off.

Urine getting into electrical outlets can create a serious risk of shock or fire, so access to these locations should be restricted. As an additional protection, electrical outlets can be protected by covering them with cling-film. Alternatively, a flap of polythene may be taped to the wall above the socket so that it drapes over the outlet and redirects urine over it in the manner of a canopy.

REPLACING FLOORING AND SOFT FURNISHINGS

If an area is persistently soiled, then urine and faeces odour will soak in and may be very difficult to remove. Consider removing carpets, curtains and soft furnishing that have been badly damaged by urine or faeces. You may be able to have these cleaned professionally.

If carpet or other flooring must be replaced due to soiling, then the floor must be scrubbed clean with a biological cleaner as above. Rotten or sodden timbers should be removed and replaced. The floor must be cleaned several times and then allowed to dry before any new flooring is put down. Paint wooden boards with varnish or gloss paint before laying new flooring over them; this helps to reduce the return of old odours.

To prevent urine from soaking through the new flooring and to prevent remaining odours from returning, it is advisable to put down a layer of thick polythene sheet in overlapping strips before laying the new flooring.

Consider putting a layer of polythene between the carpet and underlay so that any accidental soiling is easier to clean. This extra layer may be put in strategically in locations where the risk of future soiling is highest.

CONTINUING CLEANING

Once you have cleaned a particular spot once, it is tempting to leave it until the cat soils there again. In fact, this means that urine odours will continue to accumulate because one round of cleaning will never be enough to remove all of the odour.

Instead, you should clean each spot several times each week, until it has not been soiled at all for at least 3 weeks. This will remove all odours and reduce the chance of further soiling if the cat has a relapse.

ADVICE SHEET 5

CLAW MARKING

Claw marking has the functions of:

- stretching back muscles after resting
- claw maintenance and sharpening
- scent marking as a means of identifying territory to other cats.

It may also become a way for the cat to get your attention and cats will often claw the sofa right in front of you and then scamper out of the room waiting to be chased. Cats that carry out excessive clawing can become a nuisance and there are various strategies for dealing with the problem.

For some individuals, claw marking becomes a problem during periods of social tension. It will continue until the tension is relieved, so it may be necessary for your veterinary surgeon or behaviourist to carry out a thorough investigation before the problem can be resolved.

However, here is some general advice to reduce the problem of clawing.

CLAW MARKING

The natural location for this is outside the house as it is intended as a signal to other cats to warn them about the boundary of the marking cat's territory. Many gardens lack good opportunities to claw-mark but these can be easily provided. Softwood posts can be installed at the edge of the garden or small sheets of softwood can be fixed to the corners of buildings, such as sheds, with the wood grain running vertically. To determine whether a piece of wood is suitably soft for the cat to claw, try making an indentation in it with your thumbnail. If an indentation is easily made and the wood grain is wide, then the wood is suitable. As an alternative to softwood, you can use lengths or sections of natural tree-trunk that has a heavily rutted corky type of bark. It is important that the scratching posts are in clearly visible locations and not hidden out of the way. To attract the cat to scratch them, they should be rubbed against existing scratch marking locations so that some of the scent is picked up. They should then be raked vertically with a wire brush to create a few fake scratch marks.

CLAWING AFTER RESTING

When cats wake up, they will often stretch against a piece of furniture, digging their claws in and then making a few clawing movements. There is no way to displace this behaviour so it is best to install a commercially-available carpet or hessian-covered scratching post close to places where your cat rests and then scratches furniture upon waking. These can be made more attractive to the cat by marking them with heavy, vertical black lines using a permanent felt marker, and then scratching the surface with a few vertical strokes of a wire brush.

CLAWING TO MAINTAIN CLAW SHARPNESS

Upholstered furnishings and stair carpets provide perfect opportunities for cats to sharpen claws. They want a surface that will catch on the edge of the back part of the claw and then pull off any loose old nail as they wrench their claws out of the surface. Ordinary scratching posts may not provide the right kind of surface for this. Position a hessian or carpet covered post in front of the place the cat usually claws. If this does not attract the cat, then consider covering the post with a thick layer of blanket and then covering this tightly with heavy fabric. This will usually give the cat the texture it is looking for. Choose a fabric that has a strong pattern of stripes and align these vertically, or use blank fabric and make some vertical marks on it with a permanent marker.

CLAWING FOR ATTENTION

Cats often claw furniture in front of their owners as a means of getting attention. This presents problems because the cat will rapidly learn that clawing the furniture continues to get a reaction but that clawing the scratching post does not. It is therefore important to look at the cat and react when it claws the scratching posts you have provided in the house, but not when it goes to scratch a piece of furniture.

DETERRING UNDESIRABLE SCRATCHING

Once you have provided your cat with suitable substitutes, it is possible to deter them from scratching other places.

Preventing scratching of softwood (pine wardrobes, stair poles, etc.)

If the object has a varnished surface, rub down any existing claw marks and apply a treatment with commercially available wood hardener. This is a polymer which penetrates the wood and dries to make it very tough. Then apply several additional layers of high-grade varnish to the object until the surface is very smooth and hard. Test treatment on an inconspicuous section of wood before using it generally to check that the appearance of the object will not be impaired, and allow the varnish to dry completely before allowing the cats to have access to the woodwork that has been painted. You can test the surface again with your thumbnail; you should find that the surface is much harder, which will make it far less appealing to scratch.

If the object has a waxed surface, then it cannot be varnished unless the wax surface is stripped. This will almost certainly damage it. Instead, make up a mixture of solid furniture wax with a few drops of eucalyptus and citronella oil added. Apply this to the clawed area of wood as a polish. It will leave behind an odour that most cats find repellent. If this does not work, make up a preparation of solid furniture wax mixed with a few menthol crystals and several drops of eucalyptus oil and use this as a polish instead.

Soft furnishings

These can be temporarily protected with heavy-grade poly-thene sheeting, which will make the surface unpleasant to scratch. This is left in place for several weeks until the cat has switched all of its scratching to the posts and pads that have been provided.

ADVICE SHEET 6

INTRODUCING NEW CATS TO THE HOUSEHOLD

Before introducing a new cat, it is important to assess the likelihood that resident cats will accept it. An already stressed group of cats will not readily accept a new cat. Their existing problems should take priority. Improper introduction of cats carries a strong risk of fighting and long-term intolerance between them. Future stressors, such as the addition of further cats to the neighbourhood, will unmask this brooding problem, potentially to instigate spraying and inter-cat aggression. Proper introduction of a new cat is therefore very important.

General preparations for the arrival of a new cat should include:

- Providing the new cat with its own room containing a latrine, food, water and a variety of resting and hiding places. Installing a Feliway®, diffuser (CEVA Animal Health), available from the veterinary surgery, will increase the sense of familiarity and security in this location.
- Allowing the new cat to become fully confident in this new location and with all members of the family. This may take a few days, after which the cat should be eating, resting and approaching visitors to this environment normally.
- The already resident cats should be provided with several extra feeding stations, places to drink and additional places to rest and hide. A Feliway® diffuser is also useful to increase sense of security.

The new cat must then be introduced to the other cats in a series of gradual stages. Cats primarily recognise other members of their group by smell, which is why cats sometimes react oddly to their owners after they have been handling or stroking other cats.

STAGE 1: SCENT INTRODUCTION

- Prepare several disposable cloths, each labelled with a cat's name.
- Use each labelled cloth daily to collect odours from the face and flank of the cat with whose name it has been labelled. The cloths must not be mixed up and must be stored separately in plastic bags to prevent cross-contamination.
- Whenever going to greet, feed or play with the new cat, it should be briefly presented with an opposing cat's cloth to smell and investigate. The cloth should be wrapped around the person's hand. Initially this may trigger a degree of alarm (the cat may back away, hiss or freeze). At this stage, it is important not to force contact as the cat may become aggressive.
- If there are multiple cats in the household, then the resident cats should be presented with the new cat's smell, and the new cat with odours from different cats in the group.
- With repeated presentation of the cloths, the cat should ultimately ignore the odour or may react positively to it. When all cats are reacting in this way it is time to move on to Stage 2.

STAGE 2: SCENT SWAPPING

- After harvesting the odour from the cats, the cloths should be put together in a bag so that odours mix.
- This combined odour is then used in the same way as above.
- Once there is a positive reaction to this combined odour then the client should mark themselves with the mixed odour so that when the cats greet they are unintentionally self-marking with this new odour. The cloth should be rubbed on objects that the cats regularly rub against, including the owner's legs.
- Odour swapping may then switch to using a single cloth, as long as each cat accepts being rubbed with the scent from the others.
- Once all cats are accepting this new odour and are actively rubbing against the clothed hand and other objects that have been marked with the cloth, then it is time to move to Stage 3.

STAGE 3: ALLOWING THE NEW CAT TO EXPLORE

- The new cat should be allowed to explore and utilise the rest of the house while the other cats are excluded or shut in an inaccessible room. This allows the new cat to learn all of the hiding and escape places so that, as the cats meet, it does not feel vulnerable.
- Once the new cat is using the resources in the home confidently, then it is time to move on to the next stage.

STAGE 4: LIMITED FACE-TO-FACE INTRODUCTION

- The cats need to begin to see each other but without any risk of carrying out an attack. This can be managed using a glass door or mesh screen. Some child gates are made from a mesh that provides a partial barrier. Mesh barriers are best as they allow some diffusion of body odours that are involved in identification. If neither is possible, then a partly open door may be used (open wide enough for the cats to see each other but not get through).
- The cats are given food on either side of the screen at normal feeding times, or are distracted with a game.
- It is also useful to rub the door or screen with the odour from the cats so that there is maximum chance of recognition of scent.
- The cats are encouraged to play and feed progressively closer to the screen, as long as there is no aggression.

- Once the cats are showing no aggressive or fearful behaviour, they can be allowed to meet face-to-face, after an initial meeting through the door or screen.

It is important to continue mixing odours between the cats and applying their 'group odour' to the owner and common marking places in the house until the cats have begun to rub against each other or groom each other. At this point, Feliway® diffusers and other environmental changes may be taken away gradually.

The total time for the introduction process may vary from a couple of weeks to a couple of months, but there is no shortcut if harmony is to be achieved.

Index